Sensory Arts and Design

SENSORY STUDIES SERIES

Series Editor: David Howes

ISSN: 20523092

As the leading publisher of scholarship on the culture of the senses, we are delighted to present this series of cutting-edge case studies, syntheses and translations in the emergent field of sensory studies. Building on the success of the *Sensory Formations* series, this new venture provides an invaluable resource for those involved in researching and teaching courses on the senses as subjects of study and a means of inquiry. Embracing the insights of a wide array of humanities and social science disciplines, the field of sensory studies has emerged as the most comprehensive and dynamic framework yet for making sense of human experience. The series offers something for every disciplinary taste and sensory inclination.

Published Titles:

Michael Bull and John P. Mitchell (eds), *Ritual, Performance and the Senses*

François Laplantine, *The Life of the Senses: Introduction to a Modal Anthropology*

Luca Vercelloni (translated by Kate Singleton), *The Invention of Taste: A Cultural Account of Desire, Delight and Disgust in Fashion, Food and Art*

Forthcoming Titles:

Alex Rhys-Taylor, *Food and Multiculture: A Sensory Ethnography of East London*

Constance Classen, *The Museum of the Senses: Experiencing Art and Collections*

Sensory Arts and Design

Edited by Ian Heywood

BLOOMSBURY ACADEMIC
LONDON • NEW YORK • OXFORD • NEW DELHI • SYDNEY

BLOOMSBURY ACADEMIC
Bloomsbury Publishing Plc
50 Bedford Square, London, WC1B 3DP, UK
1385 Broadway, New York, NY 10018, USA

BLOOMSBURY, BLOOMSBURY ACADEMIC and the Diana logo
are trademarks of Bloomsbury Publishing Plc

First published in Great Britain 2017
Paperback edition first published 2018

Cover design: Sharon Mah
Cover image © Getty

A catalogue record for this book is available from the British Library.

ISBN: HB: 978-1-4742-8019-8
PB: 978-1-3500-8010-2
ePDF: 978-1-4742-8021-1
ePub: 978-1-4742-8020-4

Names: Heywood, Ian, 1948– editor.
Title: Sensory arts and design / edited by Ian Heywood.
Description: New York : Bloomsbury Academic, 2017. |
Series: Sensory studies series, ISSN 2052-3092
Identifiers: LCCN 2016038778| ISBN 9781474280198 (hardback) |
ISBN 9781474280211 (epdf)
Subjects: LCSH: Culture. | Senses and sensation. | Design—Psychological aspects. |
BISAC: SOCIAL SCIENCE / Anthropology / Cultural.
Classification: LCC HM621 .S464 2017 | DDC 306—dc23
LC record available at https://lccn.loc.gov/2016038778

Series: Sensory Studies

Typeset by Newgen Knowledge Works (P) Ltd., Chennai, India.

To find out more about our authors and books visit
www.bloomsbury.com and sign up for our newsletters.

To Emily and Phoebe

Contents

Figures

Notes on Contributors

Sarah Casey is an artist and lecturer in sculpture and installation at Lancaster University. She is a member of Insight, a research unit within the Lancaster Institute for the Contemporary Arts (LICA), Lancaster University. One of her core research interests is the relationship between drawing and investigative methods of other research disciplines.

Mark Clintberg is an artist who works in the field of art history. He is an assistant professor in the School of Critical and Creative Studies at the Alberta College of Art and Design. His research focuses on sensory environments and sites of hospitality in museums and galleries, collaborative practices and edible artworks.

Paul Coulton is Chair of Speculative and Game Design in the design-led research studio Imagination, part of Lancaster Institute for the Contemporary Arts (LICA), Lancaster University. He explores socio-technical issues of emerging technologies using a research-through-design approach to create speculative designs and design fictions.

Andy Darby is a PhD candidate at Lancaster University in HighWire, part of Lancaster Institute for the Contemporary Arts (LICA), Lancaster University. His research explores participatory design fictions and other co-creative methods for speculative design in the areas of human–computer interaction and futures debate.

Gerry Davies is Senior Lecturer in drawing at Lancaster University. He is a member of Insight, a research unit in the Lancaster Institute for the Contemporary Arts (LICA). He has a background in fine art practice, particularly drawing. His drawings have been exhibited in the United Kingdom, Europe, the United States and Australia, selected for survey exhibitions of contemporary drawing and shortlisted for major prizes exhibitions, most recently the Jerwood Drawing Prize 2016.

Pip Dickens is Lecturer in fine art, painting, at Lancaster University. She is a member of Insight, a research unit within the Lancaster Institute for the Contemporary Arts (LICA), Lancaster University. Her painting practice draws upon many sources from natural phenomena to the darker elements of phantasmagoria, from opacity to transparency, from rhythms within music to pattern structures in nature, from cinematic devices to literary sources.

Nick Donnelly is Professor of cognitive psychology at the University of Southampton. His research interests extend beyond the relationship of art and visual perception. They include studying how faces are processed and how we search for targets in the visual world.

Nick Dunn is Professor of urban design at Imagination, Lancaster and research director of Lancaster Institute for the Contemporary Arts (LICA) at Lancaster University. He is associate director of the Institute for Social Futures, where he also leads research on the future of cities and urbanism. His work responds to the contemporary city as a series of systems, flows and processes, and is explored through experimentation and discourse addressing the nature of urban space: its perception, demarcation and appropriation.

Beth Harland is Professor of fine art and director of Insight, a research unit in the Lancaster Institute for the Contemporary Arts (LICA), and associate member of the Institute for Social Futures, Lancaster University. She is associate editor of the *Journal of Contemporary Painting*. Her research interests include painting, temporality in art, art spectatorship and cognition.

Ian Heywood is visiting research fellow at Lancaster Institute for Contemporary Arts, Lancaster University. He has researched and published in the areas of visual art, visual culture and leisure culture. He is particularly interested in early modern art, contemporary art and their varied interpretations. He leads the Sensory Arts research strand in the Insight research unit.

Jonny Huck is a lecturer in geographical information science at the University of Manchester. His research is centred around the representation of vague geographical entities in geographical information science, novel approaches to cartography and the application of emergent technologies to geographical problems. He also maintains http://map-me.org – a freely available Participatory GIS designed to more effectively capture the vague geographical thoughts and feelings of participants – and writes the GIS blog Contact.

Naomi Jacobs is a senior research associate in Imagination, part of Lancaster Institute for the Contemporary Arts (LICA), Lancaster University. She is currently working as part of the Arts and Humanities Research Council funded Creative Exchange project. Her general research interests include knowledge exchange, interdisciplinary collaboration and digital public space: how digital technology impacts modern life and culture. She also has a background in experimental psychology.

Richard Leadbeater embarked upon a new career in academia at Lancaster University following a career in clinical medicine. His main research interests lie in the interaction between identity development and lifespan experiences and the impact that these have on the meaning of music preferences beyond adolescence. A neo-Meadian interpretation on the canon of symbolic interactionism has informed much of his current research on the trajectory of music preferences as symbolic objects of the self across the lifespan.

Alan Marsden is a senior lecturer in sound at Lancaster University and the editor of *Journal of New Music Research*. In his research he seeks to understand how listeners engage with music, and to this end he has conducted extensive research on computational models of music analysis. His other research interests include listeners' behaviour and music's contact with other sensory modalities.

Joy Monice Malnar is a licensed architect and associate professor in the School of Architecture at the University of Illinois at Urbana-Champaign. Her design work focuses on the sensory and cultural attributes of architecture. Her recent published work develops a sensory typology to assist in designing for the full range of the human senses. It moves beyond academic, phenomenological theory to present buildings designed to address cultural and environmental sustainability. Malnar is currently on the editorial advisory board of *Senses & Society*.

Linda O'Keeffe is Lecturer in sound at Lancaster University. She is a member of Insight, a research unit within the Lancaster Institute for the Contemporary Arts (LICA). She is director of the MA by Research at LICA, Lancaster University, editor of the *Interference* journal, and president of the Irish Sound, Science and Technology Association. Her interests are in sound installation, radio art, acoustic ecology, the sociology of sound, mobilities and creative methodologies in research.

Emmanuel Tsekleves is Senior Lecturer in Design Interactions at Imagination, Lancaster University. Emmanuel designs interactions between people, places and products by forging creative design methods along with digital technology. His current research also looks into how participatory design fictions can be used as a tool to provoke and generate debate around policy initiatives and emergent technology among diverse groups in the area of ageing and dementia.

Caro Verbeek is a freelance curator, a doctorial candidate at VU University Amsterdam and an embedded researcher of olfactory heritage at the Rijksmuseum, Amsterdam, and International Flavours & Fragrances, Hilversum. She teaches the course 'The Other Senses' at the Royal Academy of Art in The Hague. Verbeek has a special interest in the so-called lower senses and sensory reconstructions from the realm of history of art. She creates olfactory interventions and workshops for museums and academia.

Acknowledgments

This book had its origins in two separate sources. First, the Lancaster Institute for the Contemporary Arts (LICA) has two research units: *Insight*, which covers visual art, theatre studies, and music and sound, and *Imagination*, which deals with design. In a series of 'show-and-tell' joint research meetings it emerged that several projects were related to different aspects of the senses, not simply in the ways one might conventionally expect, given disciplinary and practical specializations. In some of our discussions new questions came to be asked about the role of the senses in the arts and design; at the same time older questions showed up in new places. These striking overlaps and initiatives were discussed within *Insight* with a view to extending areas of collaboration and exchange. It has to be said that there are today important professional and pedagogical differences between the arts and design, despite recognition of their linked history and an often porous border, sometimes crossed by ideas, styles and techniques, as well as by exceptional practitioners and teachers, from Walter Gropius to Reyner Banham. The culture and policies of LICA and its research units, alive to this situation, have sought wherever possible to promote interdisciplinary initiatives; and indeed many of the chapters in this book are jointly authored, sometimes by researchers and practitioners from what are conventionally regarded as very different fields. Certainly disciplinary differences need to be recognized where they are legitimate, but they should be questioned when they disrupt or distort ambitious research and practice. This volume represents, we believe, a distinctive and constructive example of interdisciplinary research, encompassing the arts and design, the embodied and the conceptual, as well as theory, scholarship and creative practice.

Second, having previously compiled collections on visual culture, the editor felt that we could, on the basis of our projects, make a contribution to the emerging field of sensory studies, in which leading roles are played by the journal *Senses and Society* and the Centre for Sensory Studies at Concordia University, Montreal. Eventually, with the very helpful advice of David Howes, a proposal was made to Bloomsbury for a volume in their Sensory Studies series, for which Howes is the general editor.

Eager to be as inclusive across the sensorium as possible, Howes was able to put us into contact with researchers who could extend the range of contributions. Joy Malnar, who edited the Sensory Design Reviews section of *The Senses and Society* for the first six years, in addition to authoring the leading book on sensory design in architecture, graciously agreed to write a state-of-the-art essay on the senses in architecture. We were delighted also to have contributions from Mark Clintberg, a leading theorist of the emergent field of food art, and from Caro Verbeek, who has pioneered the reconstruction of the olfactory imagination and practices of Futurism.

In addition, we would like to acknowledge support for specific chapters. Sarah Casey and Gerry Davies wish to thank Ricardo Martinez Murillo and the Cajal Institute, Madrid; Peter Matthews; Dr Lucy Lyons; Sian Bowen; The Ruskin Library and Archive, Lancaster University. Mark Clintberg's research was supported by the Hands-On Museum project under the direction of Constance Classen, which is funded by the Social Sciences and Humanities Research Council of Canada (grant no. 410-2011-2645). Paul Coulton's chapter is a reflection of his design practice in relation to the Creative Exchange project supported by the Arts and Humanities Research Council and the Engineering and Physical Sciences Research Council's project Creating and Exploring Digital Empathy. He would also like to thank a number of his PhD students for their contributions in these projects most notably Dan Burnett, Adrian Gradinar, Dave Gullick, Jonny Huck and Mike Stead. Beth Harland and Nick Donelly would like to thank the Courtauld Gallery, London, for access to the painting during their study and permission to reproduce it here. The eye movement data they report were collected and supplied by Carl Mann. They are presented here with permission and the authors acknowledge his generosity. Emmanuel Tsekleves acknowledges that Ageing Playfully was supported by the FASS-Enterprise Centre. The EPSRC Catalyst research project at Lancaster University is funded by the EPSRC, UK (Research Councils UK Grant EP/I033017/1). This work was also partly funded by the Digital Economy programme (RCUK Grant EP/G037582/1), which supports the HighWire Centre for Doctoral Training (http://highwire.lancs.ac.uk).

Finally, Ian Heywood would like to thank David Howes for his encouragement and assistance with this anthology, and Beth Harland for her support and helpful advice throughout. He would also like to thank all the contributors for their efficiency and patience.

Introduction

Ian Heywood

This anthology presents new creative and critical engagements with the senses in innovative arts and design. The chapters explore the importance of novel sensing and intelligent technologies for the human environment, and the tasks of shaping it materially, aesthetically, functionally and normatively. They also present the results of continuing reflections by artists, critics and theorists on the relationship between different senses employed by cultural artefacts, and the ways in which such artefacts give meaning to sensory phenomena and a sensory presence to meaning. The collection concentrates on design, including architecture, and the arts, specifically visual art and music, with the addition of sonic and gustatory arts. This introduction presents first a brief account of some important episodes in changing approaches to the senses in the recent history of the arts and design.[1] Its second task is to introduce individual contributions.

The senses are directly a source of stimulation, pleasures and pains, and therefore inherently important to the human organism. They are important also because it is typical of many cultural artefacts that through them sensory experience is given specific intensities and extensities, shapes and meanings. In this respect we agree with David Howes (2013) that sensory studies has two aspects. It incorporates a sensory approach to culture, the challenge here being to give full weight to the role of the senses in cultural life. It also includes a cultural approach to the senses, where this suggests setting impacts and employments of the senses in their cultural context, particularly in the ways in which they are given and contribute to shareable meanings.

It is conventional wisdom that the senses play an important role in the practices and theory of performing, musical and visual arts and in the design of artefacts and systems, large and small. The usual way to think about the function of 'leading' or 'dominant' senses here would be to consider the role of vision, hearing and touch in the experience of culture, sometimes recognizing sensory modalities in relative isolation, but at others noting how they operate in concert. Of course, the proximal senses of smell and taste, although central to aspects of cultural life, for example, in cooking and the use of fragrances in everyday and ritual settings, have frequently been taken to occupy lower positions in the sensory hierarchy of Western, and now an increasingly global, culture. The impact of historical, anthropological and cultural studies of the senses, and indeed a trans-disciplinary 'sensory turn', have ensured, however, that simplistic rank orderings have been widely and rightly questioned.[2] The result is the recent tendency to bring the supposedly inferior, less 'intellectual', senses into the scope of research and reflection, a move exemplified by the vigour and range of recent sensory studies research.[3] Of particular importance is the capacity of artefacts and events, in and through which the senses achieve prominence, to accrete, amplify and transmit meaning, including the reflexive question of the meaning of the senses themselves, their significance and place in human life.

Employment of the senses in the arts and design on the part of producers, audiences and users vary considerably, depending on intentions, interests and the level of attention achieved. That is, the nature, significance and meaning of embodied experience will vary for individuals and groups according to what they are trying to do, what aspects of the sensorium are important to their purposes, and how intently they attend to sensory phenomena. Among artists and designers, the need for reflective sensory awareness applies to conception and planning, realization and making, and to the anticipated response of those who encounter and use what the arts and design devise. Practitioners imagine and plan what the thing or event in question will look, sound, taste, smell or feel like. They grapple sensorially with materials, tools and processes to make something in the right way, to ensure it has the intended effect, and multiple sensory encounters with a model, facsimile or the real thing are often critical to evaluating its conception, progress and quality, irrespective of what other information, some of it in the form of numerical data, for example, may be available.[4]

Bringing together research interest in the senses with the concept of culture requires a familiar, unavoidable distinction between two meanings of 'culture': the anthropological and ethnographic view of culture as customs, outlooks and ways of behaviour characteristic of human groups, and a more limited focus on the skills and outcomes of intellectual, artistic and constructive making in general to which artefacts with presence, functions and meanings are central. This second notion typically attaches qualitative, normative or value dimensions to cultural activities and artefacts, be they aesthetic, ethical or political. Here we are mainly concerned with the second idea of culture, although in practice the two cannot be neatly and definitively separated.

Some of the most important episodes in the cultural history of the senses, in the context of the arts and design, have been marked by the attachment of one or other sensory mode, or a combination of them, to particular cultural values. This linking of sensory experience to wider cultural meanings and purposes has taken a number of different forms. Utopian programmes have sought to remodel sensory experience of the lived, usually urban, environment, aligning it with the demands and opportunities of modernity, while other less grandiose, often more personal artistic and design projects, have pioneered new types of sensory experience linked to cultural objects and events, including two and three dimensional works of art, performed pieces, as well as a wide range of designed artefacts, or have sought to attach new meanings to the senses, sometimes motivated by ameliorative, utopian or even revolutionary ideals. For example, consider remarks by the English critic John Ruskin in the Preface to the *Elements of Drawing*, his practical course of instruction for largely untaught working men and women, that 'the excellence of an artist, as such, depends wholly on refinement of perception' (1904: 12). He goes on to say that the aim of his course is 'a delicate method of work, such as may ensure his seeing truly' and even more pointedly that 'I believe that the sight is a more important thing than the drawing; and I would rather teach drawing that my pupils may learn to love Nature, than teach the looking at Nature that they may learn to draw' (13). Not only is Ruskin acting politically in trying to develop the sensory capacities of working people, in this case their capacity to see, thereby enriching their perceptual, cognitive and ultimately aesthetic experience, but he is also linking a specific sense to the ultimate importance, as he conceives it, of a morally edifying realism. Later in this introduction we will briefly consider other episodes in the history of the cultural meanings and employments of the senses.

Twentieth Century Visual Art and the Senses

Since the early years of the twentieth century avant-garde art movements, beginning with Dada, have sought to assault conservative tastes and conventional opinions, and to fuse advanced art with everyday life, which would be somehow revolutionized in the process. Groupings with aims similar to Dadaism have been prominent in the story of modern and postmodern art. Understanding what their ideas amount to in practice is far from simple, but the activities and views of the original Dadaist artists supply an important pointer, typically their rejection of established art institutions and forms, together with what they regarded as the single, predominating sense associated with them: sight. As part of their programme of disruptive, critical, disorienting events, assaults on what they saw as complacent, hypocritical bourgeois culture, different senses were stimulated and deprived of customary significance; for example, Kurt Schwitters' 'sound poetry', the collages of Raoul Hausmann and Hannah Hoch combining text and image, the multi-material assemblages of Johannas Badder, the music–sound pieces of Francis Picabia and Georges Ribemont-Dessaignes, and events and performances of the Cabaret Voltaire in Zurich which combined elements of music hall theatre with the political rally.

The Italian Futurists engaged in similar disruptive procedures, but famously brought multisensory experimentation to food.[5] Fillippo Marinetti's *Futurist Cookbook* was simultaneously a compendium of recipes, an attempt to modernize and liberate the Italian cuisine, an elaborate art joke and a serious political provocation. Aimed to supplant pasta, which Marinetti believed made Italians heavy, dull-witted and unsuited to the modern mechanical–electrical world, Futurist 'aerofood' was a sequence of small, light dishes prepared to emphasize touch, sound, smell as well as sight and taste. Served alongside these dishes, and meant to be stroked, were strips of velvet, silk and sandpaper.

Beyond the jokes and goading of the avant-garde, the innovative programme of art and design education pioneered between the wars by the Bauhaus represented a different proposal for a rapidly modernizing Europe, often multisensory in its methods. Aiming to bring about a series of reconciliations, of fine and applied arts, and of the independent artist, the craftsman and industrial production, it projected a new architecture for a world of machines, electricity and rapid travel. Bauhaus designers and artists set out to encourage the design of consumer goods that were functional, reliable, cheap and beautiful, and to modernize the appearance and functionality of the urban environment. Bauhaus pedagogy was rooted in the idea that there were basic, common principles of design, available as a mixture of theory and practice, which would enable a student to become proficient in all design tasks. It had on its staff artists who specialized in particular practices, for example, the painters Paul Klee, Johannes Itten, Lyonel Feininger, Wassily Kandinsky, the sculptor Gerhard Marcks and the designer and architect Marcel Brauer. Some of its teachers, however, happily spanned different practices, like the painter, sculptor and designer Oskar Schlemmer who ran the theatre workshop. Its guiding pedagogical idea was the 'total work of art', the goal of a unified, efficient, functional, attractive human environment reflecting and enhancing a distinctively modern way of life. This is necessarily in many ways a multisensory cultural and aesthetic ideal.

The famous 'basic course' devised by Itten as an introduction to key knowledge and skills for all artists and designers trained by the Bauhaus, including architects, emphasized unlocking a personal approach. Mechanical imitation of the styles of eminent artist–teachers was replaced by first-hand experience of working with a wide range of materials and techniques, which joined active exploration, experimentation and skills acquisition with increasing the quality of the student's perceptive powers. Under Itten, the students' day began with physical exercises – breath awareness and controlled, rhythmic movements, even vocal production – meant to prepare the body for creative work, part mental, part physical. What Itten called 'the law of contrast' played a large part in learning to use perceptual and manual skills. Awareness of the importance of contrasts like large–small, long–short, light–dark, thick–thin, smooth–rough was essential to successful art and design practice. For example, when they were asked to make a tonal gradation between black and white, Itten found that the best students were able to make up to forty-four perceptibly separate steps, an achievement requiring both skill with a drawing tool and a capacity to discern fine differences. Colour theory and tactile awareness were taught with a similar emphasis on contrast. Visual and tactile appreciation of rhythm in design, perhaps best understood as an aspect of a specific propriocentric sensory mode, was taught through bodily exercises akin to dance. The aim was to translate the experience of concentrated attention on flowing movement into hand and arm actions through which marks and drawings were made.

The influence of the Bauhaus on subsequent art and design education has of course been considerable, and it is evident that wide-ranging multisensory experience, often of the whole body in movement and accompanied by a mobile field of attention, was of great importance to its philosophy and pedagogy. The aim was not the avant-garde's disruption of an oppressive separation and ordering of the senses, leading to a denial of the libidinous body. Rather, it required recognizing and valuing sensory diversity, fostering the connection between manual and mental skills and the quality of perception, and putting these to work in an art and design practice oriented by a belief in progressive modernization. Unlike some other aesthetic modernizers, the artists, designers and teachers of the Bauhaus were not concerned with the wider cultural or political significance of one sensory mode against another, but the quality of concrete experience arising from multiple sensory sources was at the heart of their work.

The Surrealist movement, which began in France in the 1920s, presents a particularly complex episode in the history of modern arts and the senses. As we shall see, its attitude to sight in particular was full of tensions if not deeply contradictory. Surrealism was suspicious, sometimes notoriously hostile, to vision. Martin Jay places this antipathy within the broader current in French arts and letters he refers to as 'antiocularcentrism'.[6] Paradoxically, however, Surrealism was also strongly committed to the personal, social and artistic significance of a kind of visionary seeing, a poetics of sight.

Although often linked to Dada and its programme for a 'systematic derangement of all the senses' (Andre Breton quoted by Jay 1991: 23) many surrealist works were in sensory terms relatively conventional. Meret Oppenheim's fur-lined cup and saucer has a strong tactile impact, laced as often in her work, with sexual connotations, but well-known surrealist artists – like Hans Arp, Max Ernst, Joan Miro, Salvador Dalí, Yves Tanguy, Rene Magritte, Francis Picabia, Andre Mason and Alberto Giacometti – made what were, in many respects, traditional paintings, drawings and sculptures. Even those Surrealists who pioneered new forms of visual and graphic expression, for instance, Man Ray's rayograms and Ernst's frottage, produced images organized and presented in a way similar to mainstream drawings and prints, this despite Surrealism's ambivalence towards visual arts like painting.[7] Images were meant to bewilder the viewer, but in many cases, for example, those of René Magritte, Max Ernst and Salvador Dalí, it is often the represented thing or scene, or disrupted depictive conventions, that puzzles or confounds. Paradoxically, in order to disturb the conventions of visual representation, surrealist art often needed to refer to and rely on traditional visual languages.

For Jay the paradigmatic instance of the surrealist assault on the status of vision in the hierarchy of the senses and its capacity to produce 'order and legible space' (Jay 1991: 18), is supplied by the writer Georges Bataille, particularly in his notorious *Story of the Eye*, in which the organ of vision is submitted to a series of violent sexual degradations.[8] Jay links Bataille's mytho-poetic antiocularcentrism to the experiences of soldiers in the trenches of the First World War, the sky representing the only possible escape from lethal, traumatizing surroundings. Yet in their public quarrel, Bataille accused Breton of forging an idea of vision which he compares to that of a celestial 'supereagle', an Icarian figure rising high above the earth in order to bring down the lesser imperial eagle of 'authoritarian idealism'. Bataille's preferred image is Karl Marx's 'old mole' of *The Eighteenth Brumaire*, a representation of a revolutionary movement burrowing and snuffling in the dark earth, amid the rejected, profaned, polluted material that so engaged him.

At times, then, surrealist attitudes appear prejudiced against the visual arts, something of an irony given the later prominence of photography and cinema in the movement's reputation and legacy. The paradigmatic locus of this aspect of the surrealist imagination is the dark labyrinth, not the lucid order of recessive perspectival space. It ultimately conveys a tropical preference for blindness, and for the auditory and the literary, over the visual.

The regime of ocularcentrism described by Jay is, however, anything but the simple dominance over Western culture of one idea of vision. As he points out, its resilience is due to the way different concepts of vision can replace others subject to criticism.[9] For example, the Surrealists rejected both the idea of intellectual intuition – speculative, philosophical seeing in the mind of clear and distinct concepts, which runs from Plato to Descartes and Hegel – but also the positivist belief that reliable knowledge must be based in replicable empirical observation, paradigmatically the sober visual inspection of objects as they are. Yet there can be found in Surrealism a contrary, more positive attitude to vision, enthusiasm for another mode of seeing, the idea of visionary illumination. Jay provides copious examples, which include that of the 'innocent eye' of the child, the imagery of dream and fantasy, and the chance glimpse, characteristic of urban street life, that reverberates in memory and the psyche.[10] The valorizing of the *coup d'œil*, the glance that misses nothing, is related to this other strand of surrealist thinking, which distances itself from ordinary and scientific seeing but recruits another idea of vision for poetic ends.

It is often said that the Surrealist programme sought to engineer a 'revolution of everyday life' by releasing the powers of desire and imagination supposedly blunted and distorted by prevailing bourgeois rationalism. Surrealist works tried to bring to consciousness repressed psychological drives, to explore supposedly unprofitable mental states and present quasi-philosophical puzzles about the relationship between language and meaning. They were meant to disturb rather than to supply 'aesthetic' sensory pleasure. While often seen as being in open revolt against ordinary existence, obsessed by dreams, fantasies and the unconscious, mature Surrealism also devised ideas and techniques – collage, frottage, the 'exquisite corpse', *coulage* – meant to release the 'miraculous' locked up in everyday life, bringing to light its mysteries and beauties. Surrealists held that the poetic dimension of everyday life was elusive because of the routine, taken-for-granted way in which ordinary things and events are habitually experienced. Poetic vision, the perceptual element of what Michael Sheringham (2006) calls 'surrealist visuality', is blunted in part because of the dominant idea of what it is to see and be seen. The exploration of reverie and parataxis was already largely familiar in the literary arts, hence the Surrealists' interest in writers and poets like Charles Baudelaire, Stéphane Mallarmé and Guillaume Apollinaire. Following in the wake of these explorations, surrealist practice emphasized the value of strong sensory impressions lodged in a receptive short-term memory, which could then mingle freely with images and ideas, giving rise to a prose poetry of sensations.[11]

As fashioned in the techniques of artists like Max Ernst, the surrealist gaze is meant to liberate ordinary vision from its conventional habits and impairments, allowing us to see 'this life'. Apprehending the real in this way, being open to what is already there, but remains veiled, has what Fernando Gil calls the 'force of the self-evident' (Sheringham 2006: 83); it has a 'hallucinatory' character. While the truth of evidence lies in sensory experience, enabling the thing to 'show' itself as it is, the senses are not passive but exert an active, shaping force. Paradoxically, for surrealist poetics, attention is effortful and constructive, 'producing' self-evidence through a 'perceptual and linguistic process' (84).[12]

Visual Arts: Post-War Developments

During the second half of the twentieth century the visual arts diversified rapidly, initiating more sensory experimentation. Avant-garde, anti-commercial movements like Fluxus inherited something of the Dada outlook, adding to its engagement with sound and music new forms like performance, mail art, and the making and using of simple, enigmatic objects (Fluxkits) that featured in their events and festivals. Fluxus artists routinely ignored what they felt to be arbitrary boundaries between media and their associated sensory modes, pioneering new kinds of sensory dissociation.[13] Radical movements like those of Art Povera expanded the range of sculptural materials with new tactile qualities, while land artists like Richard Long, Nancy Holt and Robert Smithson took sculpture out of the gallery, often expanding its scale and impact so greatly that bodily movement and a wide sensory range were required to experience it properly.

The scope and significance of the sensory impact of visual art underwent further changes with the advent of feminist, body and performance art. The consumption of food by artists and collaborators featured in works by Barbara T. Smith, Bobby Baker and others, although the symbolism of food seems to have mattered more than its strictly sensory aspects.[14] In one type of body art it became common to submit the body of the artist to stress, discomfort or even pain, and introduced anxiety or distress into the experience of the audience. For example, in *Rhythm 0* Marina Abramović encouraged spectators to use 'instruments of pain and pleasure' directly on her body. Feminist body art in the 1970s and 1980s explored different aspects of the female body in relation to patriarchy, as well as different, emancipatory kinds of sensuality.[15]

Installation art is associated with such a wide range of artefacts, presentational modes and audience experiences that generalization about its sensory dimensions is virtually impossible. Frequently, however, sight, touch and hearing were engaged, often in ways that surrounded, submerged or even assaulted the spectator. The idea of 'immersive' works introduced a distinction between spectacles to look at and situations to be experienced. Thus, for example, in his 2006 *Test Site* at Tate Modern, London, Carsten Höller exposed his public to the disorienting thrill, for Höller an 'inner spectacle', of headlong movement down an enclosed, twisting slide down between several floors of the building.

With its often philosophically and politically inclined criticism of formalist, commoditized and connoisseurial art, Conceptualism attempted to distance itself from taste, aesthetic pleasure, romantic notions of expression, and the alleged special imaginative gifts and refined skills of the artist-craftsman and creative prodigy. There was a heavy reliance on texts, analytical and critical rhetoric, prosaic documentary photographs and austere, unembellished objects. The influence of semiotics and poststructuralist ideas on later, less doctrinaire conceptual styles so prominent in art since the 1980s has tended to privilege 'reading', the intellectual interpretation of what are in essence 'texts', as a form of access to works of art superior to any sensory mode, whether singular or multiple. Yet a formal, distinctly aesthetic dimension often lingers because conceptual artists, in their efforts to securely identify their works as texts, impose on their artefacts exacting, if frugal, perceptual assumptions about the appearance of writing.[16]

The multiplicity of postmodernist works, attitudes and doctrine is so diverse that generalizations are even more hazardous. We can say, however, that while much postmodern art exploited the sensory experimentation of earlier avant-garde and oppositional movements, the significance of the senses was not usually at the centre of its concerns. Damian Hirst's most famous pieces, for example, are in sensory terms familiar: large, heavy vitrines echo the accoutrements of a natural history museum, displays of pharmaceuticals have a bright clinical presence, and his diamond encrusted skull could be a high-end jewellery-shop fitting or an archaeological treasure displayed under museum conditions. Despite their feistily kitsch content and surface sheen, the sculptures of Jeff Koons are formally and perceptually conventional, some of them even requiring plinths. Like Hirst's best-known works, their scale, opulence and brash vulgarity, amplified by their sculptural connotations, mark them out as polished visual spectacles, designed to stupefy or disconcert. Their sensory presence is largely instrumental, the means by which the work reflects back to the viewer a suave cultural vacancy.

One exception to postmodernism's apparent lack of concerted interest in the senses is the philosophy of Gilles Deleuze, a leading influence on postmodernist theory.[17] Deleuze's *Francis Bacon: The Logic of Sensation* and parts of *Difference and Repetition* set out a novel and radical view of the relationship between sensation and the arts. Deleuze contrasts works of art he admires with the targets of his critical philosophy: the order and stability of bourgeois life, the deadening routines of everyday existence, the pervasive influence of political and cultural power that limit disruptive emancipatory creativity, personal and collective. Culture itself was seen by Deleuze and many post-war French theorists as a series of essentially repressive representational systems, manifested in *doxa*, common, taken-for-granted opinions and the mythologies or ideologies locked into the meaning of everyday words and images. For Deleuze, the task of critical philosophy is to seek out subversive moments when the fixing and ordering powers of routine-signifying practices came unstuck. These unsettling occasions represent an opportunity to encounter the formless, liberating force of desire, the other, the unrepresentable process of becoming itself. Art is a place where the fault lines, folds or tensions in the smooth surface of everyday reality appear, and the need to make art arises for those who sense something 'unbearable', but also something beyond the suffocating banalities and imperious facts that pass for the meaningful conditions of life. What matters to art is a type of construction: 'We paint, sculpt, compose, and write with sensations. We paint, sculpt, compose and write sensations' (Deleuze 1994: 166). Despite their differences, the arts seek to produce a 'bloc of sensations, a pure being of sensations' (167). The artist needs to escape from familiar 'lived perceptions', ideas of fixed, known, easily representable and recognizable objects on the one hand and equally familiar states of the passive subject affected by sense data on the other. While in much visual art there is a resemblance between image and visible aspects of the world, something Deleuze seems to value, the work must assert its priority, its independence: 'The smile on the canvas is made solely with colours, lines, shadow and light' (166). Deleuze insists that art 'undoes the triple organization of perceptions, affections, and opinions in order to substitute a monument composed of percepts, affects and blocs of sensation that take the place of language' (176). The work's ability to preserve is thus inextricable from its capacity, as a structured group of sensations, to achieve independence from the everyday conditions of its production, be these a recognizable object or event or the perceptual state of a receptive subject. This is what Deleuze calls 'the logic of sensation'.

Deleuze offers interesting insights into the work of the painter Francis Bacon and elsewhere into film, but in addition he provides a philosophical framework within which sensation, desire and the body are given a fresh meaning and increased importance. In this his work resembles the phenomenological approach of Maurice Merleau-Ponty. Like Ruskin, they are thinkers who link the senses and cultural phenomena in which they are activated, both contributing and receiving meanings, to philosophical, ethical, political and aesthetic ideas and values.

To conclude, within the multiplicity of contemporary art practices can be found vigorous deliberate and unintended experiments with sensory modalities, touching on synaesthesia, corporealization (and decorporealization), fragrance, prosthetics and robotics.[18] Recently (2015) London's National Gallery has seen *Soundscapes*, an initiative that invited visitors to 'Hear the painting. See the sound'. Musicians and sound artists were asked to select a painting from the collection and respond by composing a new piece of 'immersive' and 'site-specific' music or sound art in response.

Also in 2015 Tate Britain hosted *Sensorium*. In this exhibition, again described as 'immersive', four paintings from the collection 'inspired sounds, smells, tastes and physical forms'. Physiological audience responses were detected and recorded by 'sophisticated measurement devices', with the aim of stimulating a broader multisensory experience of what is still a predominantly visually oriented gallery.

Critical responses to these and other multisensory explorations have been varied. The multisensory artwork is no more guaranteed success or importance than the products of any other approach. Nevertheless, prompted by sensory curiosity, imaginative restlessness, new technological opportunities and continuing reflection in the arts on the significance and value of embodied experience, it seems highly likely that such projects will continue to flourish.

Design

The study and practice of design covers both broad object types, for example, those associated with graphic, product and engineering design, and a narrower range of objects and areas of application, for example, fashion, fabric and game design. To its traditional concern for the functional, aesthetic and economic aspects of the things it creates or modifies has been added a focus on meaning or rhetoric. Some approaches to design practice have also changed their scale of application, encompassing not just specific object types but large collections of objects and functions, extending for example to the urban environment and even to the design of immaterial 'systems' or 'policy'. Any intentional activity that produces something new or that modifies an existing artefact can be said to involve design, and so many manifestations of design have important sensory consequences or implications.

The competing histories of design each provide different slants on the sensory aspects of design practice. As we have seen in the case of the Bauhaus, early modernist design was preoccupied by the relationship between form, to which aesthetic appearance and sensory experience – predominantly visual and tactile – contributed, and function, the object's capacity to perform its intended purpose effectively and efficiently, the subject of rational, practical evaluation and judgement. This gave high modernist design artefacts a classically unadorned look as designers searched for the 'type-forms' of goods in everyday use, redesigning and simplifying chairs, tables, telephones and so on. For example, Marcel Breuer's *Chair B33* (1927–28) was meant to be a 'clear, logical form based on rational principles', and as such 'styleless', independent of particularities of time and place.[19] Made of simply bent tubular steel and canvas, it is elegant, airy and portable, offering elemental visual, tactile and temperature contrasts between shiny metal and dark, stretched fabric. For some of its critics, Bauhaus high-mindedness and the aesthetic tenets of modernist design represented the imposition of an arbitrary taste for geometric forms buttressed by a bossy, prescriptive view of how modern men and women should live and what they should enjoy. The enduring popularity of modernist design classics and of a 'modernist style' suggests, however, that their appeal is not the result of a passing fad for geometrical minimalism or for goods signifying a doctrinally pure progressive outlook.[20]

'Consumer-led design', in some ways a radically different approach to modern design, began to emerge in the United States in the 1930s with a change in the focus of large industrial companies producing goods for mass markets. Up to this point their focus had been on continual technical improvements and increasing efficiency of manufacture, which stimulated sales by reducing the unit costs of highly standardized goods.[21] The new outlook, prompted in part by fears that sales and process would drop once a given market reached saturation, emphasized frequent stylistic modifications, often of negligible or no functional importance but perceivable and significant to consumers. While other more recent approaches – for example, participatory or co-design and green or sustainable design – do not exclude artefactual pleasures and meanings, they are particularly important for consumer-led design.

Product designers did not ignore the potential for the sensory properties of consumer goods to be directly enjoyed. For example, Raymond Loewy comments on the inviting curves of the 'Hobbleskirt' Coca-Cola bottle of the 1930s:

> The sensory aspects of the normal human being should be taken into consideration in all forms of design. Let's take the Coca-Cola bottle,

> for instance. Even when wet and cold, its twin-sphered body offers a delightful valley for the friendly fold of one's hand, a feel that is cosy and luscious. (Loewy 1951: 297)[22]

The many and varied sensory pleasures offered by designed objects should not be underestimated. As already noted, because the senses are a natural source of pleasures and pains they are necessarily important to the human organism. In the context of arts and design how, from an audience's or user's point of view, a cultural product looks, sounds, smells, feels or tastes is a perennial concern. Sometimes these features need to be considered separately, sometimes together.

Attempting to understand the aesthetic dimensions of sensory experience, and allowing 'aesthetic' to mean sensory experiences that human beings find pleasant, neutral or unpleasant, experimental psychologists have sought to identify broad perceptual principles or mechanisms. If these principles are rooted, as they are claimed to be, in psycho-physiological processes of the human organism, it would be plausible to suppose that they have already been understood intuitively by artists and designers. Validated and illuminated by experimental, psychological research, however, they can be self-consciously applied.[23]

This body of research suggests that important perceptual features need to be discernable in order to arouse pleasure or displeasure. They can be made to stand out from a confusing welter of detail by contrast, a long-recognized design principle already encountered in relation to Bauhaus pedagogy. Once different experiential elements are identified they are often grouped according to similarity, a tendency particularly marked within single sensory modalities. Hence, the grouping of features with similar or related functions is common in aesthetic practices.

Balance or harmony between discernably different features is often perceived as pleasurable. Shapes, forms and compositions based on the golden section, as well as symmetry, have supplied perceptibly balanced arrangements. Preferred proportionality also seems to be strongly medium specific. Another principle relevant to sensory preference is unity in diversity, that is, arrangements of multiple sensible features that appear to 'hang together'. Simultaneous awareness of high levels of multiplicity and complexity, together with strongly unifying grouping, appears to match interest or arousal with intelligibility and reassurance and so provides pleasure.

For experimental psychology the meaningful properties of objects are subjective. That is, an artefact looks or sounds up-to-date or typical or strange because of a judgement or interpretation made by the user about perceivable features. Objects recognized as familiar or as prototypical of things of a certain sort are often rated pleasurable, perhaps because the cognitive processing necessary to reach this judgement seems to reach a satisfying conclusion. An object can be perceived as particularly exciting and resolved because it successfully exaggerates key, prototypical features, the well-known 'peak-shift' principle. With objects perceived to be 'honest', overt properties provide relevant, reliable information. For example, a ceramic cup conveys information about drink temperature while a polystyrene container does not.

While repetition and familiarity are widely conducive to aesthetic pleasure, there are also contrary principles like novelty and originality. The results of experiment and innovation may be stimulating and exciting, but they also risk appearing strange, ugly or unintelligible. Researchers have found maximum preference for 'intermediate' levels of perceived originality, somewhere between complete familiarity and extreme novelty. Repeated exposure to new sensory experiences often seems necessary before they become enjoyable.

Returning to consumer-led design, it was recognized in the 1930s that value could also be added to essentially similar products by 'eye appeal'. Attractiveness need not depend entirely on aesthetic pleasure but could also come from the incorporation of an appropriate message about the tastes, standing and outlook of the product's possessor. If Whiteley (1993) is correct, the emergence of contemporary design begins with a shift from a hedonistic or aesthetic view of sensory experience to a concern with the capacity of sensory experience offered by designed artefacts to convey social meaning. Out of the process of mobilizing the sensory so that it conveys a story about ownership, taste and imagined identity develops 'the outlook of the market economy, and this ideology forms the very basis from which our contemporary design emerges' (14).

Efforts to stimulate the desire to consume are part of a familiar story with important economic and social consequences.[24] In order to create demand for new products before old ones were worn out, designers, marketers and advertisers had to work together to create new wants, not merely for cheaper and functionally superior products but for the accoutrements and signs of lifestyle identity, with visual and other sensory features functioning as social signs. While it is undeniable that the look of modernist design can signify lifestyle, outlook or status, nevertheless its theory and practice uphold quite different values, and if consistently carried out according to these fundamental principles, it departs radically from consumer-led design. Whiteley's alternatives to what he calls consumerist design – green and sustainable design, matched by responsible consuming – typically put moral, political and ecological principles at the forefront of their concerns, not sensory or aesthetic qualities, although this is not to say that they ignore them entirely.[25]

While the lifestyle semiotics of the consumer-design approach persists, much contemporary design incorporates the somewhat broader idea of planned perceptual qualities conveying a meaning of some kind. Social signification can be one among several such meanings. More important in specific cases could be the capacity of the artefact's form and appearance to suggest actions relevant to its use, sometimes referred to as 'affordances'.[26] For example, the simple, horizontal door handle can invite both the correct hand position and its downward movement. Other meanings will often be, however, rhetorical attempts to persuade the purchaser or user that a product is connected to desired values or purposes. Design rhetoric in this sense, creates the 'ethos' of an object by incorporating a 'sign value'. For example, the supposed ethical practices of coffee bean suppliers or the performance and orthopaedic advantages of a new running shoe are meant to give products an edge in competitive markets where meaning can matter just as much as price or functionality.

Marshall McLuhan's famous distinction between 'hot' and 'cool' media (McLuhan 1964) highlighted the importance for media like film, photography, radio and the lecture of a predominating single sense and their low levels of audience participation, whereas for media like television, cartoons and the seminar more than one sense and active participation were often called for. When McLuhan wrote this original definition he considered television a cool medium, although nowadays it would more likely be considered towards the hot end of the spectrum, along with interactive media such as video games. 'Hot' and 'cold' with respect to media thus turn out to be, as McLuhan intended, not static definitions but dynamic concepts. As technology moves towards creating more multimodal and multisensory experiences this idea provides a useful lens for considering what type of interaction is desired. For example, is a designer trying to create something that will conjure up vivid perceptions and give information quickly, or is the aim to facilitate less hurried, more detailed and nuanced exploration? For a number of designers, the ubiquity of screens and screen interface technology and the attendant eclipse of materials and material properties have reached some kind of limit, and there are signs of a revived interest in sensory contact with material things, a more embodied idea of experience.

Music and Sound Culture

A history of Western and global music and musicology from a sensory point of view is beyond the scope of this introduction. From the point of view of a sensory approach to sonic arts, however, it would be useful to outline the appearance in the early years of the twentieth century of atonal composition, together with Theodor Adorno's notorious critique of a 'decadent' musical culture, and the emergence, through technological innovations and artistic experiment, of sound culture.

Classical and popular music, as well as jazz, are structured around tonality, a system of notes – sounds with a definite pitch and duration – organized so that one tone is central, with other notes forming a hierarchy around it. The music composed between 1903 and 1925 by Alban Berg, Arnold Schoenberg and Anton Webern, members of the Second Viennese School, was a response to what they saw as a creative crisis in late-romantic music. Rejecting tonality, they were guided by sometimes highly abstract principles and systems, which they saw as authentic, necessary developments in musical structure. For the unconverted, however, the results can sound not like music but jangling, random noise. While the 'difficulty' of much modernist art has diminished over time, this perception – in effect a judgement based on a discrepancy between what is heard and the sensory and emotional pleasure expected of music – has for many remained stubbornly in place.

Adorno, a philosopher and critic, but also a pupil and friend of Alban Berg, gives a controversial interpretation of this and other changes in musical form and its context. His ambitious social theory of music culture is about the historical fate of the senses, and in particular what happens to ways of actively or reflectively attending to sensory experience – seeing as opposed to looking, hearing rather than listening – in the transition from industrial to consumer capitalism. In 'On the Fetish Character of Music and the Regression of Listening' Adorno adapts Marx's critique of 'commodity fetishism' applying it to cultural goods and music in particular. Marx argued that the money and markets of capitalism convert the things produced by human beings to meet human needs into commodities, goods and services bought and sold on a market. The value of a commodity is established either in terms of other goods that can be exchanged for it or its monetary value or price. In this process the human characteristics and worth of the thing – its sensuous materiality, its capacity to contribute to the meeting of human needs and the quality of life – disappear into an exchange value universally mediated by monetary worth.

According to Adorno, in classical Greece music was understood to have the capacity to both excite violent emotions and to calm them, preoccupations vividly present in the myth of Orpheus. Up to the advent of mature capitalism music retained these dimensions, and was able periodically to function critically by expressing and endorsing sensuality and spontaneity against the social imperatives of uniformity and self-discipline. It represented and projected a kind of subjective freedom held up against the demands of inequitable necessity. Yet the greatest music also incorporated a utopian moment of synthesis, an image of happiness and fulfilment.

> Not only does the musical synthesis preserve the unity of appearance and protect it from falling apart into diffuse culinary moments, but in such unity, in the relation of particular moments to an evolving whole, there is also preserved the image of a social condition in which above those particular moments of happiness would be more than mere appearance. (Adorno 1991: 28)

For Adorno, under mature capitalism all forms of music become commodities, designed artefacts whose sensory characteristics and meanings are determined increasingly by their capacity to achieve monetary value. The sensory allure of the commodity is not incorporated simply to make it attractive but in order to disguise its real nature as abstract exchange value.

Adorno argues that the production and reproduction of music under modern conditions – in the concert hall and recording studio, in distribution and broadcasting – is typically a process of simplification and homogenization. Emphasis is added to some features and passages to create palatable sonic morsels like prominent melodies, lavish musical colour and drama. The contribution of parts to the whole is de-emphasized, resulting in conglomerates of sensual richness and structural impoverishment. The 'culinary' pleasures of music divert listeners from realizing and exploring more deeply what is missing from contemporary life, denying them dissatisfaction and critique. Art's 'promise of happiness' was a fitfully anticipated hope of resolution, in which sensory pleasure was accompanied by intellectual awareness of the distance between desire and the conditions of its ultimate satisfaction. Yet at this point in its history neither the genuinely hedonistic nor critical possibilities of music are possible. The sonic *bonne bouche* and the need to be readily recognized as belonging to one or other familiar genre deprive music of the capacity to be disruptive and strange. For Adorno, even the purported musical novelties found in jazz and pop are merely dissimulated familiarity. Recognition and repetition dominate what Adorno calls 'regressive listening' to highly standardized products. Against this background only an austere denial of debased musical pleasures in the interest of the quasi-autonomous demands of musical structure retains some validity, something Adorno found in atonal composition. Although condemned by critics from the political right and left as exaggerated, sweeping and elitist, Adorno's is an important critical analysis of the connection between art's sensory pleasures and meanings and the changing ways in which cultural forms can be technologically and economically produced, reproduced, distributed and commercialized.

Although music is constituted by sounds, the idea of sonic culture suggests the possibility of works having some of the characteristics of music but without being music in the conventional sense. It is almost as if sound, in order to be perceivable as such, needs to be released from its employment in music. Audio culture, which has emerged over the past half century as a result of the work not just of musicians, composers and sound technologists but also of artists from a variety of backgrounds, is defined by attention to 'sonic substance, the act of listening, and the creative possibilities of sound recording, playback, and transmission' (Cox and Warner 2004: xiii). Interest in extending the boundaries or questioning restrictive definitions of music has often come from trained performers, theorists and composers. Other contributors have been engaged primarily with the development and exploration of sonic technologies, devising new sound-producing equipment and modifying existing instruments, for example, Harry Partch's percussion instrument *Cloud Chamber Bowls* and Conlon Nancarrow's designs and works for player-piano. Trained as a radio engineer, and working directly with sound material instead of notation and scores, Pierre Schaeffer used emerging recording devices to expand the range of expressive sounds available to composers and performers beyond those available through traditional musical instrumentation.

Perhaps the best known twentieth-century figure linking sound culture with experimental music is John Cage, whose influences came from a wide variety of sources, including Western classical music, Indian philosophy and Buddhism, and whose innovations include musical indeterminacy, aleatory composition, electro-acoustics and advances in 'prepared' instrumentation. His most famous piece, *4' 33"*, was a performance of the absence of deliberate 'musical' sound. The point of the piece is not, however, a polemical or theoretical challenge to ideas about the identity of music or its sensory seductions, but rather to encourage awareness of whatever sounds are present in the environment around the performance. In ways similar to Ruskin's exercises in visual acuity, Cage is seeking to stimulate listening and careful attention to the fabric of daily life.

An important aspect of recent sound culture has been the impact of technology for recording, producing, modifying and disseminating sound. McLuhan famously forecast that the advent of electronic media would see the displacing of predominantly silent and visual forms of communication in favour of media offering multisensory, immersive experiences (McLuhan and Powers 1989). More recently others have argued that sound recording supplants the visual and intellectual predominance of score-based Western classical music, democratizing sonic culture and making the 'ear' more prominent. The tape recorder and more recent computer devices have made it easy for music production to bypass traditional instruments, skills, contexts of performance and even sounds. All this has been expanded and enhanced by the appearance of digital technology. Yet possible uses of this technology are enormously diverse, and the tension remains between new forms of 'music' and pieces in which sound, and its cognates, silence and noise, are evident and given significance in their own right.

Turning now to the individual contributions, the chapters in Section 1 are concerned with relationship between the sensory aspects of the arts and design, the contemporary urban environment and new technologies.

As darkness falls, vision's limited powers makes other senses more prominent. The multisensory romance of the city at night conjures up images of chance encounters and unfamiliar or eerie sights and sounds. In 'Shadowplay – Liberation and Exhilaration in Cities at Night' Nick Dunn considers the experiential, methodological and artistic possibilities offered by nocturnal walking in the contemporary city, contributing to an anthropology of the city at night. In the process, Dunn revisits the 'nocturnal palimpsest', with its tropes of flight and freedom, of clandestine activity and exotic sensory encounters. The linking of the city at night with cultures of disaffection has a long history, from Charles Baudelaire's nineteenth-century evocation of the 'spectacle of Paris' to the art and literature of Surrealism, Situationism and psychogeography in the twentieth century. In the twenty-first century, the city as a setting for nocturnal wandering has begun to change dramatically. Although sober citizens often avoid some areas after dark, and there night's shadows can still avail privacy or threat, elsewhere there have been sustained attempts at surveillance and control usually to reduce the visible signs of criminality, disorder and poverty, and to engineer an optimally efficient consumer-oriented environment. Reflecting on the emergence of the 'digital panopticon', Dunn assesses the potential of digital mediation, its distractions and constraints, but also finds continued opportunities for deviance, resistance, reflection and creativity.

In 'The Role of Playfulness and Sensory Experiences in Design for Public Health and for Ageing Well' Emmanuel Tsekleves and Andy Darby describe and evaluate a collaborative research project aiming to produce a playfully interactive walking trail offering new opportunities for enjoyable, casual physical activity in one of Lancaster's parks. Working with the local community and the Lancaster City Council, and following a co-design process, a number of interactive and multisensory schemes for casual play were proposed, examined and evaluated with potential users. The study describes how, following extended user engagement, visitors to this urban park were given the opportunity to design and interact virtually and physically with purpose-built games and experiences via Near Field Communication technology, including the making of a large hybrid wind chimes and a xylophone artefact providing physical and digital experience. The case study highlights the importance for scheme users of sensory and bodily play that is perceived as 'enjoyable' rather than as highly strenuous and demanding.

Naomi Jacobs and Jonny Huck, in 'Can We Give Ourselves Extra Senses? Exploring Sensory Augmentation', describe a design project aimed to assess the technological augmentation of senses relevant to navigation, and in particular whether current directional technology is able to facilitate a 'sense of direction'. Their case study uses a first-person experiential methodology to explore the question of what a new sense might feel like. That is, how would the provision of an extra directional sensibility impact upon a mobile experience of the landscape, particularly if this is in addition to the standard range of senses? Jacobs and Huck's project was designed to assess the extra-sensory augmentation provided by the wearable *Northpaw* navigation device. Technology like this can be attached to the body but the information it supplies is not necessarily experienced *through* the body, thus producing embodied cognition. Jacobs and Huck ask whether available technology has this capacity to supply an integrated, subliminal 'sense of direction', and, if so, how this could influence a user's feeling for space and place? In addition, a digital public space created and available through portable devices now surrounds much physical space, raising questions about access to it and its eventual effects on other modes of awareness.

In 'Sonifying Memory: Creative Approaches to Representing Socially Constructed Soundscapes', Linda O'Keeffe examines an artist residency at the Leitrim Sculpture Centre, Ireland, that culminated in the construction of a solo exhibition in 2014. The work was an attempt to represent artistically the soundscape memories of a collection of five older adults who had lived in or near the Smithfield area of Dublin from the 1940s, and sonic data collected by eighty-four teenagers living in or around Smithfield today. These participants were part of a large research project, examining the co-construction of an urban soundscape. In particular, the study interrogated the potential of sound to shape communities' perception of place. Further, the research found that the users of space play a part in its co-construction, not in an actual physical re-design but in re-imagining spatial use and meaning through the deployment of their own sounds. Discussing the relationship between academic research, creative practice and a process of co-design, O'Keeffe sees the project as an examination of sound as a social construct within the context of an urban location having a history as well as a specific social and cultural character. However, in reimagining the findings as a work of art new ideas and questions emerged about how one can represent sensory knowledge through creative practice. The chapter looks at both collection methods and some of the findings from the research, and how these were translated into a sound installation.

The contributions to Section 2 critically appraise conventional views of the significance of the so-called proximal or lower senses in art and culture, advocating a more inclusive approach to historical evaluations and contemporary curating. They also evaluate current trends in architecture from a sensory point of view and argue that an art form, in this case music, apparently dominated by one sensory mode frequently shows the capacity vividly to evoke others.

In 'Scented Colours: The Role of Olfaction in Futurism and Olfactory (Re-)Constructions', Caro Verbeek argues that the sense of smell was a source of inspiration, as well as a means of expression, to European visual artists at the *fin de siècle*. The by-then deteriorating position of sight as the noblest of senses was under attack by artists searching for a less intellectual, more direct and corporeal way of engaging a wider, less uniformly bourgeois audience. Artists such as F. T. Marinetti and Marcel Duchamp turned to olfaction as a means of achieving this end. Especially during the interwar period, Futurists, Dadaists and Surrealists organized scented dinner parties and performances, and created aromatic toys and perfumed sculptures. Unfortunately most of these events and objects are by now inodorate, lost or were never recorded. Therefore part of the methodology of the innovative research reported in Verbeek's chapter involves the reconstruction of these art historical scents, in collaboration with International Flavours & Fragrances, a major producer of these products, and heritage institutions, such as the Rijksmuseum (Amsterdam) and Villa Rot (Burgrieden). Behind the specific project is the hope that it will once again be possible to 'get in touch' with this volatile heritage. The main question explored in the chapter is, however, what does it actually mean to perceive scents of the past?

Mark Clintberg reminds the reader that while the sense of taste has long been used as a convenient metaphor for aesthetic acuity in the fields of art history, connoisseurship and philosophy, and has been applied to the apprehension of artworks in museums, visitors to such environments have generally been required to appreciate exhibitions primarily through the sense of sight, leaving their literal, gustatory sense of taste at the museum entrance. In his chapter, 'Museums of Good Taste, Artworks of Good Taste: Gastronomic Contemporary Art', he argues that today's art museums are going through a radical sensory shift, whereby the non-visual senses, and taste in particular, are entering the gallery, taking on much more than metaphorical significance. The chapter discusses the increasing number of gastronomic art practices making their way into museums and galleries, and explores the changing philosophical terrain first used to block such gastronomic experiences from the museum. Focussing his discussion on the work of Felix Gonzalez-Torres and Rirkrit Tiravanija, Clintberg shows the gustatory sense has vibrant artistic potential that is being used to celebrate taste, as well as a capacity for the expression and exchange of social and cultural meaning. Taste, argues Clintberg, should now be recognized not as offering merely proximal and so restricted experience, but as a sense affording rich aesthetic contemplation and important cultural meanings.

Joy Malnar uses the occasion of the 2015 Chicago Architecture Biennial competition to assess the state of today's architecture, specifically when judged from the point of view of sensory and bodily embedding of people in places and with nature. She argues in 'The 2015 Chicago Architecture Biennial: The State of Sensory Design' that competing designs for the lake-front 'kiosks' largely failed to improve the built environment of Chicago's Lake Michigan waterfront, and therefore contributed little to what should be an open, accessible, richly enjoyable public space. Due to the structure of the competition itself, departures from the competition brief and a lack of intimate knowledge of and engagement with the Chicago location, as well as a lingering 'ocularcentric' outlook still found in today's echoes of architectural modernism, the kiosks, or rather what in reality became pavilions, were all too often primarily things to be viewed, despite more ambitious interactive and ecological intentions. Advocating an expanded notion of design embracing experiential, symbolic and ecological aspects, Malnar believes that public architecture should seize the opportunity to foster a multisensory awareness of, and an embodied engagement with, the natural and human environment, and in this way contribute to the enjoyment and well-being of a diverse citizenry.

The capacity of music to transport the hearer to another 'place', an attractive or yearned for 'affective environment' with sensory aspects, has been widely discussed, a phenomenon that applies also to other kinds of art. In 'Music: Seeing and Feeling with the Ears', Alan Marsden and Richard Leadbeater propose that the imaginative destination is not simply sonic in character, but exhibits other kinds of objects and events, appearances and textures, a 'deeper' sensory and emotional manifold contributing to the intuition of an imaginative world in which to 'be' differently. They focus on sensations reported to be integral to the experience of music, not to the context of listening. Of particular interest are listener descriptions of the intrinsic character of a piece of music as 'dark', 'light' or 'hard', terms which have a distinct sensory aspect. Drawing on extensive database records of interviews, as well as original research into the reception of music, Marsden and Leadbeater investigate this idea of the multi- or metasensory character of the experience of art works able to transport their audience. This alternative reality accessible through music is available to all the senses, not just through hearing. It does not demand sensory specialization, yet appears to be richly sensuous.

Finally, the essays in Section 3, explore visual and tactile responses to original paintings as opposed to reproductions, the challenges to interface design offered by virtual objects and screen access, and the strategies of artists confronting invisible or barely visible subjects. They also review 'opticality', a concept widely disputed by different approaches to the status of the visual, and the reality of the painter's studio, whose multisensory aspects are arranged to serve the needs of a bodily and material practice.

Beth Harland and Nick Donnelly, in 'Art Spectatorship and the Senses: An Eye Movement Analysis Exploring the Experience of Viewing Paintings and Reproductions', interrogate the significance of apparently fine sensory differences between viewing reproductions of paintings and viewing the things themselves. Image reproduction has expanded our knowledge of the world's great art collections, but the nature of the experience when viewing a reproduction as against an actual work is altered. Images evoke a range of sensory, emotional and cognitive experiences that go beyond the merely visual. In particular, paintings displayed in galleries are presumed to hold pre-eminence for spectators over reproductions of them. We might be said to engage a range of senses in a more active manner in the presence of a painting. The pre-eminence of the original emerges in the availability for inspection of information about physical relief that we can add to the colour, texture and form information available in both paintings and reproductions. This study of Manet's *A Bar at the Folies Bergere* in the Courtauld Gallery, London, by a team of artists and psychologists using eye-tracking technology, explores whether the availability of relief information changes the pattern of fixations for spectators viewing the picture. Four expert and four novice spectators viewed the original painting in situ, and sixteen novices viewed a to-scale reproduction of the picture. All spectators had their eye movements recorded as they verbally described the image and their response to it. Harland and Donnelly summarize their findings and shed light on the importance of the perceptual properties of the original for different aspects of the viewing experiences of novice and expert groups.

The arrival of different kinds of communicative, 'intelligent' and interactive technologies, some of which are being embedded in a wide range of ordinary, everyday objects, the so-called Internet of Things, is changing the landscape for design practice, argues Paul Coulton in 'Sensing Atoms and Bits'. While traditional product design was guided by functionality and aesthetics, clues or 'affordances' about its potential use were often incorporated into the object. Both designers and users had the chance of evaluating practical hypotheses about the purpose and functions of a product through direct sensory information, but this is not the case with virtual objects accessed through screens. Hence, the notion of affordances, classically understood as opportunities for specific uses and employments objectively present in things themselves, confronts fresh problems in a world accessed through screens. While relatively recently the Internet was a place to be visited, now, argues Coulton, it is 'where we live'. He describes some of these new technologies and the concepts and terminology that are being developed by designers and theorists in order to understand the opportunities and challenges they represent, for example, new object types like gizmos, spimes and biots. He discusses the design of a 'physical playlist', a novel 'intelligent' hybrid object which is physical, shareable and can be made personal, the 'information bandwidth' of different sensory channels, and a difference between sensing and perceiving which he believes may be of increased importance to designers as they confront and devise a new reality of 'atoms and bits'.

Sarah Casey and Gerry Davies's 'Drawn Away From Vision: Encounters with the Unseen' examines strategies used in drawing to capture information at the edge of, and even beyond, the scope of vision. Using historical and contemporary examples they discuss the responses of artists who draw when efforts to capture and convey visual information face serious challenges, either because the subject is unavailable to normal vision or when practices of observation have become highly problematic, for example, in conditions of darkness. Ranging across scientific and fine art traditions they explore the appeal to other senses supplementary to vision in order adequately to convey experiences that are fugitive, bewildering or unfathomably intricate. The chapter analyses how artists have challenged their graphic competencies, identifying where traditional methods help and where they break down. The works of Thomas Harriot, Robert Hooke, George Stubbs, the extraordinary drawings of the seventeenth-century portrait miniaturist Johannes Thopas, and the nineteenth- and twentieth-century biological illustrations of Ramon y Cajal and Camilio Golgi provide important historical examples. Turning to the strategies of contemporary artists engaged with the unseen or the invisible, Casey and Davies examine a number of innovative contemporary drawing practices. Lucy Lyons' work is concerned with what lies at the edge of vision, while Claude Heath and Peter Matthews grapple with phenomena that are invisible or indistinct, appealing instead to other senses, touch in the case of Heath, and the sense of bodily immersion for Matthews. Their discussion of the drawings of Sian Bowen also concerns the salience of tactility, with intricate marks tracing the contact of the drawing instrument with paper, recalling the articulacy of tactile gestures. They suggest how this tactile plenum invokes a kind of perceptual silence.

Critical debates about modern and postmodern visual art have repeatedly taken up the idea of 'opticality'. In 'From Impressionism to Opticality: An Episode in the Sensory History of Art', Ian Heywood revisits important episodes in these debates in order to clarify and separate different interpretations of this idea, and evaluate its implications for the study of sensory culture. Specifically, it is argued that Greenberg's idea of opticality seeks to encapsulate, but ultimately confuses, two different notions. The first, for which Greenberg has been justly criticized, is a restrictive teleology that seeks strenuously to isolate and decontextualize vision. The second, informed by Greenberg's acute critical analysis of the late paintings of Paul Cézanne, brings to light a fundamental historical aspect of the relationship between vision and touch, and between illusion and frank materiality in modern painting, a nexus with important philosophical and cultural implications. The latter are discussed with reference to Robert Pippin's recent revision of Hegelian aesthetics, and a comparison with other accounts of pictorial modernism, and in particular an interpretation of the philosophical significance of the sensory and material aspects of Paul Cézanne's late painting given by Merleau-Ponty and Martin Heidegger.

In 'A Choreography of the Senses – The Painter's Studio', Pip Dickens explores how the studio environment is organized and used to control the impact of sensory experience on the practice of painting. While vision has, necessarily, a leading position in the painter's studio, the receptivity of other senses contributes other kinds of awareness, sometimes required by or helpful to the embodied business of making pictures but at others distracting and unwanted. The close connection between painting practice and touch is well known, but, suggests Dickens, the supposedly less relevant senses of sound and smell also belong to the multisensory studio environment. In addition, Dickens considers the repetitive, rhythmic movement of the artist around the studio and his or her gestures in front of the work as the elements of a kind of integrated proprioceptic awareness. The widely discussed phenomenon of 'flow' or 'being in the zone' also attests to a qualitative dimension to self-perception of bodily movement. Dickens proposes that a 'choreography of the senses' is what the studio enables, allowing specific sensory inputs to be turned on or off, amplifying some and quieting others, in relation to the demands of the activity or work taking place.

In conclusion, while contemporary art and design have important historical and professional differences, and host within them many contrasting approaches, the research and creative practice reported in this collection suggests significant areas of overlap, some historical, some more recent in origin and others emerging now. One such area is a continued recognition of the ways in which acute awareness of the presence and action of the sensory aspects of arts and design artefacts is essential in thinking about their effects and meanings for users and audiences. The capacity to work sensitively and creatively with sensory experiences of different kinds remains essential to arts and design education, training and practice. While the rise of 'digital culture', the Internet of Things and screen-based interaction has attracted considerable attention, the challenges and opportunities of sensory, embodied experience for designers and artists remain, albeit in ways modified by the economic and social embedding of computer technologies in everyday life.

Hopefully, the collection also makes evident what can often be the false polarity between cultural artefacts in which one sense appears to play a leading role and artefacts which are ostensibly multisensory and immersive. Several factors may be involved. First, recent neurological research has revealed how different sensory modalities are closely connected in what is called 'multisensory integration'. It may therefore be extraordinarily difficult, not to say unnatural, for human beings rigorously to isolate one sense from another. Second, what the modal anthropologist François Laplantine (2015) calls 'sensory thinking' is surely the core of arts and design practices. Close attention to and analysis of these practices and their outcomes reveal that intense creative work with and through the medium of one sense almost invariably spills over into other modalities. Senses misbehave, they refuse to be regulated, confined and split off. When separated they call out, appeal to and echo one another. Sometimes the empirical absence of a particular mode of sensory experience, notably touch and sound in the context of the visual arts, creates reverberations which, although they can only be given visual expression, are nevertheless profoundly important to the experience and meaning of a work.

The chapters in this book also make clear that the sensory aspects of the arts and design are not addressed finally to the receptive but isolated individual as sources of hedonistic pleasure with a capacity for market exploitation or social control. As Laplantine argues, and as the history, outlook and working practices of the arts and design attest, the 'mind' should not be seen as property of the brain once it has reached a certain level of neurological complexity, but as flowing out and back through the body into the social and cultural world. The arts and design typically supply concrete vitality to cultural forms but also offer critical, sensory reflection on their meaning and qualities. This is perhaps the right way to understand what John Berger is trying to get at in remarks about the results of sustained sensuous thinking in the paintings of Matisse and Velazquez. What Matisse sought to express through his passion for 'pure colour' was not so much the pleasures of bourgeois opulence but ' "the nearly religious feeling" he had towards sensuous life' (Berger 2015: 279), its universality and value. In Velazquez's paintings of Phillip IV's court jesters and buffoons, infinitely distant from run-of-the-mill royal portraits, is a kind of self-possession. While the face of Juan Calabas is 'flickering with laughter', his eyes are 'impassive'. The buffoons are not absent from themselves, in the theatricality of their court role or in mental confusion, 'they simply find themselves – after the laughter – beyond the transient' (136). Yet in visibly claiming for themselves the dignity of self-possession they also confront, and prompt in the viewer, an awareness of the difficulty and fragility of this achievement, and with it the question of the place and significance of the senses and the body under modern conditions.

Notes

1 For a larger historical canvas, see Classen 2014.
2 Howes 2013.
3 For example, see the Sensory Studies website, and its reviews and reports of publications: http://www.sensorystudies.org/ (accessed 17 October 2016). See also the journal *Senses and Society*: http://www.tandfonline.com/toc/rfss20/current/ (accessed 27 October 2016).
4 This kind of attention usually applies even to 'conceptual' work positioning itself in opposition to what is seen as an exaggerated or unwarranted interest in sensory experience. Conceptual art has its distinctive 'aesthetic'.
5 See Christine Poggi's convincing and salutary correction of standard views of Futurism: Poggi 2009.
6 See Jay 1991: 15–38, which formed the basis for the fourth chapter of *Downcast Eyes* (Jay 1993).
7 See Breton (2002), *Surrealism and Painting*. There is insufficient space to discuss Surrealist photography, but see Krauss's strenuous efforts to narrow the gap between Surrealist photography and Derridean ecriture (Krauss 1981), Sherringham's balanced account (Sherringham 2006) and Jay (1993: 26–27). For Surrealist cinema, see Richardson (2006), Matthews (1971) and Kovacs (1980). Also Jay (1993: 27–30)
8 See also his essays on Dalí and Vincent Van Gogh in *Visions of Excess*: 'The "Lugubrious Game"' and 'Sacrificial Mutilation and the Severed Ear of Vincent van Gogh', respectively.
9 Jay, 'Scopic Regimes of Modernity Revisited' in Heywood and Sandywell 2014.
10 See Jay 1992: 23.
11 Sheringham observes that for Breton special moments of perception can reveal a 'connection between life as something given (rather than earned), and individual subjectivity as something virtual rather than circumscribed' (Sherringham 2006: 70).
12 See also Sheringham's discussion of the 'philosophy of self-evidence' (2006: 85–86).
13 See Higgins 2002. Also Higgins, 'Art and the Senses: The Avant-Garde Challenge to the Visual Arts' in Classen 2014, volume 6.
14 See Barbara Kirshenblatt-Gimblett, 'Playing to the Senses: Food as a Performance Medium', *Performance Research* 4(1) (1999): 1–30.
15 See Jeanie Forte, 'Women's Performance Art: Feminism and Postmodernism', in *Theatre Journal* 40(2) (May, 1988): 217–235.
16 See the discussion of Hans Haake in Bois 1993: xvii–xx.
17 See Sauvagnargues 2013 and Heywood 2002.
18 See Caroline A. Jones 2006.
19 See Whiteley 1993.
20 In architecture broadly 'modernist' styles still thrive; for example, see two recent winners of the Royal Institute of British Architects' annual Sterling prize, the Marburg Museum of Literature (Germany) and the Sainsbury Laboratory in Cambridge (UK). Broadly modernist design styles are also found in many domestic consumer products, for example, the IKEA range and in many more expensive brands.

21 Some historians of design give paramount importance to approaches largely determined by consumer behaviour, and oppose this directly to a design history focused on the ideas of a few, visionary designers. See Woodham 1997.

22 Passage quoted by Schifferstein and Hekkert in Bacci and Melcher 2001: 543.

23 See Schifferstein and Hekkert in Bacci and Melcher for a useful summary of this body of research. Also Schifferstein and Hekkert 2007 for an application to product design in particular.

24 A high level of consumer spending, as opposed to saving, has long been seen as critical to the health of market economies. Easy credit led to increasing levels of household debt in advanced economies. US household debt rose from nearly zero in the 1950s to $13.8 trillion in 2008, before declining to $11.85 trillion by 2012 (www.businessinsider.com/ny-fed-q1-2015-household-debt-2015-5, accessed 2015). In the United Kingdom it rose rapidly until levelling off in 2007 but reaching £1.452 trillion at the end of September 2015 (themoneycharity.org.uk/money-statistics, accessed 2015).

25 'Green' architecture has been widely attacked for its supposed neglect of aesthetic principles by the architect Peter Eisenman, but defended by Lance Hosey (2012) among others.

26 The term was coined by the psychologist James J. Gibson in 1977; see his *The Ecological Approach to Visual Perception*. Affordances are 'action possibilities' objectively present in the environment whether or not agents actually recognize them as such.

References

Bacci, F. and D. Melcher (eds) (2011), *Arts and the Senses*. Oxford: Oxford University Press.

Bataille, G. (1985), *Visions of Excess: Selected Writings, 1927–1939*, edited and introduced by Alan Stoekl, translated by Allan Stoekl with Carl R. Lovitt and Donals M. Leslie, Jr. Minneapolis: University of Minnesota Press.

Berger, J. (2015), *Portraits: John Berger on Artists*, edited by Tom Overton. London: Verso.

Bois, Yves Alain (1993), *Painting as Model*. Cambridge MA: MIT Press.

Breton, Andre (2002), *Surrealism and Painting*, introduction by Mark Polizzotti. Boston: MFA Publications.

Classen, C. (ed.) (2014), *A Cultural History of the Senses*, vols. 1–6. London: Bloomsbury.

Cox, C. and D. Warner (eds) (2004), *Audio Culture: Readings in Modern Music*. New York: Continuum.

Gibson, James J. (1986), *The Ecological Approach to Visual Perception*. Hillsdale NJ: Lawrence Earlbaum Associates.

Heywood, I. (2002), 'Deleuze on Francis Bacon'. In *A Companion to Art Theory*, edited by Paul Smith and Carolyn Wilde. London: Blackwell.

Heywood, I. and B. Sandywell (eds) (2014), *Handbook of Visual Culture*. Oxford and London. Berg/Bloomsbury.

Higgins, H. (2002), *The Fluxus Experience*. Berkeley: University of California Press.

Hosey, L. (2012), *The Shape of Green: Aesthetics, Ecology, and Design*. Washington, DC: Island Press.

Howes, D. (2013), 'The Expanding Field of Sensory Studies'. Available at http://www.sensorystudies.org/sensorial-investigations/the-expanding-field-of-sensory-studies/ (accessed June 2015).

Howes, D. and C. Classen (2014), *Ways of Sensing: Understanding the Senses in Society*. London: Routledge.

Jay, M. (1991), 'The Disenchantment of the Eye: Surrealism and the Crisis of Ocularcentrism', *Visual Anthropology Review* 7(1) (Spring): 15–38.

Jay, M. (1993), *Downcast Eyes: The Denigration of Vision in Twentieth-Century French Thought*. Berkeley: University of California Press.

Jones, Caroline A. (ed.) (2006), *Sensorium: Embodied Experience, Technology and Contemporary Art*. Cambridge, MA: MIT Press.

Kovacs, S. (1980), *From Enchantment to Rage: The Story of Surrealist Cinema*. Cranberry: Associated University Press.

Krauss, R. (1981), 'The Photographic Condition of Surrealism', *October*, 19 (Winter): 3–34.

Laplantine, F. (2015), *The Life of the Senses: Introduction to a Modal Anthropology*, translated by J. Furniss. London: Bloomsbury.

Locke, J. (1689/1964), *An Essay Concerning Human Understanding*. London: Fontana/Collins.

Loewy, R. (1951), *Never Leave Well Enough Alone*. New York: Simon and Schuster.

Matthews, J. H. (1971), *Surrealism and Film*. Ann Arbor: University of Michigan Press.

McLuhan, M. (1964), *Understanding Media: The Extensions of Man*. New York: McGraw Hill.

Poggi, C. (2009), *Inventing Futurism: The Art and Politics of Artificial Optimism*. Princeton: Princeton University Press.

Richardson, M. (2006), *Surrealism and Cinema*. Oxford: Berg Publishers.

Ruskin, J. (1904), *The Works of John Ruskin, The Elements of Drawing*, volume XV, edited by E. T. Cook and Alexander Wedderburn. London: George Allen.

Sauvagnargues, A. (2013), *Deleuze and Art*, translated by Samantha Bankston. London: Bloomsbury.

Schifferstein, Hendrick N. J. and P. Hekkert (2007) (eds), *Product Experience*, San Diego: Elsevier.

Sennett, R. (1990), *The Conscience of the Eye: The Design and Social Life of Cities*. London: Faber and Faber.

Sheringham, M. (2006), *Everyday Life: Theories and Practices from Surrealism to the Present*. Oxford: Oxford University Press.

Spark, Penny (2013), *An Introduction to Design and Culture: 1920 to the Present*. London: Routledge.

Whiteley, N. (1993), *Design for Society*. London: Reaktion Books.

Woodham, J. M. (1997), *Twentieth Century Design*. Oxford: Oxford University Press.

Part 1

Sensory Arts and Design, New Technologies and the Urban Environment

1

Shadowplay – Liberation and Exhilaration in Cities at Night

Nick Dunn

> In wide arcs of wandering through the city
> I saw to either side of what is seen,
> and noticed treasures where it was thought there were none.
> I passed through a more fluid city.
> I broke up the imprint of familiar places,
> shutting my eyes to the boredom of modern contours.
>
> (A. A. Dun 1995: 9)

Introduction – Stepping into the Uncanny

Architecture is often understood to be the concrete facts of the built environment, material assemblages that enable us to approach the city as both subject and object of narrative and interpretation. It is at once personal, borne of lived and detailed experiences, yet also universal, sometimes shared by many over its lifespan. As Aiden Andrew Dun's quote at the beginning of this chapter suggests, there is much that goes unnoticed in the city, especially in the interstitial and liminal spaces that are often overlooked. Our bodies easily conform to the familiar places of routine, and exploring the urban landscape outside of our regular patterns of movement means we can experience revelatory discoveries and create 'spatial stories' (de Certeau 1984: 115–122). So as much as we inform it, architecture in turn shapes us, to paraphrase Jonathan Raban's *Soft City*. However, this chapter will seek to explore a different and less familiar side of our cities, that is, during those hours when the daylight has gone. Over the last few years I have spent a considerable amount of time walking through and around various cities at night.[1] I wish to propose that perhaps the primacy of architecture is not its body in light but is to be found within the itinerant, fleeting shawl of darkness that recasts our built environment and senses away from the dominance of the visual towards a multisensory experience. For at night our visual abilities are attenuated, placing greater emphasis on what we hear, smell, taste and touch. During nocturnal hours the transition and time in our cities also becomes elastic and foggy, distinct in many ways from the space and place of everyday life. Behavioural patterns, regimented and routine, result in our movements inscribing various lines (Ingold 2007) upon our built environment, creating vectors (Gatt 2013) that may become residual in memory even if they are fleeting in terms of time. This chapter will draw on empirical data and personal experience in order to contribute to an understanding of the anthropology of the nocturnal city. It will seek to elucidate on the ongoing entanglement that occurs at the boundaries of body and urban landscape: day and night; space and materiality.

Journeys of the night have been the subject of contemporary depictions (Sandhu 2007), while walking as a methodology (Sinclair 1997; Careri 2001) has been recently reclaimed by various artists, writers and architects. As such, much romance has also been ascribed to nighttime peregrinations, the disclosure of clandestine operations and liminal actors, illicit encounters and the foreboding unknowns. Walking around the centres and hinterlands of cities at night, however, and the reality experienced may be far less spectacular and sensational than first assumed, at least initially. Instead of the gory 'horrorshow' of casual violence in the manner of *A Clockwork Orange* or the neon-lit carnal machine consummations of J. G. Ballard, urban landscapes at night provide intricate though frequently subdued sounds and sights. Unlike walking in the daytime, at night the city blends our different senses together into an often highly arresting quale. Indeed, to go out into the night, especially on one's own, is a decisive act. Walking is a primary measure of the urban landscape since it reaffirms our relationship to place and movement through space. Therefore, to do so at night means that our footsteps assay the blurred boundaries between essences of place and their attributes distinct from the daylight hours. Before we examine the contemporary urban night further, it is worth at this point to retrace some of the steps of those before us to understand where some of our attitudes towards the night originate.

Nocturnal Palimpsest – Those That Came Before

The history of civilization may also be understood as the history of cities, played out across a very long timeframe. The story of our relationship with cities has become increasingly relevant as more and more of us live within urban landscapes. Certainly we know that during the last decade a profound shift occurred around the globe (UNFPA 2007) insomuch that more people now live in urbanized areas than at any previous time in human history, a pattern that seems likely to continue for the foreseeable future.

Parallel to this account of our existence is an alternative history: the story of our relationship with the night, our fears, struggles and perceptions of the dark. Bound into this narrative are all our attempts to vanquish it and ultimately conquer our nocturnal environment through illumination, to exert artificial and manmade control over circadian rhythms. There is a long history of night travels as integral to cultures within darkness, the nocturnal hours sheltering the shady worlds of miscreants, shift workers and transgressors. Night by its very definition contrasts day, summoning notions of darkness and fear.

Indeed, in stark contrast to our contemporary view of it, in the past, rather than falling, night was understood to rise. As A. R. Ekirch (2005: xxxi) has noted, '[T]he darkness of the night appears palpable. Evening does not arrive, it "thickens."' This smothering of the landscape as the firmament of night condensed provides understanding as to perhaps why it has sometimes been referred to as man's first necessary evil, our oldest and most haunting terror. In his 1757 treatise, *A Philosophical Enquiry into the Origin of Our Ideas of the Sublime and Beautiful*, Edmund Burke claimed that darkness remained, as always, 'terrible in its own nature.' Throughout history, the nocturnal accomplice of darkness has cast the shadowy hours of evening and early morning as a time and space during which our rational thought could be circumvented by fear, our understanding of routine and environment be skewered by transgressions, and our innermost sanctums be invaded by unwanted guests, imaginary or sometimes deadly real. Locked doors, shuttered windows, rituals, prayers and protective charms worn to evade capture by the long claws of the night were just a few of the preventative interventions to secure one's sleep and family.

Despite this proliferation, rather than because of such measures to counter the perceived impending nightly devastations, the night did not typically bring forth ominous, even fatal, clashes of uncompromising individuals or groups, but enabled more discretely clandestine histories: times, places, spaces where human expression was not as easily subjected to the scrutiny of daytime. It is well known that up until the late seventeenth century, most people had two sleeps, with a distinct interval. Modest but highly valued freedoms from the bonds and worries of daily life could be found here. This period within the sleeping pattern was typically used for prayer, writing, sex or visiting neighbours, but the practice quickly diminished with the industrialization of cities and attendant changes in working patterns and artificial illumination, which disrupted our natural behaviour and body rhythms. As Bryan D. Palmer (2000: 9) has observed, beliefs and concerns regarding the unsettling nature of night have been metaphorically entwined through the arts, further propagating the negative aspects of darkness alloyed to cultural and social practices throughout history:

> peasant dissidents and witches in the moment of feudalism's dissolution; pornographers, libertines, monsters and Jacobin conspirators in the Age of Revolution; pirates and slaves in the ascendency of mercantile

> capitalism; debased trades and dishonorable work, the sociability of the tavern and the fraternal order, the dangerous classes of the Industrial Revolution; . . . cultures of erotic, musical, cinematic and poetic disaffection, many of which consolidate in capitalism's mid-twentieth-century epic of conformity's success, Cold War America; and the ravages of the oppressed and dispossessed in the inner cities of late capitalism's material and cultural chaos.

This leads us towards more familiar territory, the contemporary urban landscape at the beginning of the twenty-first century. Considerable attention has been given to the city and urbanism through a wide spectrum of analytical and critical lenses since issues and problems concerning these unwieldy subjects are highly complex.[2]

Digital Panopticon – What Is There Left to Feel?

The burgeoning interest in cities as places for happiness (Montgomery 2013); wealth (Glaeser 2011); social cohesion or fear (Minton 2009); or positive transformation (Hollis 2013), amongst many other perspectives, in recent years has cast them to the forefront of public consciousness through considerable debate and conjecture in the mainstream media. Cities have long been acknowledged as *the* confluence of human activity, especially commerce and capitalism, but more recently they have become the new ground for a different and frequently much more subtle type of exploitation. In this construct, venture capitalists, economists and politicians, among others, recalibrate the failing rhetoric of accelerated neoliberal capitalism into a more fluid, pervasive and insidious site for business. The message is clear if not explicitly tattooed across the built environment: without expenditure you are rarely welcome.

And this does not even account for how things change at night, which brings forth further and amplified issues of security and safety. Indeed, the threat of night has also been legislated against; as a cover it has been historically assailed by the intrusions of light (Schivelbusch 1995), and more recently the proliferation of technologies illuminating its dark corners and opening it up to the glare and stare of surveillance and scrutiny. Towards the end of the twentieth century, Jean Baudrillard (1993: 44) would summarize the disappearing qualities of the night in terms of universalizing loss, the bland homogenizing of humanity and history thus: 'Ours is rather like the situation of the man who has lost his shadow: either he has become transparent, and the light passes right through him or, alternatively, he is lit from all angles, overexposed and defenceless against all sources of light.'

This loss is not simply personal as an infringement on privacy, but also has a huge environmental cost. Efforts to protect our night skies through official organizations and community groups and reclaim the wonder of the galaxies and the highly affective chiaroscuro of moonlight have become a significant and growing concern (Attlee 2011; Bogard 2013). The plight of tens of thousands of birds trapped in the 9/11 memorial, *The Tribute in Light* in New York, is a high profile and extreme example (Talanova 2015) of a situation caused by artificial lighting in cities replicated elsewhere around the globe. In the urban landscape after dark, the question may no longer be what spaces we wish to engage with, but *when* are they? Of course, most cities are rarely plunged into complete and utter darkness and when they are it is usually due to a huge power failure, which has strong negative associations from the critical, such as the impact on emergency services, to the perceived. Much more typical and familiar to us in an urban context are the ochre glow of streetlights and neon refractions of our cityscapes. Even in those parts of the city with the greatest light pollution, the absence of people can be a strange and exhilarating experience. However, to use artificial lighting to simply enable night to function in a similar manner to day is also to tamper greatly with distinctive characteristics. Schlör (2013: 242) points towards the fundamental essence thus: 'The night tells one how the city really is, how "the whole" functions; and secondly, night, and only night, represents the presence of the past, the myth, in the city of the present.' It is this conjuring of memory, presence and attention that nightwalking provides that makes it such a deep and multisensory experience.

Beyond the confines of daily tasks there is the emergence of a desire to claim back the night, away from the data deluge of email accounts, social-media prods and attention-leeching digital devices, towards the experiential qualities of the here and now rather than the tenuous and distant. It is this recent shift in our relationship with our immediate surroundings that has become highly mediated rather than attentive. This position is further supported by Patrick Keiller (2013: 135) who laments the loss of our important and interwoven relationships with the urban landscape: 'Instead, in the UK and elsewhere, cities might now be distinguished not so much by the merits of their spatial form, their society, culture, and so on, but by how successfully they negotiate continual social, economic and technological change.'

Spatial conventions and rules are relaxed if not completely abandoned as night falls, appropriation of urban space occurs in the deep pockets of the city away from natural surveillance or the scanscape of CCTV cameras. New rhythms slowly build as the impetus for occupying nocturnal margins spreads across the urban landscape. The palimpsest of the city's surfaces is added to with graffiti tags, throw-ups and pieces, while the furtive glances buried in deep cowls elicit the adrenaline pump of those immersed in the edges of normative society, at least during these hours. For the night brings with it personal transformation alongside that of the city – as our identities blur and shift, different traits simultaneously folding in and unfurling in relation to the crepuscular environment. Our internal weather system changes, increasingly attuned and tethered to our immediate surroundings.

Out there is the endless possibility of night stretching out in every direction, in here the varying thoughts and emotions gently ebb and flow around in response to the body's changing isotherms and sensations. So how to make sense of the nocturnal urban landscape?

Making Sense of the Contemporary Cityscape

The banality of the reconstruction of many post-war European cities coupled with wider societal optimism in technologically driven futures prompted a surge of numerous architecture groups, such as Archigram, Archizoom and Haus-Rucker-Co among many others, to develop new ways of conceiving architecture and apparatus for mediating between the body and the built environment. The latter's *Environment Transformer* project of 1968 proposed 'technoid helmets that expand horizons optically, abduct their wearers to a visual course of new perspectives on the urban surroundings' (Blomberg 2014: 32). Although such novelty and experimentation prevails in architecture education and research, this fascination with spatial equipment to speculate and understand the world around us has a long history. Its value, as Geoff Manaugh (2013: 27) explains, is that 'given the right instruments, humans gain access to and, more importantly, begin to interact with entire systems of objects and landscapes that were present all along but had otherwise been physically undetectable, camouflaged or hidden against an inhuman context or background.'

There appear to be two potential fields of influence at play here. First, the fragmentation of urban space which, far from the order and legibility we may anticipate, has become complex and unintelligible (Jacobs 2002). This has led to a tendency to overlook the ordinary and commonplace, yet vital, aspects of the contemporary city. Second, the parallel aspect of the increasing emphasis on data to help us navigate and understand our cities (Offenhuber and Ratti 2014). The ability of mobile devices to provide us with continuously updated and typically accurate information about our surroundings can be very useful, especially for those uncomfortable with or seeking knowledge of new places. However, such interfaces also filter our relationship with cities, gently and surreptitiously nudging us towards particular locations of a place based on an aggregation of data mining and stored personal preferences. Perhaps of greatest concern in the context of this chapter is that such devices are highly distracting. They reduce discovery and encounter through a mediated experience. This is something most of us are fully aware of yet we find it very difficult to resist, the impact of which is enormous since our lives become saturated with 'representations' (Crawford 2015). Rather than enter the complex and broad argument about the relationship of mobile technology and its influence on us, whether for good or ill, to which others have devoted entire books if not complete oeuvres, let us just put the smartphone down for a minute, or even better turn it off.

How to make sense of any city, let alone at night when our reliance on the visual is at best diminished if not completely misleading? Wayfinding, that is, locating and orientating oneself in the built environment, is an essential part of placemaking. However, our understanding of cities does not necessarily easily correlate to the formal descriptions offered by plans and cartography. Walter Benjamin describes this disorientation between the actual experience of the city and its many representations thus:

> Now the city turns into a labyrinth for the newcomer. Streets that he had located far apart are yoked together by a corner like a pair of horses in a coachman's fist. The whole exciting sequence of topographical dummies that deceives him could only be shown by a film: the city is on its guard against him, masks itself, flees, intrigues, lures him to wander its circles to the point of exhaustion. But in the end, maps and plans are victorious: in bed at night, imagination juggles with real buildings, parks, and streets. (2005: 24)

In recognition of these phenomena and in order to better understand it, Kevin Lynch undertook pioneering research on how individuals perceive and navigate cities. His 1960 seminal work, *The Image of the City*, explained that people understood their built environment via cognitive maps that enabled them to recall the information of the urban landscape using particular elements. Of course, the nocturnal city does not necessarily provide the same degree of familiarity and congruence. Quite the opposite due to our overreliance on the visual, which, once diminished, may cause considerable alarm and discomfort. As Anthony Vidler (1992: 167), discusses, the threat of dark space is frequently perceived as the harbinger of the unseen and unnerving, 'space is assumed to hide, in its darkest recesses and forgotten margins, all the objects of fear and phobia that have returned with such insistency to haunt the imaginations of those who have tried to stake out spaces to protect their health and happiness.' Uncoupling fear and darkness is no mean feat, especially given the portrayal of cities at nighttime which, whether fictional or factualized, is often dramatic and threatening. Yet, there is little evidence to support that this depiction directly correlates into crime statistics (Felson and Poulsen 2003). On the contrary, the greater the build-up of surveillance technologies in our cities, the increase in our feelings of anxiety and fear since we enter 'the prosthetic paradox' (de Muynck 2004). Instead, it is worth reconsidering our perception, as in Minkowski (1933) and Callois (1987: 72), darkness is not the simple absence of light, 'There is something positive about it. While light space is eliminated by the materiality of objects, darkness is "filled," it touches the individual directly, envelops him, penetrates him, and even passes through him.' So how best to measure ourselves against the domain of the nighttime city? Juhani

Pallasmaa writes of the porosity between the urban landscape and the body, a relationship in flux:

> I confront the city with my body; my legs measure the length of the arcade and the width of the square; my gaze unconsciously projects my body onto the facade of the cathedral, where it roams over the mouldings and contours, sensing the size of recesses and projections; my body weight meets the mass of the cathedral door, and my hand grasps the door pull as I enter the dark void behind. I experience myself in the city, and the city exists through my embodied experience. The city and my body supplement and define each other. I dwell in the city and the city dwells in me. (2005: 40)

It is evident that materials temper our relationship with the environment physically but also physiologically. Therefore, while architecture is undoubtedly a spatial art, it may also be understood as a temporal one. The architect Peter Zumthor (2006: 13) writes about our perception of atmosphere through a highly developed emotional sensibility: 'Not every situation grants us time to make up our minds on whether or not we like something or whether indeed we might be better heading off in the opposite direction.' Such emotional sensibility is somewhat heightened in the nighttime city when our eyes are less reliable as a means to make sense of what surrounds us. In addition, the city itself changes in character: reconfiguring itself as the architecture morphs and melds. At night the whole city can become spolia for new monuments. But a nagging question recurred when presented with the opportunity to talk about my research in cities at night, that is, *how* to record this experience, the nature of which can be so elusive (Figure 1.1)?[3]

Initial perambulations led me to explore different ways to document and map my nightwalks. The first few weeks of walking were simply that, walks without purpose as I generally stayed away from bright lights and went in no particular direction, allowing the mood and weather of each walk to guide me. Upon returning home, I would think about the walk undertaken and note any points of interest. After a month or so of this, I experimented with different methods of collection, trying to capture the experiences as I walked, whether through sound recordings, short films or photographs (Figure 1.2). In all cases, the same problem, albeit with varying degrees of frustration, emerged. First, whenever I engaged in a technique, no matter how unobtrusively I sought to employ it, the very act of doing something related to the walk rather than being immersed in the act itself detracted significantly from the experience. Second, the addition of any equipment was cumbersome, not so much physically but certainly psychologically as it changed where I walked and the reasons for doing so. It brought unnecessary and often unwarranted suspicion on my motives, not always ideal given others for whom the night may provide something else.[4]

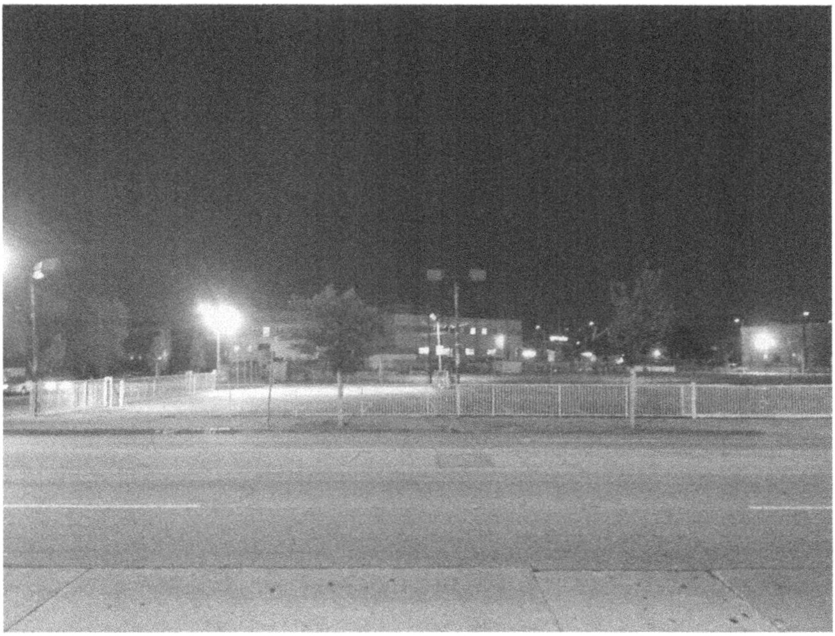

FIGURE 1.1 *Ghost urbanism, Hollywood, Los Angeles*, Nick Dunn, 9 April 2013. The ethereal and uncanny nature of an urban landscape dominated by automobiles during the day which is completely emptied out at night, that is, a distinct 'lack' of presence is palpable when physically there, but it is difficult to convey through visual material. Photo by Nick Dunn.

Similarly, attempts to use notation and sketches (Figure 1.3) were also relatively unhelpful in either describing what was experienced or ensnaring the often disparate and fleeting qualities of nightwalks in the city. Although I persevered with various maps, developing a form of shorthand notation for recording aspects, rhythms and encounters of various sorts, they still did little to evince what had transpired (Figure 1.4).

In the end, words were the least subdued way of conveying my night-walking. This is a difficult territory to enter in itself, a field of very rich and potent writers spanning a long line that has woven around philosophers, poets, psychogeographers and many more (Beaumont 2015). However, the abstraction proffered by words is useful as a device since it at once enables the detail of the walk to be explained while not relying on the visual. Furthermore, the very act of writing in this context is the tracing of a narrative that not only enables the reader to *project* (as opposed to see) their own interpretation and purview upon the text description, enabling her or him to construct a world on top of it, but it also facilitates the writer to bridge between the multisensory experience of the spatial practice and the elusive qualities of darkness in the city. It is these rich, otherworldly qualities of the everyday environment cast into shadow that stir 'the whole fauna of human

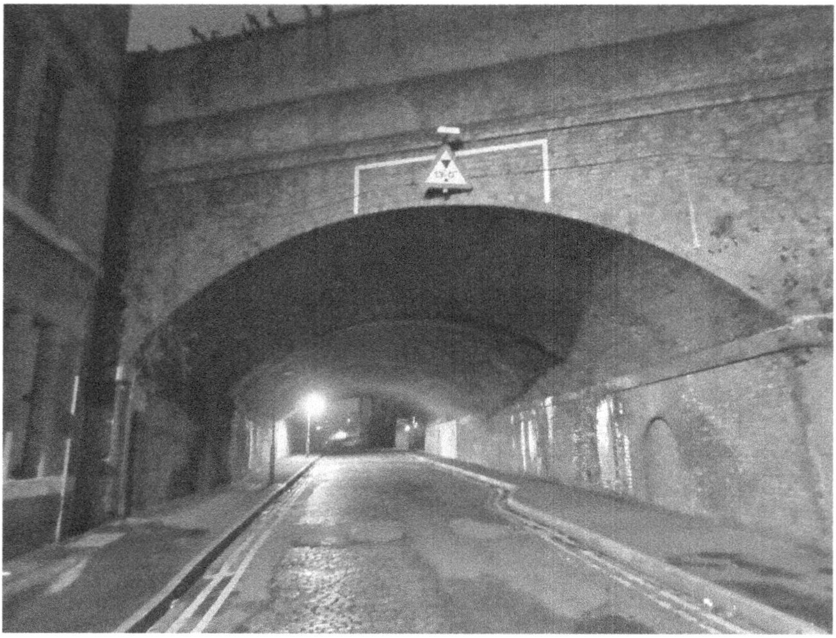

FIGURE 1.2 *Homeward bound, Chapel Street, Salford*, Nick Dunn, 26 January 2014. In the nocturnal hours, the absence of urban life and the shawl of darkness and shadows recasts the built environment, some buildings and structures lose their definition, melding and morphing into one another while time becomes elastic and foggy. Photo by Nick Dunn.

fantasies' that Louis Aragon identified, which 'drifts and luxuriates in the dimly lit zones of human activity, as though plaiting thick tresses of darkness' (1994: 13). By way of example, the following passage is an extract from one of my walks taken on 26 January 2014:

> *The night stretches before me. The background slish of traffic on the Mancunian Way overhead as I emerge, walking slowly from the subway, ears prickled by the smashing of glass somewhere behind. This is Manchester on a cold and wet winter night where the opacity of the city's infrastructure loses its gravity and melds toward the neon and sodium morse code above. Indecipherable messages, these ghost texts to unknown gods and spirits hang in the air like stolen thoughts from another time – the lost future that got delayed, tied down in the bondage of bureaucracy, boredom and blame. But now the shouting is all over. Instead, this award-winning concrete serpent remains frozen against asphalt forever, undulating between buildings and woven across the landscape. My left foot skids on the masticated remains of a club flyer chewed by rain and indifference. Where now for the secret, the quiet and contemplative?*

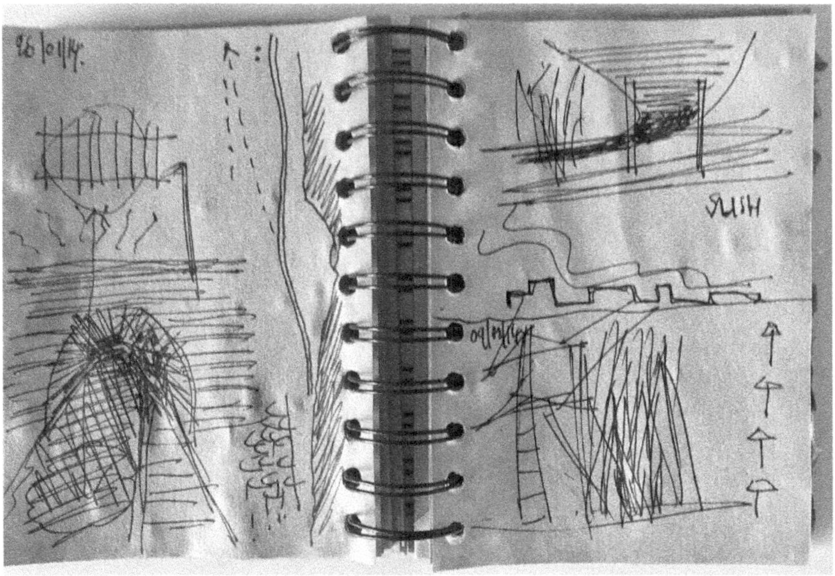

FIGURE 1.3 *Sketchbook pages, 26 January and 9 February 2014.* One double-spread from numerous notepads, sketchbooks and loose leaves of paper that illustrate quickly produced drawings. The left-hand page and top of the right-hand page were done during a nightwalk, while the image on the bottom of the right-hand page was made through recollection when I had finished another nightwalk. Photo by Nick Dunn.

Onward and up the ramp which, glistening in the wet, looks like the runway to the Beetham Tower beyond, its red lights stretching out the astral plane of the city into something significant in height if unknown in character. The decrepit shadows of Little Ireland, Engels' long since vanished horror, squalid memories held in brick and mortar hang around these streets. Slinking down alongside the culverted Medlock, the repressed industrial memories of yesteryear flow underneath hundreds of sleeping students in their castle. The dank walls of the railway viaduct run to an open mouth, the archway littered with jetsam from last night's gigs and clubs, shorn from revellers in the witching hour. Geometric fungi courtesy of the street artist Truth adorn the underbelly of the arch, somewhat tarnished and stained by the weeping brickwork after rainfall.

I am now spat out into the meniscus of Whitworth Street as it bends against the Bridgewater canal. Turning right, upward to where Oxford Street and Road kiss between The Grand Old Lady and eclectic baroque of the Refuge Assurance Building, crenellated walls run down major vistas into the city. Not tonight though. Instead, a quick retrace finds me down by the water, murky grey-brown lava, sludging past unnoticed

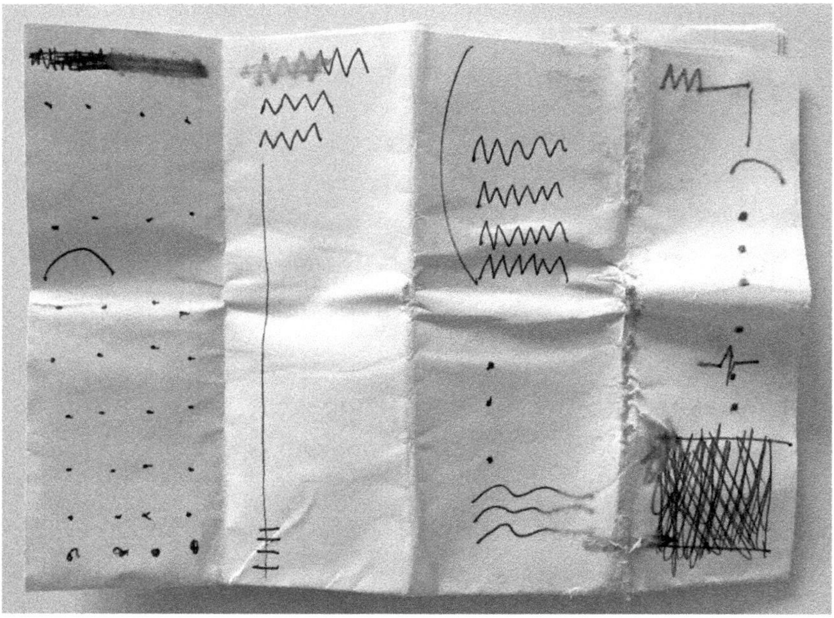

FIGURE 1.4 *Pocket Map, 20 February 2014.* An example from my extensive collection of maps made during nightwalks. Throughout the last several years I have experimented with different forms of mark making and notation to denote various aspects of the nocturnal city, such as rhythm, texture, enclosure, density, etcetera. Some were made during the walk itself, including those scribbled within the confines of a large, damp, coat pocket (several of which have perished through saturation), while others were produced through memory and reflection. Photo by Nick Dunn.

behind the blank looks of apartments and offices. Under the bridge and along the path the buildings loom inwards, a scrum of architecture leaving the constricted sky a mere navy-black bruised ribbon above.

So here I am again, a nocturnal dowser, summoning the ghostly streams of the city – palimpsestic phantoms interned in asphalt and brick lie doleful and bereft of any awakening. Flowing along the canal path, figures ahead once merged are now fleeting as new unions separate then disappear upon my footsteps. A young man with streetlamp jaundiced eyes piercing the shadows weighs up options and chances, then knocks a bottle over harrying to street level and the carn(iv)al atmosphere above. Onward and inward through the city's guts, bellicose rumblings overhead and muffled snippets of the urban corpus waft in and out of audibility. Walking down here is like sloshing through molasses save the stench – which is acrid rather than sweet – with each footstep thick as it pushes into the dark, tinged with apprehension. Slowly ascending from this underworld, I hear the stray clatter of heels and voices braying for carriages several streets away. The sterility of Piccadilly Gardens, neutered public space at its most banal, nullifies thought and reflection.

Engulfed in stone and turf platitudes even the typically lachrymose fountains can shed no more at this hour. The eels of the tramlines course in studied curvature towards Shudehill, but the gravity of Market Street draws the feet down its incline toward the pillar box at Corporation Street. That open-mouthed witness to the IRA bomb on 15 June 1996 no longer silently screaming in red but quietly memorialized in gold. Here the burnished image of the city in the aftermath of restoration and pre-millennial development can only reflect back its own emptiness. To my right, the reconstituted Sinclair's Oyster Bar and The Old Wellington Inn, themselves not saved from the traditional butchery that once resided here, now grafted together perpendicular to one another.

The downward pull continues over the River Irwell, that molten mirror that both divides and stitches Manchester and Salford. The ancestral home of Celts and Romans long since passed through, the landscape at this hour has a meagre and disparate tribe of weary pleasure-seekers, looking for the embers of another party with just a few cigarette fireflies to animate their own waggle dance. Turning left down Chapel Street, Suprematist sculptures of light pin down roller shutters, bins and fences. Furtive side streets back away into the shadows, the cold air palpable and heavy in my lungs. Fragmented and resuscitated post-war dreams of inner city ring roads sweep my direction back toward the city with its four-lane impasse but it cannot compete with the punctuated industrial rhythms of the Victorian railway bulking onward to my right. The arches, far from being voids, seem to be moulds for urban aspic; holding detritus, snuffling sounds, papers and plastics in a choreomania beyond my translation. It must be past 5am by now, time to head home through sodium-fused suburbs.

The Anthropology of the Nocturnal City

If we look more closely at the nature of walking, we may be able to understand something more fundamental about this frequently underappreciated spatial practice. As stated earlier, walking is a primary measure since it reaffirms our relationship to place and movement through space. Understanding our relationship with the city and the effects it has upon our bodies is key. This interdependence between our anatomy, its senses and the urban landscape did not escape the attention of Henri Lefebvre. In his seminal work, *The Production of Space*, he explains why this reciprocity is vital to spatial practices and, therefore, the production of alternative ways of being in the city:

> The genesis of a far-away order can be accounted for only on the basis of the order that is nearest to us – namely, the order of the body. Within the body itself, spatially considered, the successive levels constituted by the senses (from the sense of smell to sight treated as within a differentiated

> field) prefigure the layers of social space and their interconnections. (1991: 405)

The history of human activity is intrinsic to our primary form of motion, whether as migrations, pilgrimages, pleasure or protest; it has been fundamental to our being present in the world and connected to the landscape. It seems evident that in our era of rapid technological development, the attentive and deeply situated relationship we may have with our urban landscape is easily lost. Writing about lines, Tim Ingold (2007: 75) refers to the distinction between the *walk* and the *assembly*, where the latter version is fragmented rather than the trace of a continuous gesture. When trying to work out how best to represent my own nocturnal peregrinations, this also raised complex issues about the methods I might use to document my activities as discussed in the previous section. Walking at night, wayfaring within the semi-familiar or unknown, rethreads us back into the urban fabric. This is no simple task since our experiences of cities are increasingly mediated, tethered as we are to mobile devices and networks that draw us away from the tangible. Our contemporary 'fear of missing out' intertwined with instant and incessant social media represents an end of absence (Harris 2014). However, we may wish to reconsider what we really give our attention to as Zygmunt Bauman has suggested:

> Contrary to an impression made common in the modern era, procrastination is not a matter of sloth, indolence or lassitude; it is an active stance, an attempt to assume control over the sequence of events and make that sequence different from what it would be were one to stay docile and unresisting. (2000: 134)

From this perspective walking at night, therefore, may be understood to be a subtle act of resistance towards the limits of the day-to-day. Why should this matter? Intrinsic to a withdrawal from our environment is a decline in our first-hand awareness and knowledge of place and each other, with digital proxies seemingly telling us everything and nothing due to the abundance of information but a lack of direct, physical connection *and* attention to context. This relates to anthropological work on vectors since they are inherently motile and point towards the ongoing shifting effects of relationships (Gatt 2013). To reclaim some of what may be lost, walking into the night can be a recalcitrant act against the confines of the daily grind, a means of exfoliating the worries and weight of familiar roles and responsibilities. But I suggest it is much more than this. Instead, to venture into the night, to enter its thickness and go beyond its apparently opaque limits, is to sense a broader world comprised of challenges to our curiosity and experiential moments of infinite diversity. The city at night may evolve into the *terrain vague*, described by Levesque as:

> an indeterminate space without precise boundaries . . . a place . . . outside the circuit of the productive structures of the city, an internal,

> uninhabited, unproductive and often dangerous island, simultaneously on the margins of the urban system and a fundamental part of the system . . . the counter image of the city, both in the sense of a critique and a clue for a possible way to go beyond. (2002)

Richard Sennett (1994: 15) goes so far as to argue that urban space has largely become 'a mere function of motion', engendering a 'tactile sterility' which in turn leads to a pacifying of the body. Sennett contends that the imperative to minimize disruption and distraction for pedestrians and drivers – to keep them focused on shopping, working and playing in preferred ways – means that movement is typified by rapid transit without arousal. In addition, the alluring qualities that drew our attention to the urban night throughout history are rapidly becoming an endangered species, caged and commoditized in commercial situations. Yet there still remains plenty of opportunity to explore the space within cities that, after all, is not a void, a neutral container or passive background for things to happen. Quite the contrary, it is a living entity. Sanford Kwinter (2010: 74) describes space as 'a participant, an unstable and unpredictable process that both harvests and produces reality on the run.' Understood in this way, the structures of daytime can quickly break down at night, especially since our visual cognition attenuates and we may place greater reliability on the aural, olfactory and tactile, perhaps also the gustatory. Furthermore, the impact of materiality upon the sensory experience of walking becomes heightened and nuanced as place impresses itself on the pedestrian body and vice versa.

Conclusion

Walking in urban landscapes at night directs our attention towards the experiential qualities of the *here* and *now* in our immediate surroundings rather than the tenuous and distant. As Georg Simmel noted, the 'boundary is not a spatial fact with sociological consequences, but a sociological fact that forms itself spatially' (1997: 143). To go out walking into the night is a decisive act against boundaries both perceived and concrete. The management of urban space typically restricts the sensual world, limiting the body's experience of pungent smells, rough textures and distressing sounds within spatial envelopes. Given that so much of our interaction with each other in the daytime is predicated on the visual, the denial of this at night, both optically (how our eyes work) and practically (there are typically not as many people around), means that we have to find new ways of connecting with and discovering our environment. Many aspects of the city that seem preordained during the day are open to interpretation at night – we become our own cartographers, forging maps from fused and complex sensory experiences rebalanced from daylight's prejudices. Being present and directly experiencing through the spatial practice of walking is essential to uncovering a different understanding of our built environment that contradicts such manufactured smoothness. Considered in this manner, walking at night may be understood as an inscriptive practice, enriched with the potentialities that Bergson here describes:

> There do not exist *things* made, but only *things* in the making, not *states* that remain fixed, but only states in the process of change. Rest is never anything but apparent, or rather, relative. The consciousness we have of our own person in its continual flowing, introduces us to the interior of a reality on whose model we must imagine the others. (2012 [1913]: 188)

Walking in cities at night, therefore, enables us to reconnect with the city and give things our undivided attention, a welcome respite from the ongoing erosion and subdivision of our time and sense of belonging in the world. Moving, quite literally, out of the glare and stare of our commoditized and highly structured days and into alternative modalities within the shadows of our cities may be one of the few truly beautiful and sublime practices available to us.

Notes

1 This initially began as an approach to address a chronic inability to sleep and, having not found other ways of encouraging rest, I took to the streets. At first I walked extensively around my neighbourhood in south Manchester, but gradually my perambulations became longer and led me further afield. It is a practice I have continued.
2 In the United Kingdom, for example, the Governmental Office for Science's Foresight: Future of Cities project examines the challenges and opportunities facing cities over the next fifty years. Available at https://www.gov.uk/government/collections/future-of-cities (accessed 12 September 2015).
3 This work was first presented as part of the *Sensing Architecture* symposium held at the Royal Academy of Arts, London, on 29 March 2014.
4 Interestingly, much is written about the various vices of cities at night, but in my experience I very rarely encountered illegal activity but instead tended to meet the homeless people who were typically accommodating and curious to talk about what I was doing, if not occasionally bemused or amused by it.

References

Aragon, L. (1994), *Paris Peasant*. Translated and introduction by S. Watson Taylor. Boston, MA: Exact Change.
Attlee, J. (2011), *Nocturne: A Journey in Search of Moonlight*. London: Hamish Hamilton.
Baudrillard, J. (1993), *The Transparency of Evil: Essays of Extreme Phenomena*. London: Verso.
Bauman, Z. (2000), *Liquid Modernity*. Cambridge: Polity.

Beaumont, M. (2015), *Nightwalking: A Nocturnal History of London*. London: Verso.
Benjamin, W. (2005), 'Moscow'. In M. W. Jennings, H. Eiland and G. Smith (eds), *Selected Writings. Volume 2, part 1, 1927–1930*. Cambridge, MA: The Belknap Press of Harvard University Press.
Bergson, H. (2012), *The Creative Mind: An Introduction to Metaphysics*. New York: Dover Editions.
Blomberg, K. (2014), *Haus-Rucker-Co: Architekturutopie Reloaded*. Köln: Verlag der Buchhandlung Walther König.
Bogard, P. (2013), *The End of Night: Searching for Natural Darkness in an Age of Artificial Light*. London: Fourth Estate.
Bressani, M. (2015), 'Light into Darkness: Gaslight in Nineteenth Century Paris'. In S. Isenstadt, M. M. Petty and D. Neumann (eds), *Cities of Light: Two Centuries of Urban Illumination*. Oxon: Routledge, pp. 28–36.
Burke, E. (1757), *A Philosophical Enquiry into the Origin of Our Ideas of the Sublime and Beautiful*. Available at http://www.gutenberg.org/files/15043/15043-h/15043-h.htm (accessed 12 September 2015).
Callois, R. (1987), 'Mimicry and Legendary Psychasthenia'. Translated by J. Shepley. In A. Michelson, R. Krauss, D. Crimp and J. Copjec, *October: The First Decade*. Cambridge, MA: The MIT Press.
Careri, F. (2001), *Walkscapes: Walking As an Aesthetic Practice*. Barcelona: Gustavo Gili.
de Certeau, M. (1984), 'Spatial Stories'. In *The Practice of Everyday Life*. Berkeley: University of California Press, pp. 115–122.
Crawford, M. B. (2015), *The World Beyond Your Head: On Becoming an Individual in an Age of Distraction*. London: Penguin.
Dun, A. A. (1995), *Vale Royal*. Uppingham: Goldmark.
Ekirch, A. R. (2005), *At Day's Close: A History of Nighttime*. London: Weidenfeld & Nicolson.
Felson, M. and E. Poulsen (2003), 'Simple Indicators of Crime by Time of Day'. *International Journal of Forecasting* 19: 595–601.
Gatt, C. (2013), 'Vectors, Direction of Attention and Unprotected Backs: Re-specifying Relations in Anthropology'. *Anthropological Theory* 13(4): 347–369.
Glaeser, E. (2011), *Triumph of the City: How Our Greatest Invention Makes Us Richer, Smarter, Greener, Healthier, and Happier*. London: Penguin.
Harris, M. (2014), *The End of Absence: Reclaiming What We've Lost in a World of Constant Connection*. London: Penguin.
Hollis, L. (2013), *Cities Are Good for You: The Genius of the Metropolis*. London: Bloomsbury.
Ingold, T. (2007), *Lines: A Brief History*. London: Routledge.
Jacobs. S. (2002), 'Shreds of Boring Postcards: Towards a Posturban Aesthetics of the Generic and the Everyday'. In Ghent Urban Studies Team *Post Ex Sub Dis: Urban Fragmentations and Constructions*. Rotterdam: 010 Publishers, pp. 15–64.
Keiller, P. (2013), *The View from the Train: Cities and Other Landscapes*. London: Verso.
Kwinter, S. (2010), *Requiem: For the City at the End of the Millennium*. Barcelona: Actar.

Lefebvre, H. (1991), *The Production of Space*. Translated by D. Nicholson-Smith. Oxford: Blackwell.
Levesque, L. (2002), 'The "Terrain Vague" as Material – Some Observations'. Available at http://www.amarrages.com/textes_terrain.html (accessed 17 September 2015).
Manaugh, G. (2013), *Landscape Futures: Instruments, Devices and Architectural Inventions*. Barcelona: Actar.
Minkowski, E. (1933), 'Le temps vécu'. *Etudes phénoménologiques et psycho-pathologiques*, Paris, pp. 382–398.
Minton, A. (2009), *Ground Control: Fear and Happiness in the Twenty-First-Century City*. London: Penguin.
Montgomery, C. (2013), *Happy City: Transforming Our Lives through Urban Design*. London: Penguin.
de Muynck, B. (2004), 'The Prosthetic Paradox'. *Angst & Ruimte / Fear & Space*. Rotterdam: NAi Publishers, pp. 8–15.
Offenhuber, D. and C. Ratti (2014), *Decoding the City: How Big Data Can Change Urbanism*. Berlin: Birkhäuser.
Pallasmaa, J. (2005), *The Eyes of the Skin: Architecture and the Senses*. New York: John Wiley.
Palmer, B. D. (2000), *Cultures of Darkness: Night Travels in the Histories of Transgression*. New York: Monthly Review Press.
Raban, J. (1974), *Soft City*. London: Hamish Hamilton.
Sandhu, S. (2007), *Night Haunts: A Journey through the London Night*. London: Artangel and Verso.
Schivelbusch, W. (1995), *Disenchanted Night: The Industrialization of Light in the Nineteenth Century*. Berkeley and Los Angeles: University of California Press.
Schlör, J. (2013), *Nights in the Big City*. Translated by P. G. Imhof and D. R. Roberts. London: Reaktion.
Sennett, R. (1994), *Flesh and Stone: The Body and the City in Western Civilization*. London: Faber.
Simmel, G. (1997), 'The Sociology of Space'. In D. Frisby and M. Featherstone (eds), *Simmel on Culture*. London: Sage, pp. 137–185.
Sinclair, I. (1997), *Lights Out for the Territory*. London: Granta Books.
Talanova, J. (2015), '9/11 Tribute Lights Briefly Shut Off after Birds Get Trapped'. *CNN*. Available at http://edition.cnn.com/2015/09/12/us/9-11-tribute-lights-off/ (accessed 14 September 2015).
United Nations Population Fund (UNFPA) (2007), *State of the World Population 2007: Unleashing the Potential of Urban Growth*. UNFPA: New York.
Vidler, A. (1992), 'Dark Space'. *The Architectural Uncanny*. Cambridge, MA: The MIT Press, pp. 167–175.
Zumthor, P. (2006), *Atmospheres: Architectural Environments – Surrounding Objects*. Berlin: Birkhäuser.

2

The Role of Playfulness and Sensory Experiences in Design for Public Health and for Ageing Well

Emmanuel Tsekleves and Andy Darby

Introduction

Play is one of the main drivers of human cultural development. It has been the topic of research across different areas including psychology (Berlyne 1969), learning (Singer 2013), marketing (Huotari and Hamari 2012), child development (Barnett 1990), ethnography (Gaver et al. 1999), human–computer interaction (Kuts 2009) and game design (Deterding et al. 2011). Play and playfulness encourage exploration and creativity, and stimulate social interaction and competition. Play often provides satisfaction through a direct reward for one's successful actions and, most importantly, entertains and allows us to 'escape' from the realities of everyday lives. This chapter presents and discusses the value and role of playfulness in its bodily and sensory aspects for the design of activities and interventions situated in urban spaces and aimed at public enjoyment and ageing well. After a discussion of related work, the authors present the Active Parks case study, which aimed at co-designing a playful, tangible health trail in a public park in order to engage sedentary and older park users in casual physical activity. The design process followed consultation, and the playful proof-of-concept prototypes developed offered several valuable insights as to the design of similar playful activities in public urban spaces. Following the lessons learnt from the case study and the study of the relevant literature, the authors offer three key values and eight practical recommendations on the design of playful experiences for public health and ageing well in urban spaces.

Related Work

There are several definitions of 'playfulness'. The most common ones widely accepted in the literature define 'playfulness' as a dispositional tendency to engage in play (Van Vleet and Feeney 2015) or the pre-disposition to frame (or reframe) a situation in such a way as to provide oneself (and possibly others) with amusement, humour and/or entertainment (Barnett 2007). Play and being playful is how we first experience the world around us (Barnett 1990), losing ourselves in play, whether it was creating a make-believe world, throwing a ball between classmates, or teasing and role-playing with friends. Unfortunately, as we grow older we tend to distance ourselves from playfulness and get locked into the linear, problem–solution, adult mindset. As Stanley Hall put it, 'We do not quit playing because we grow old, we grow old because we quit playing' (1904: 235). Although playfulness is traditionally associated with children, it is equally significant for adults. Van Vleet and Feeney (2015) identify in their review of the literature the importance of play behaviour and playfulness in adulthood and the need for more research in this area.

Playful design, the mapping of playful experiences from games or toys to other non-game-context experiences, has gained interest in recent years (Walsh et al. 2010). Although it has been a subject of research (Bekker et al. 2010; Ferrara 2012; Deterding et al. 2013; Salah et al. 2014), it has not been explored as widely in the area of health and ageing well, and more precisely in engaging adults and older people with physical activity. There is a body of research evidence (Staempfli 2007; Proyer 2014a; Proyer 2014b; Mahdjoubi and Spencer 2015) which suggests that playfulness can contribute to healthy ageing by stimulating higher levels of cognitive functioning related to positive emotions, well-being, intrinsic life goals and coping with stress. Furthermore, playfulness, via its link to promoting an active way of life (as a health-oriented behaviour), might also be associated with greater levels of physical activity (Proyer 2014b; Mahdjoubi and Spencer 2015). In addition to this, play is an inherently human aspect that stimulates well-being (McGonigal 2011), especially when presented in the form of playful interactions – interactions that incorporate elements of fun and play (Salah et al. 2014) – as they encourage and facilitate environments where users are more interested in enjoying themselves than they are in achieving a specific task (Dekel et al. 2005). Environments such as public spaces (e.g. parks, squares, etc.) are ideal for this due to their interactive nature and because they are designed to be looked at, walked in and used by many people on a daily basis (Dekel et al. 2005). Hence the development of ambient play environments provides an opportunity to design and develop playful interactions to stimulate social and physical play (Bekket et al. 2010). This is further reinforced by the design of tangible play artefacts, where physical artefacts are electronically augmented and enhanced to trigger various digital events (Nam and Kim 2011; Salah et al. 2014). The blending of tangible (physical) and digital elements have recently grown in popularity within video games and toys too, with physical game pieces becoming a popular addition to traditional digital games.[1] The reason behind this lies in the qualities only found when interacting with physical objects, namely the multisensory experience from handling a physical object – experiencing texture, shape, weight, colour, size – something that one cannot simply discover from intangible digital artefacts. Multisensory stimulation has been found to be of therapeutic value for people with dementia (Baker et al. 2001; Dias de Macedo et al. 2015) and Parkinson's disease (Suteerawattananon et al. 2004; Jiang and Norman 2006) as well as for supporting healthy ageing (Mora 2013; Park and Bischof 2013). Although tangible play artefacts have been found to have the potential for providing innovative ways for children to play, learn and exercise (Price et al. 2003; Bekker et al. 2014), they have not been explored much with adults and in particular by older adults.

A number of tangible urban play artefacts have been developed which offer playful experiences. These focus on encouraging exploration and discovery of urban spaces in a leisurely and playful manner by connecting the digital (mobile phones with wireless network technologies) with the physical world (e.g. buildings, city landmarks), reporting positive results in increasing people's engagement with such experiences (Iguchi and Inakage 2006; Rashid et al. 2006; Vogiazou et al. 2006). Romero et al. (2010) have employed playful experiences in care homes for older people, which has shown promise with regard to user engagement in physical activity. In Bristol, the Watershed – a social enterprise and registered charity – has developed in collaboration with other civil and technology partners the world's first playable city, creating a framework by which to think differently about the city and generating a social dialogue by creating shared experiences through play (Watershed 2015). Although Playable City does not place a focus in health, it provides an interesting example of adult user engagement through tangible playful interactions in an urban environment (de Lange 2015). Other projects focusing on playful designed artefacts for health include the *Kwiek* and the *Piano Staircase*. *Kwiek* is an urban exercise route implemented around de Eerdbrand, an elderly care facility in Eindhoven, the Netherlands, aimed at healthy ageing (*Kwiek* 2013). It uses existing and other specially designed street furniture and infrastructure. For instance, it turns a lamp post into a spot to stretch shoulders, a bench into a place to exercise your legs and bollards to slalom around. The specially designed symbol tiles on the pavement mark where and what kind of exercise one could perform, directing users to the next exercise and communicating the whole route. Although no formal study of the effectiveness of the route has been reported in the literature, it forms a useful example of how street infrastructure can be turned into a playful tool for supporting exercise for an ageing population.

In the *Staircase Piano* the stairs of the Odenplan metro station in Stockholm, Sweden, were transformed into a giant functioning piano keyboard – much like the piano made famous in the Tom Hanks movie *Big* (1988). Applying pressure on each step sounds a musical note. This playful artefact encouraged commuters to opt for the intriguing new stairway and to enjoy making musical movements as they moved up and down the scale, and facilitated social interactions along with physical exercise (Peeters et al. 2013). Volkswagen, which funded the project, found 66 per cent more people than normal chose the musical stairs over the escalator (Bates 2009). However, no information on the evaluation methodology and the sample size was given. In light of the above, it emerges that there is a great and growing potential for playfulness to be employed in the design (playful design) of tangible (physical–digital) artefacts and interventions for engaging people, especially an increasingly ageing population, in physical exercise and socializing in urban environments in a leisurely manner. Although only a handful of recommendations have been offered for the design of playful experiences and interactions, all of them focus on the design of playful experiences for children and most are provided purely for the purposes of entertainment (Korhonen et al. 2009; Shackell et al. 2009; Bekker et al. 2014; Tieben et al. 2014).

The Active Parks Project

The following section presents a single case study which has employed playful design to engage older people in taking exercise and co-creating with other people. The Active Parks Project (March–September 2014) aimed at co-designing a concept for an interactive 'health trail' in a green space to explore the effects of playful interactive experiences on the casual physical activity of park users in Ryelands Park, Lancaster, UK. In a series of co-design workshops with local residents (n = 25, age = 40–70, average age = 60), the Lancaster City Council and the National Health Service, Lancashire Public Health, a number of ideas and concepts were developed which informed the design proposition of the health trail and offered new ways of motivating and engaging in physical activity specific to the locals who frequented the park. Active Parks employed a co-design process (Sanders and Stappers 2008) along with qualitative research ethnography methods (namely observations, interviews and focus-groups) for data gathering. Interviews were conducted with project stakeholders (n = 3), workshop participants (n = 5) and user testers (n = 12) of the two prototypes developed. Thematic analysis was employed for data analysis (Gibbs 2007), where all data collected are involved in a process of identifying themes throughout, using coding, indexing and categorizing towards emerging themes. During the second co-design workshop the data were grouped and themes emerged (presented in the next section) which were finally synthesized by the workshop participants into a shared vision: 'A

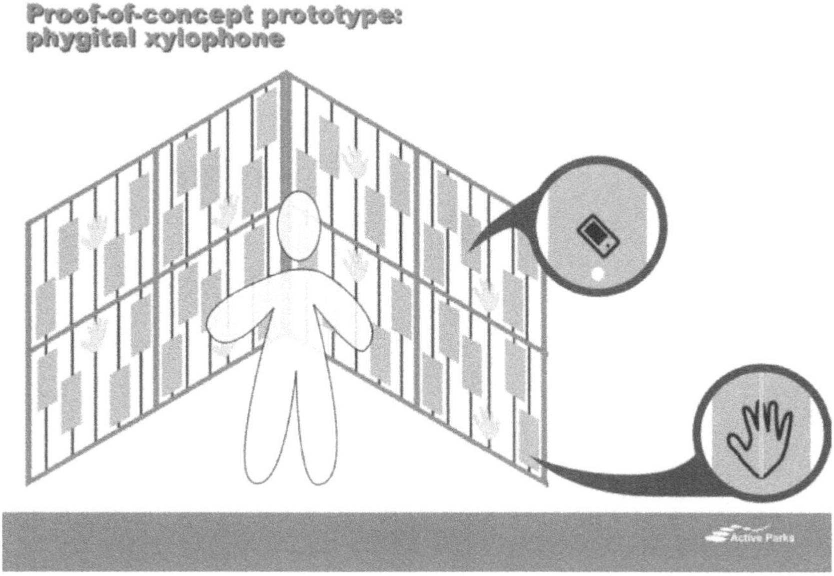

FIGURE 2.1 *The initial design proposal of the xylophone artefact, which was a result of the co-design process and data analysis.*

community space with fun and activities safe for everyone to enjoy.' This vision was the guiding force behind the ideas generated and the rapid prototypes created by the end of the second workshop.

The team chose to realize the 'xylophone' concept put forward by participants. It was felt that this idea represented a single interaction that could be part of a larger series of interactions as part of a 'health trail'. It also encompassed all the key values and themes identified by co-designers in the workshops and enabled shared play, tactile and audio stimulation (see Figure 2.1). Two proof-of-concept prototypes were realized to illustrate the possibilities of playfulness in engaging people with physical activity in public urban spaces and to explore how it could be used and implemented in public urban environments. Both prototypes were built at large scale and employed conductive technology.

The first prototype was constructed with a mobile Near Field Communication (NFC) interface and a conductive touch interface based on a MaKeyMaKey4 microcontroller. The touch interface allowed people to play the prototype like a music instrument (see Figure 2.2). For the mobile interface, users could choose to play freestyle or follow the mobile instructions that indicated which numbers to tap next (see Figure 2.3). Using this function with the mobile phone, users could play the notes for 'Twinkle, Twinkle Little Star'.

The second prototype was developed based on the feedback received from the testing of the first. This time the NFC interface was dropped and

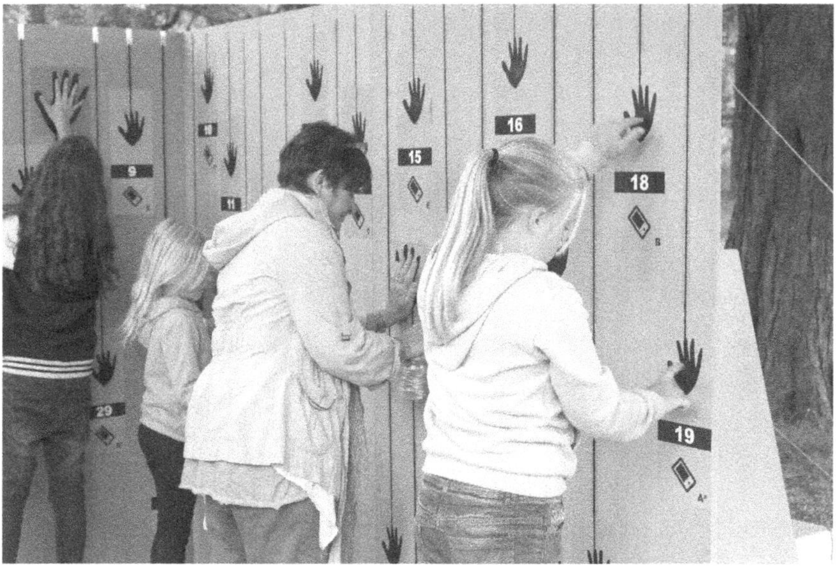

FIGURE 2.2 *Users interacted with the touch interface of the xylophone by putting their fingers or hands on the conductive painted touch points.*

only the conductive touch interface was used. Copper was employed as an alternative conductive material. The form of the prototype gained more attention this time and a free-standing structure was designed and built incorporating a wooden frame as the base, thirteen copper pipes for conductivity and to case the wires and thirteen acrylic globes covered with some copper tape for the touch elements. LED lights were added and they provided visual feedback in addition to sound when users touched the interface (see Figure 2.4). The two prototypes were pilot tested and evaluated on site in Ryelands Park (n=150, age 4–80), and in Lancaster city's central square (n=350, age 2–80).[2]

The co-design process identified key values for the project. It was important that the interactive health trail followed those values and enabled the local community to engage in exercise in a playful manner. Ten key themes have been identified from the analysis of the focus-group data and workshop activities. These are: playfulness, intergenerational use, shared activities, social interaction, local engagement, community friendship, physical wellbeing, outdoors exercise, a sense of fun and a showcase to others. Enjoyment and playfulness were considered as key contributors to engaging people in the first place and to keeping the motivation going.

There was a shared feeling among participants that the interactive trail should not be presented as a health intervention but as a playful activity linked to leisure. The idea of an adult playground became popular. Participants referred to games, fun and play and presented examples of activities from their childhood that combined play with exercise, such

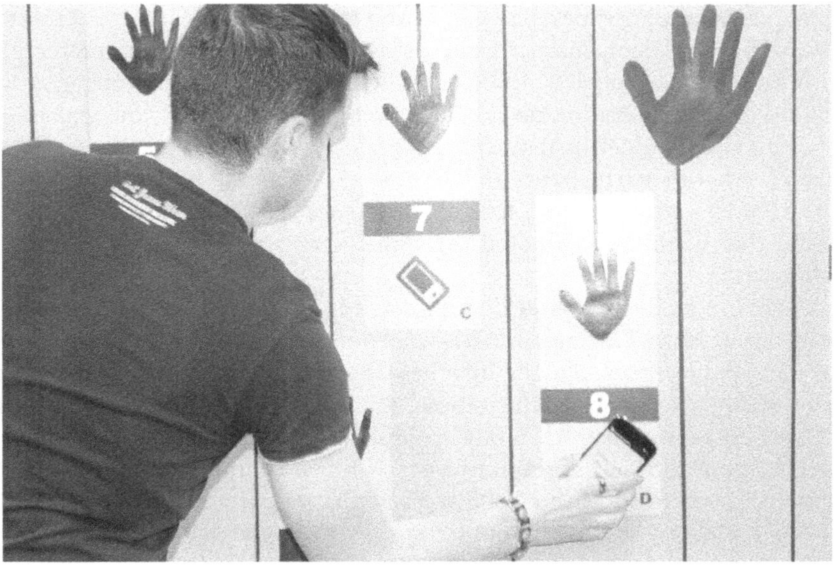

FIGURE 2.3 *A user interacting with the mobile (NFC) interface of the xylophone by using the phone to touch the artefact.*

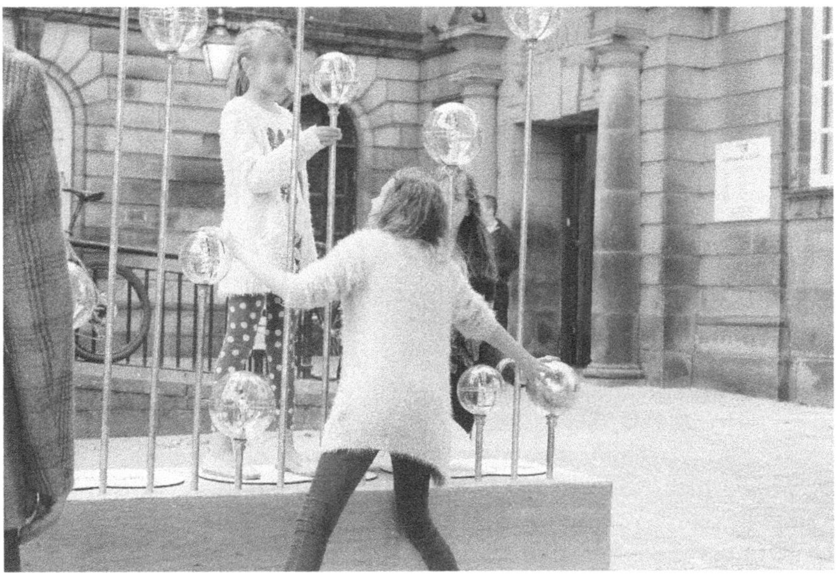

FIGURE 2.4 *The second version of the xylophone prototype with lights being added on the design.*

hopscotch, skipping ropes, ball games and treasure hunt. All these activities have several common characteristics, such as physical exertion, interaction with tangible play objects and simultaneous stimulation and engagement of several senses. As the discussion developed, a concept emerged for a large playful musical instrument situated in the park. This concept was taken further by participants and developed into a tangible artefact. Music was proposed here as a tool for collaborative play and multisensory interaction that could be facilitated through a large musical play object in a public space.

Thematic analysis was also employed for the data emerging from the prototype testing. The main themes were non-age-specific playfulness, multisensory experiences, playing together, fun and joy, exploring and experimenting, toys for adults, inclusiveness, connectedness and music and lights.

The first prototype tested both a conductive interface and an NFC-based interface, but the lack of responsiveness with the phone as an NFC reader made the experience cumbersome. Participants preferred the immediate feedback and tactile sensation of the conductive approach. It was observed that by using their hands when interacting with the conductive interface of the xylophone, users could concentrate more on the play activity and engage their senses of touch, sight and hearing equally and in a coordinated way as opposed to focusing on a mobile phone screen. The sense of touch (touching the painted hands on the xylophone to play music) seemed to be very strong and well explored by participants of all ages.

Participants also commented on the collaborative affordance of the conductive approach to interacting as opposed to the solo mode of the mobile interaction. Users who had not previously met explored the prototype together, linking hands to create conductive human chains. The experiences of connecting with the play object and music but also with other people through physical touch were highlighted by users and observed by the research team.

Each of the prototypes showed that the simplest of playful interactions appear to stimulate casual physical activity among a wide range of users and, in addition, observation of usage indicated that they might offer opportunities for interaction. The theme of play, playfulness and fun kept appearing in both the interviews but also feedback left by participants at the graffiti walls (see Figure 2.5). This was linked by several people with exercise and stretching. It is also interesting to note that a desire for easy playfulness over exertion was evident among some users. This led to the artefact being referred to by users as the 'musical bench'.

The importance of music was also highlighted by several participants, linking it with motivation for exercising and as an inspiration tool for more play and discovery. The playful interaction acted as a leveller with even accomplished musicians finding the musical element challenging but fun. The aesthetic effect was viewed as surprising and unusual.

The second prototype developed the concept to include motivating feedback from lights and a new physical design that acted as a bench, light

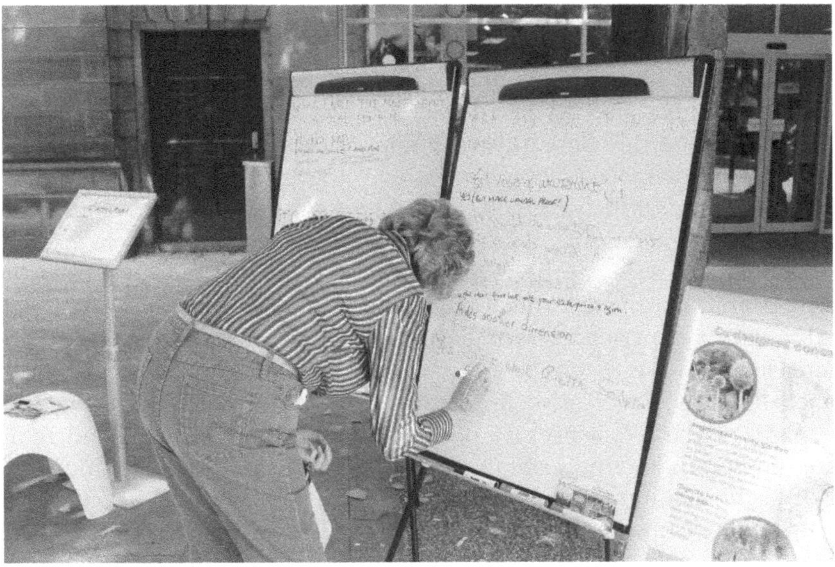

FIGURE 2.5 *User feedback was collected in a creative manner on graffiti walls.*

source and activity in the park space. Participant requests for a visual feedback, along with the audio and tactile feedback, indicated the value of multisensory engagement for play. Participants also provided ideas for turning it into a more playful artefact. Several of these suggestions revolved around a musical 'Simon says' type of game, in which one player would play several tunes in turn while the other person had to recall and replay them, increasing the number of tunes and covering the distance each time. It was also observed that in the second prototype that included the lights, several participants created their own playful ad hoc games where a player would have to follow the sequence of lights the previous person played.

Discussion and Recommendations

From the themes that emerged and lessons learnt from the Active Parks case study, as well as the review of the literature on play and playfulness, we present and discuss three core values and eight associated recommendations for the design of playful experiences for public health and for ageing well. The three core values are: playfulness as a means of stimulating physical exercise; inclusiveness, leading to fun ways of keeping active for all participants; and connectedness, through which physical and mental play can bring people together.

There are fun ways of keeping active, and playfulness is a key to engaging both sedentary and older people in casual physical activity. Exercises incorporated within a playful environment (an interactive toy or artefact) can greatly increase people's physical exertion through multisensory stimulation. To maximize engagement with physical activity and exercise, it is important that fun and play are highlighted, and that the artefact is not only designed but also presented as a play and leisure activity, rather than a health or medical-related intervention. With these findings in view, we make the following recommendations.

Recommendation 1: Emphasize fun and play experiences over health or medical intervention.

Such experiences can be made more enjoyable through multisensory interactions that involve touch, audio and sight. Being able to offer several sensory experiences will further captivate user engagement and increase the sense of joy, sensation and thrill (Korhonen et al. 2009). Shackell et al. (2009) also highlight the value of engaging users with as many of the five senses as possible and through natural and fabricated material. Having artefacts designed on a large scale is important in order to facilitate and encourage moment and physical exertion (see Figure 2.6). As movement (upper/lower and/or full body) is the key here, the size and scale of the playful artefact should be carefully designed to embed motion as a core element in the experience of play. Advice should be sought at this stage from health professionals and selected movements and exercises incorporated in a playful manner. Rewards for movement (especially large, more complex ones) should be given through the provision of multi-stimulus feedback, including visual, audio and tactile ones.

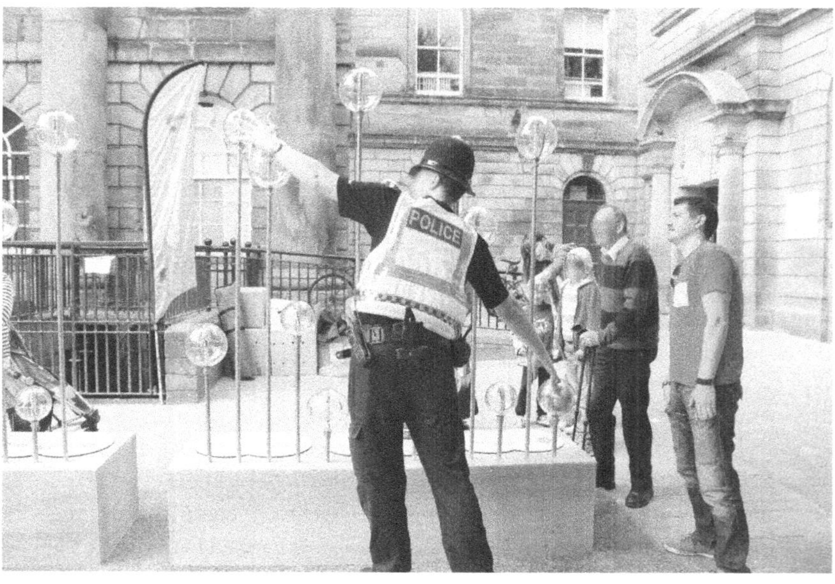

FIGURE 2.6 *The large scale of the artefact required even the tallest of users to move and stretch.*

Recommendation 2: Aim for large-scale multisensory designs and provide multi-stimulus feedback.

Key facilitators for play are generative artefacts or toys. These are play activities and experiences that encourage the creative expression of their users. Unlike games that are very structured and in which every possible choice and interaction is well defined by designers, play activities and toys are generative and open-ended. There are several options and paths that the user can explore. This encompasses important values for the design of successful play experiences for public health. First of all, being generative means that users can create their own rules and games for play, therefore discovering each time a different experience and hence being encouraged to revisit and keep moving/exercising. Bekker et al. (2014) refer to this as open-ended play, and Tieben et al. (2014) describe it as emergent play. For instance the generative design of the xylophone artefact in the Active Parks Project encouraged users to invent and play their own games of 'Simon Says', 'Follow the Light', and so on (see Figure 2.7). Second, being open-ended means that the game or play experience is never truly over, unlike a game where you stop when you reach a win or lose position. It is up to the players to decide when to stop and come back again to continue or switch to a newly created game, very much like a toy where children make up different rules of play. Third, being generative facilitates creative expression and stimulates additional feelings of sensation, accomplishment and pride in oneself. In the case of Active Parks, audio was employed as the element that facilitated creative exploration of music generation.

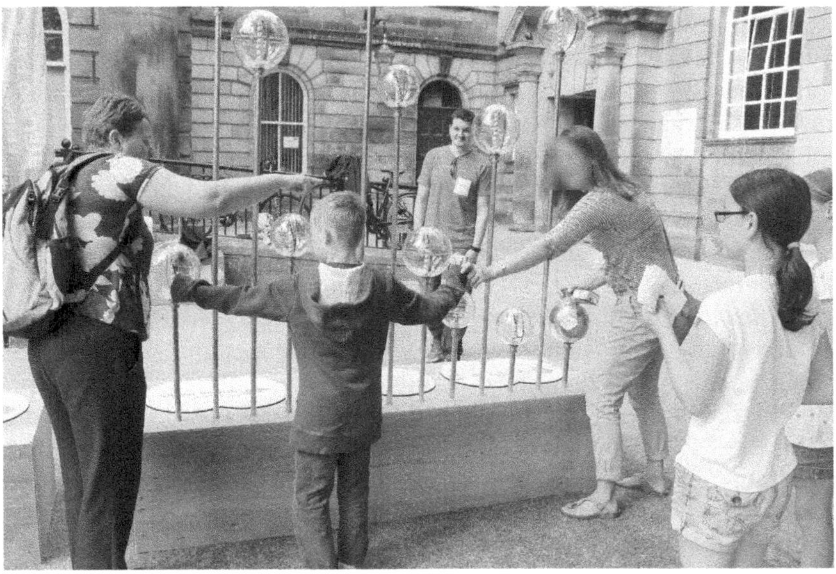

FIGURE 2.7 *Users created their own rules and games when playing with the artefact.*

Recommendation 3: Make play open-ended, generative and explorative very much like a toy.

Offering an external reward for an activity (such as vouchers, points, etc.) provides a strong social signal that the activity in question is not worth doing for its own sake. For example, if engaging in exercise for a specific amount of time lowers your health insurance premium or entitles you to a shopping voucher, this creates the misconception that exercising is a chore or merely a means to other ends. One of the key differences and benefits of play versus games is play's internal rewards system, which arises from the positive emotions that emanate from engaging in it. Emotions like spontaneity, joy (Barnett 1990) enjoyment, curiosity, social interaction (Kuts 2009) discovery, relaxation, sensation, thrill (Korhonen et al. 2009), challenge, exploration, expression, fantasy (Korhonen et al. 2009; Kuts 2009) and humour (Barnett 1990; Korhonen et al. 2009) should be augmented throughout the design of the playful artefact to tap into intrinsic motivation.

Recommendation 4: Aim for intrinsic rewards and tap into users' intrinsic motivation.

The second value stressing inclusiveness is very important and is a prerequisite for artefacts and interventions installed in a public urban environment. As such artefacts aim at being made available they should be inclusive and accessible by everyone who uses the space. They should not cater for a specific age group and their interaction affordances should offer participation to everyone. This is where the technology and interaction mode utilized should be made very easy to use and ideally without the need to read instructions. Again, provision of different types of feedback can augment this. An opportunity for the designer to make a link between the play and spaces can be incorporated in the design process resulting in an artefact that creates a visual or cultural link with the place in which it is installed or the play experiences it offers. Active Parks employed conductive technology for engaging with the artefact as it was seen as a more natural way of interaction and it also meant that it was cheaper to implement and everyone in the park could use it with little or no instruction. The mobile interaction was dropped during the design of the second prototype as there were issues around accessibility. Not everyone in the park owned or was confident in operating a smartphone.

Recommendation 5: Link spaces and play and make it an inclusive design through tangible play.

Currently, the vast majority of playful experiences and activities available in public spaces are aimed mainly at young children. Evidence provided by the literature (Staempfli 2007; Proyer 2014a, 2014b; Mahdjoubi and Spencer 2015) highlights the benefits and importance of playfulness for adults and for ageing well. In addition, the Active Parks case study revealed that playfulness is ageless and, in fact, the older the user the more they will be immersed in play (see Figure 2.8). Data from the interviews, observations and graffiti wall provided a clear suggestion of the value of playfulness for adult and older users in terms of engagement, social interaction and as a tool for escape and release from the realities of daily living.

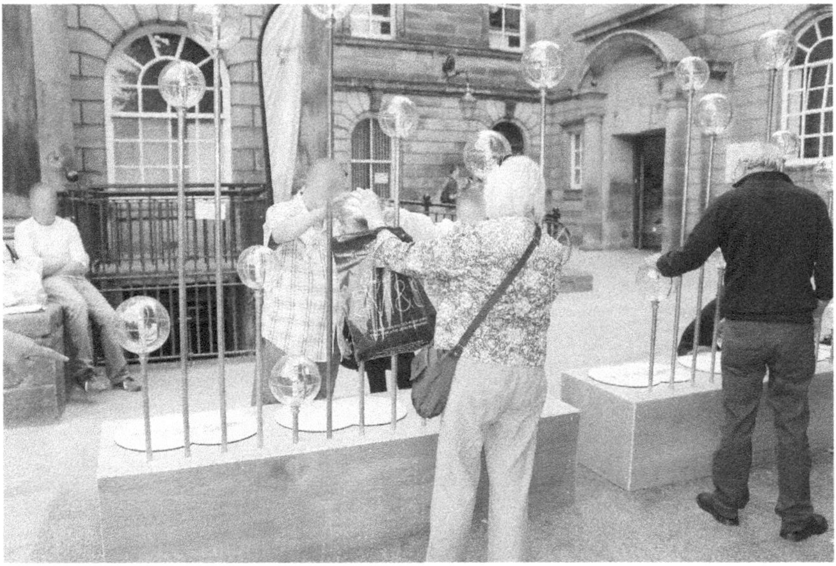

FIGURE 2.8 *Playfulness is ageless; the older the user, the more they engaged with play.*

Recommendation 6: Remember that playfulness is ageless.

Designing playful experiences and activities that would successfully engage adults and older adults in a public setting is however much harder when compared to designing for children. A key prerequisite for engaging in the first place and then being immersed in play is the creation of what is known as the 'magic circle' (Huizinga 1964) in which players may feel safe, resourceful and empowered within that moment and space of the game (Salen and Zimmerman 2003). The concept of 'the magic circle' can be gathered from the way young animals and children engage in play too. They play when they see their parents around monitoring the environment, thus taking care that no outer threat is present. In Active Parks, for instance, this was achieved through both the visual and aesthetic design of the play activity, which portrayed a level of both play but also science (through the lights and copper structure). In addition to this, the use of the synthetic turf grass around the artefact (see Figures 2.7 and 2.8) created a visual signpost of the play space where engaging with play activity was expected and was in a safe place to do so, thus creating the 'magic circle'. Once people were in that space they were expected to engage in play and felt safe as everyone else was doing the same without the fear of criticism or ridicule although this was placed in a public space.

Recommendation 7: Create a 'magic circle' and a safe space for play and exploration.

Having an artefact designed for a public space provides the designer with a challenge and an opportunity for creating new, and enhancing existing,

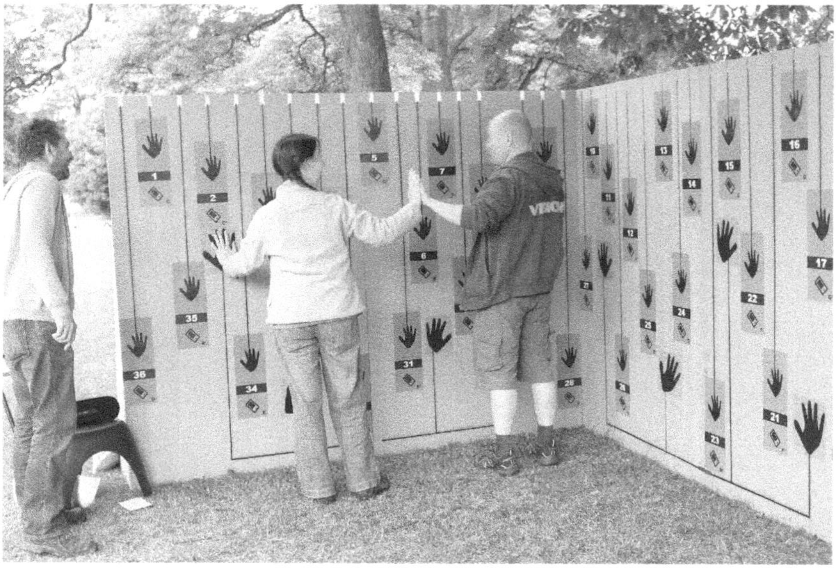

FIGURE 2.9 *Encouraging connectedness through physical touch and play.*

social interactions. Connectedness forms one of the key values for humans, as we are social beings. Play is an inherently social activity. Facilitating social interactions is a key prerequisite for successful play space design (Shackell et al. 2009). Following these two principles, it is crucial for play activities designed for open urban and public spaces to include artefacts that embed the value of connectedness. This can be manifested both in terms of the physical but also the cognitive and emotional. The former can be accomplished through the design of tangible artefacts that have affordances and employ technologies that encourage and require physical connection for play; for example, in Active Parks the use of conductive technology and the placing of play elements further apart encouraged physical touch for play (see Figure 2.9). In terms of the latter, this can be achieved through the design of the play activity where collaborative play reduces cognitive load and increases feelings of sensation, fellowship, sympathy and accomplishment, hence our final recommendation, hence our final recommendation.

Recommendation 8: Design tangible artefacts that embed the value of connectedness by offering affordance for connecting people together physically or through play

Conclusion

Although there is a lack of research in the area of playfulness in public health and for ageing well, the field is gaining momentum. The benefits of play and playfulness in increasing our well-being and social interaction and with respect to the quality of the ageing process have been discussed above. A case study has been presented, providing guidance on the design of tangible playful experiences for health and ageing well in public urban places. The lessons learnt from the case study and the literature review have led to eight practical recommendations for the design of playful experiences for public health. These have been encompassed within three core values. The first value provided addresses the core qualities of play and how to implement these into a designed, ludic artefact; the second value highlights inclusiveness in the design of playful experiences for health in public spaces; the third value touches on connecting and bringing people together through tangible play. We also conclude that several of the prerequisites defined by Shackell et al. (2009) in the Play England report, although aimed at the design of successful play spaces for children, can be applied to adults with some level of modification. This is the first paper to propose practical recommendations for the design of playful experiences and activities for public health and for ageing well. We envisage that this would form a basis of guidance and inspiration for designers, communities and health professionals who wish to employ a playful lens for the adoption and promotion of physical activities in public and urban spaces.

Notes

1 See http://uk.ign.com/articles/2014/02/07/skylanders-in-top-20-game-franc hises-ever-175-million-toys-sold (last accessed 15 October 2015). See also http://www.engadget.com/2015/01/15/people-love-nintendo-amiibo/ (last accessed 12 October 2015).

2 See http://imagination.lancs.ac.uk/Active_Parks and http://www.makey-makey.com/ (accessed 17 October 2016).

References

Baker, R., S. Bell, E. Baker, J. Holloway, R. Pearce, Z. Dowling and L. A. Wareing (2001), 'A Randomized Controlled Trial of the Effects of Multi-Sensory Stimulation (MSS) for People with Dementia'. *British Journal of Clinical Psychology* 40(1): 81–96.

Barnett, L. A. (1990), 'Playfulness: Definition, Design, and Measurement'. *Play & Culture* 3: 319–336.

Barnett, L. A. (2007), 'The Nature of Playfulness in Young Adults'. *Personal Individual Differences* 43: 949–958.

Bates, C. (2009), 'Scaling New Heights: Piano Stairway Encourages Commuters to Ditch the Escalators'. http://www.dailymail.co.uk/sciencetech/article-1218944/Scaling-new-heights-Piano-stairway-encourages-commuters-ditch-escalators.html (accessed 5 October 2015).

Bekker, T., J. Sturm and B. Eggen (2010), 'Designing Playful Interactions for Social Interaction and Physical Play'. *Personal and Ubiquitous Computing* 14(5): 385–339.

Bekker, T., L. de Valk and B. Eggen (2014), 'A Toolkit for Designing Playful Interactions: The Four Lenses of Play'. *Journal of Ambient Intelligence and Smart Environments* 6(3), 263–276.

Berlyne, D. (1969), 'Laughter, Humor and Play'. In G. Lindzey and E. Aronson (eds), *The Handbook of Social Psychology*. 2nd ed., Reading, MA: Addison-Wesley Publication Company, 795–852.

Bischof, G. N. (2013), 'The Aging Mind: Neuroplasticity in Response to Cognitive Training'. *Dialogues Clin Neurosci* 15(1): 109–119.

Dekel, A., Y. Simon, H. Dar, E. Tarazi, O. Rabinowitz and Y. Sterman (2005), 'Adding Playful Interaction to Public Spaces. Intelligent Technologies for Interactive Entertainment'. *Lecture Notes in Computer Science* 3814: 225–229.

Deterding, S., D. Dixon, R. Khaled and L. Nacke (2011), 'From Game Design Elements to Gamefulness: Defining "gamification" '. In *Proceedings of the 15th International Academic MindTrek Conference: Envisioning Future Media Environments (MindTrek '11)*. New York: ACM, 9–15.

Deterding, S., S. Björk and L. Nacke (2013), 'Designing Gamification: Creating Gameful and Playful Experiences'. *CHI'13 Extended Abstracts on Human Factors in Computing Systems*, 3263–3266.

Dias de Macedo, D. C. Anthony and C. W. Picanço-Diniz (2015), 'Beneficial Effects of Multisensory and Cognitive Stimulation in Institutionalized Elderly: 12-Months Follow-Up'. *Clinical Interventions in Ageing* 10: 1351–1360.

Ferrara, J. (2012), *Playful Design: Creating Game Experiences in Everyday Interfaces*. Brooklyn, NY: Rosenfeld Media.

Gaver, B., T. Dunne and E. Pacenti (1999), 'Design: Cultural Probes'. *interactions* 6(1): 21–29.

Gibbs, G. (2007), *Analyzing Qualitative Data*. London: Sage.

Hall, G. S. (1904), *Adolescence: Its Psychology and Its Relations to Physiology, Anthropology, Sociology, Sex, Crime, Religion and Education*. New York: D. Appleton.

Huizinga, J. (1964), *Homo Ludens; A Study of the Play-Element in Culture*. Beacon Press.

Huotari, K. and J. Hamari (2012), 'Defining Gamification – A Service Marketing Perspective'. In *Proceedings of the 16th International Academic MindTrek Conference*. Presented at MindTrek'12. New York: ACM, 17–22.

Iguchi, K. and M. Inakage (2006), 'Morel: Remotely Launchable Outdoor Playthings'. *Proceedings of 2006 ACM SIGCHI International Conference on Advances in Computer Entertainment Technology (ACE '06)*. New York: ACM, Article 35.

Jiang, Y. and K. E. Norman (2006), 'Effects of Visual and Auditory Cues on Gait Initiation in People with Parkinson's Disease'. *Clinical Rehabilitation* 20, 36–45.

Korhonen, H., M. Montola and J. Arrasvuori (2009), 'Understanding Playful User Experience through Digital Games'. In *Proceedings of the International Conference on Designing Pleasurable Products and Interfaces*. New York: ACM, 274–285.

Kuts, E. (2009), 'Playful User Interfaces: Literature Review and Model for Analysis'. In A. Barry, K. Helen and K. Tanya (eds), *Breaking New Ground: Innovation in Games, Play, Practice and Theory: Proceedings of the 2009 Digital GamesResearch Association Conference*, London, September 2009.

Kwiek (2013), Kwiek: Urban Exercise Route. Available at http://kwiekbeweegroute.nl/ (accessed 10 October 2015).

de Lange, M. (2015), 'The Playful City: Play and Games for Citizen Participation in the Smart City'. *Scientific Report.* COST TU1306 STSM report. Utrecht University.

Mahdjoubi, L. and B. Spencer (2015), 'Healthy Play of All Ages in Public Open Spaces'. In H. Barton, S. Thompson, S. Burgess and M. Grant, (eds), *The Routledge Handbook of Planning for Health and Well-Being.* London: Routledge, pp. 136–149.

McGonigal, J. (2011), *Reality Is Broken: Why Games Make Us Better and How They Can Change the World.* New York: The Penguin Press.

Mora, F. (2013), 'Successful Brain Aging: Plasticity, Environmental Enrichment, and Lifestyle'. *Dialogues Clinical Neuroscience* 15(1): 45–52.

Nam, T. and C. Kim (2011), 'Design by Tangible Stories: Enriching Interactive Everyday Products with Ludic Value'. *International Journal of Design* 5(1), 85–98.

Peeters, M., C. Megens, E. van den Hoven, C. Hummels and A. Brombacher (2013), 'Social Stairs: Taking the Piano Staircase towards Long-Term Behavioral Change'. In *Persuasive Technology.* Springer Berlin Heidelberg, pp. 174–179.

Proyer, R. (2014a), 'Perceived Functions of Playfulness in Adults: Does It Mobilize You at Work, Rest, and When Being with Others?' *Revue Europeenne De Psychologie Appliquee* 64(5): 241–250.

Proyer, R. (2014b), 'Playfulness Over the Lifespan and Its Relation to Happiness'. *Zeitschrift Für Gerontologie Und Geriatrie* 47(6): 508–512.

Rashid, O., W. Bamford and P. Coulton (2006), 'PAC-LAN: Mixed-Reality Gaming with RFID-Enabled Mobile Phones'. *ACM Computers in Entertainment* 4(4): 1–17.

Romero, N., J. Sturm, T. Bekker, L. de Valk and K. Sander (2010), 'Playful Persuasion to Support Older Adults' Social and Physical Activities'. *Interacting with Computers* 22: 485–495.

Salah, A., B. Schouten, S. Göbel and B. Arnrich (2014), 'Playful Interactions and Serious Games'. *Journal of Ambient Intelligence and Smart Environments* 6(3): 259–262.

Salen, K. and E. Zimmerman (2003), *Rules of Play: Game Design Fundamentals.* Cambridge, MA: The MIT Press.

Sanders, E. B.-N. and P. J. Stappers (2008), 'Co-creation and the New Landscapes of Design'. *CoDesign: International Journal of CoCreation in Design and the Arts* 4(1): 5–18.

Shackell, A., N. Butler, P. Doyle and D. Ball (2009), *Design for Play. Design for Play: A Guide to Creating Successful Play Spaces.* Play England. Nottingham: DCSF Publications.

Singer, E. (2013), 'Play and Playfulness, Basic Features of Early Childhood Education'. *European Early Childhood Education Research Journal* 21(2): 172–184.

Staempfli, M. B. (2007), 'Adolescent Playfulness, Stress Perception, Coping and Well Being'. *Journal of Leisure Research* 39(3): 393–412.

Suteerawattananon, M., G. S. Morris, B. R. Etnyre, J. Jankovic and E. J. Protas (2004), 'Effects of Visual and Auditory Cues on Gait in Individuals with Parkinson's Disease'. *Journal of Neurological Science* 219: 63–69.

Tieben, R., J. Sturm, M. M. Bekker and B. A. M. Schouten (2014), 'Playful Persuasion: Designing for Ambient Playful Interactions in Public Spaces'. *Journal for Ambient Intelligence and Smart Environments* 6(4): 341–357.

Van Vleet, M. and B. Feeney (2015), 'Play Behavior and Playfulness in Adulthood'. *Social and Personality Psychology Compass* 9(11): 630–643.

Vogiazou, Y., B. Raijmakers, E. Geelhoed et al. (2006), 'Design for Emergence: Experiments with a Mixed Reality Urban Playground Game'. *Personal and Ubiquitous Computing* 11: 45–58.

Walsh, R., M. Boberg, J. Arrasvuori, H. Korhonen and T. Walsh (2010), 'Introducing Game and Playful Experiences to Other Application Domains through Personality and Motivation Models'. 2nd Int IEEE Consumer Electronics Society, Games Innovation Conference, pp. 1–8.

Watershed (2015), Playable City. Available at http://www.watershed.co.uk/playablecity/overview (accessed 10 October 2015).

3

Can We Give Ourselves Extra Senses? Exploring Sensory Augmentation

Naomi Jacobs and Jonny Huck

Senses are our way of engaging with the world around us, taking input from our environment and incorporating it into our understanding. We are all familiar with the 'five senses' of taste, touch, sight, smell and sound. However, the environment contains a great deal more information than is available to these five. Some of this information we might already be able to incorporate into our experience through less traditional 'senses' such as proprioception (knowing where parts of our body are), but still more is beyond our normal experience. The 'sensors' which come as standard in our bodies have limitations, but these might be overcome by the use of technology, through which we might develop a much wider range of sense capabilities.

In this chapter we will explore possibilities of designing technology to extend the way we experience the world around us, not just through readouts and static information relayed from external sensors and filtered through our conscious awareness, but what happens when these information sources become more integrally incorporated into our experience. To reflect on this, this chapter reports and reflects upon a case study that uses a first-person experiential methodology to explore whether design and technology can be used to enhance our sensory experience. Through this, we consider what a new sense might *feel* like. This is itself a sensory metaphor; we are exploring the lived experience of incorporating new sensory data to our construction of the world around us. The area chosen to explore this is direction and navigation. Although being able to orient and navigate is not usually considered a separate sense, we do speak of a 'sense of direction'. This may not simply be a metaphor. Awareness of our spatial location is a potential area for sensory extension, as explored below.

Technology as Part of Our Sense of Self

Information forms a large part of our experience of the world. Our five standard senses take input about light waves (sight), vibrations (sound/touch) or chemical stimuli (smell/taste) and our brains translate this and extract meaning that is relevant for our experience, creating our perceptions of the world. 'From the moment we are born until we die, our sensory system is feeding our brain vast amounts of information' (Cochrane 1997: 112). However, an important aspect to note is that we do not indiscriminately take all input from our senses, assemble it in some internal representation and then interpret our experiences based on that. It now seems clear that our conscious minds disregard much of the input that arrives via our senses. Andy Clark posits that direct perception itself (rather than a complete picture) is what creates our mental representations; that 'we create inner states that simultaneously describe partial aspects of the world and prescribe possible actions and interventions' (1996: 50–51). In other words, we build our perceptions of the world based on the information that is relevant to decisions that we need to make and actions we intend to take. Though other information may be available, it only becomes incorporated into our perceived worldview when it might be relevant to our behaviour. While we think we 'see' a complete picture of the world around us, this is an illusion conjured by our brains creating a 'memory' of the outside world based upon what it expects to be there (O'Regan 1992). This can be demonstrated by experiments in which, for example, participants are asked to read a screen of text that changes based on their visual fixation; their gaze is tracked and words outside of the visual field (where they are focussing at any one particular moment) are replaced by gibberish (Churchland et al. 1994). The reader cannot 'see' the way the text changes, and perceives the full page of text to be there in peripheral vision at all times, even if they are told the nature of the experiment. The critical thing that allows this to work is that the text changes are made in the gap between visual fixations while the eye is in motion; the brain has no input during this time and so fills in the gaps based on expectations.

Even in creating this selective picture of the world, however, we are limited by the capabilities of our biological senses. These limits may vary between individuals, or at different stages of life. For example, the ability to hear higher pitches declines with age, through sensorineural age-related hearing loss known as presbycusis. Genetic variation between individuals can lead to impairments in sensory ability, such as inherited colour blindness, but also enhancements. An example of this can be seen in the work of the artist Concetta Antico[1] who has tetrachromacy – four types of colour receptor cells in her eyes rather than the normal three, or the two seen in some forms of colour blindness. She is able to perceive a far wider range of colour, and uses this to enhance her art.

Almost since the earliest days of human culture, technology has been used to affect and enhance our bodies' capabilities. The earliest clothing can be dated, through a variety of evidence (from stone-scraping tools, to the evolution of body lice) to between 83,000 and 170,000 years ago, and would have played a vital role in temperature regulation and protection, allowing our species, *homo sapiens*, to spread across the entire globe into climates quite unlike the African regions of our origin. Technologies to enhance our sensory capabilities beyond the existing limits of our bodies are nearly as ancient. Examples in vision alone cover everything from the telescope to eyeglasses; these not only correct degraded vision but also allow enhanced abilities in those who otherwise would be restricted in the limits of their sight. In this way, technology can complement our bodily senses and extend them.

Technology attached to our body, and which becomes a fundamental part of our daily lives, can become incorporated into our bodily schema – in a way feel like 'part' of your body, and an extension of your senses. An example of this can be found in the reactions to those who wear wrist watches. The following was a comment spontaneously made on Twitter, but it reflects a common phenomenon which many readers may be familiar with:

> I left my watch at home & it's really, really bothering me. I feel really, profoundly uncomfortable. Like I've lost a finger. @thejimsmith,[2] 5 November 2014

This is possible because of the close association between our brains and the tools and technology that we use. The incorporation of external factors into our sense of self happens because of the way that our experience is created from interactions between our mind, bodies and environment, enabled by the immense plasticity of our neural architecture. This can be seen through examples of those whose brains show physiological differences relating to use. This includes those who learn new skills, for example, London taxi drivers, whose brains can be seen to be visibly affected by learning 'The Knowledge' of London's streets (Maguire et al. 2000). The converse can also be seen in individuals whose brains show physical differences but overcome these to replicate functions seen in a fully developed brain. For example, in 2014, a twenty-four-year-old woman in China was discovered to have a large portion of her brain, the cerebellum, missing since birth. She had been living a relatively normal life, functioning with only limited impairments such as delayed speech and walking (Yu et al. 2015). Her brain appears to have compensated for her lack in early development, repurposing other areas to undertake the functions that the cerebellum would usually be vital for.

This flexibility allows adaption of the ways that sensory input is processed. Visually impaired people can use clicking as a form of sonar to 'see' their environment, and it has been shown that this skill can be learned by anyone (Teng and Whitney 2011). Our brains quickly adapt when the input does not match what is 'expected'. Jan Degenaar (2014), for example, undertook an experiment into spatial vision that included the wearing of inverting glasses which swap the left/right axis of vision. He found that after a significant period of wearing the glasses (123 hours) he was able to correctly locate objects in space without thinking about it and react naturally to their position despite his altered perception. David Eagleman, who is currently conducting work in sensory substitution vests, sums it up thusly: 'My view is that the brain is a general-purpose computational device . . . You could take any kind of data stream and the brain will figure it out. I consider it the biggest miracle no one's heard of' (Li 2015).

Theories of embodied cognition suggest that it is by interaction with the physical world that our mind is built, and our senses are critical to this (Wilson 2002). Human brains are highly specialized not for particular inputs or experiences, but to adapt to whatever is required. This also includes using external objects as extensions of our cognitive system, such as writing down numbers in order to do complex calculations, or rotating puzzle pieces to see how they fit rather than doing the rotation mentally. We offload some of the work from our brains to the world around us. This can even include other people. Clive Thompson (2013) describes how couples may not make the effort to recall information that they know their spouse will remember 'for' them, a process known as transactive memory. As technology, and in particular digital technology, becomes more complex, it may be that we are increasing the amount of cognitive effort that we are transferring out of our brains.

Some people are concerned that reliance on technology is damaging our capabilities, for example, Nicholas Carr (2010) argues that there may be trade-offs in letting technology do the work for us, in effect that we might be 'getting dimmer'. By automating cognitive processes, he suggests, we may be getting 'worse' at them, and that by the crutch of technology our brains are no longer used to functioning in the way that they might have had to previously. However, the theory of embodied cognition suggests this has always been the case, and that our evolutionary history is based upon the incorporation of tools and external support to our cognitive models through brain plasticity. There is however a question of how this incorporation of technology changes our behaviour and the ways in which we live our lives – either by replacing or improving abilities which are damaged or degraded, adding new ones that did not previously exist, or even giving us new cause to reflect on the way that we have previously done things without the benefit of the technology. This is particularly the case with regards to technology which affects our senses, our bodies, and our physical interaction with the environment around us.

Transhumanism and the Extension of a Direction Sense

Prostheses which replicate lost bodily function are becoming ever more complex. Beyond correcting vision we can now regulate heartbeat with pacemakers, provide cochlear implants to correct hearing loss and replace missing limbs with prosthetics that incorporate nerve endings so they can be moved 'by thinking' (Sofge 2015). Some prosthetics, however, may even enhance human abilities beyond normal functionality, for example, bionic limbs specifically designed for functions such as rock climbing (Kiss 2015). When Oscar Pistorius entered the Olympics with his 'Cheetah' prosthetics, there was controversy because evidence suggested they gave him a competitive advantage over non-amputee athletes.[3]

To consider what additional senses might be added to our repertoire with the aid of technology, we can look to the animal kingdom for inspiration. Many species have superior or alternative sensory capabilities to humans, such as the superior discernment of smells that a dog possesses, or the ability some animals have to see colours beyond those that we are able to, such as ultraviolet or infrared. If we could provide a way for our eyes to interpret these colours, could we enhance our vision to see more colours?

There are several animal species which possess magnetoreception, the ability to sense where the magnetic north is. This is most well studied in birds, and there is now some understanding of various mechanisms that are used to sense the magnetic field including magnetite particles in an organ in the beak, and a 'chemical compass' in the eye (Wiltschko and Wiltschko 2005). Although there is some research which suggests that humans, too, may have this ability (Baker 1987), there has to date been little evidence found for any biological mechanism by which this might function, and it does not appear to contribute to what is colloquially known as a 'sense of direction'. Some research has experimented with artificially inducing magnetoreception, most commonly as a navigational aid for those who are visually impaired (Adame et al. 2013).

Erik Jonsson (2007) proposes that way-finding is made up of two factors, direction frame and dead reckoning. Direction frame is described as an internal sense of 'north', and seems to be related to the ability to maintain an ongoing track of objective direction based on relative orientation. He describes experiences where people with a highly attuned sense of direction can become 'displaced' in relation to their experience of where north 'should' be, getting lost because they are following an incorrect internal calibration. He relates an uncanny feeling of 'rotating 180 degrees' when in such a circumstance he realized his mistake and the world reoriented. This demonstrates that this 'sense' is relative rather than absolute directionality. It also does not appear to be possessed by everyone to the same degree. Jonsson suggests that it is less common in those who live in modern urban environments.

The research described here therefore attempts to look at whether the direction 'sense', which appears to be based on internalization of location tracking and relative direction frame, can be augmented by extra sensory information about the true orientation by artificially providing magnetoreception. We will focus on the process of embodied cognition, asking whether such a novel sensory input can be 'internalized' and sensed or felt rather than accessed consciously and reflectively as might be information given by a map and compass.

Experimental Intervention: Methodology

This chapter is examining sensory experience and how it might feel to have changes made to sensory capacity through augmentation, and therefore a first-person experiential methodology was chosen. Three tasks were designed in order to provide a baseline measure of navigational ability and grounds for personal reflection, followed by repetition of the tasks with the addition of the technological intervention, and qualitative experiential data collected. In the following text, where the first-person singular is used, it relates to the experience of the first author of this chapter.

The experiment was conducted in three stages: Stage 1, the baseline evaluation of navigational experience and ability with no augmentation device; Stage 2, the use of an off-the-shelf device for magnetoreception; and Stage 3, the use of a bespoke adaptation of this device with repetition of the evaluation tasks conducted at the initial baseline. The evaluation tasks are described below:

Task 1 – Map reading

The subject was taken to a novel location and given a map with two locations marked: the current position (A) and the destination location (B). The task was to make the journey between the two, and examined map-reading and the ability to orient on a map and relate it to location in order to find a route.

Task 2 – Route tracing with no map

The subject was taken to a novel location (A) then driven to a second novel location (B) within a complex road network (an estate of interconnected streets). The task was to make the journey back to location A on foot, without the aid of a map. The option was given to either retrace the driving route or find a different, more direct route.

Task 3 – Route finding with no map

The subject was taken to a novel location (A), then directed on foot to a novel location (B) via an indirect route. The task was to return to location A using the shortest route.

In order to accurately record the route taken during each task, an off-the-shelf mobile mapping and data collection app (Fieldtrip GB[4]) was used, which created GPS-traces of the walking routes that could then be plotted onto a map using standard GIS software.

Experimental Intervention: Stage 1 (Baseline)

Taking part in this experiment prompted introspection and reflection on the act of navigation and direction finding. Even completing the baseline tasks, with no technological intervention prompted extra attention to be paid to the surroundings because of the expectation of the need to remember the route:

> *At several points I was aware that under normal circumstances, this would be the time I would take out my phone and consult Google maps. This was particularly true where I was being asked to find my way back from somewhere that I didn't recognise and where I had no idea of the road layout or of how far from my destination I was.*
>
> *I have never considered myself particularly good at navigation and direction finding, so I was greatly surprised to find that all three tasks were completed successfully.*

Task 1: Map reading

Location (A) was at a dead end in a small housing estate, consisting of many small interconnected roads and footpaths, and the map provided did not immediately make it clear how or if each set connected.

> *I decided to act as I normally would if I were travelling from one place to another, and take the 'straightforward' route on the larger roads – that had a smaller number of places where I would have to make a choice as to which direction to take.*

Following the map was a continuous process of checking and rechecking while travelling down the route as marked.

> *At the very beginning of the route I wasn't entirely confident that I knew where I was on the map, and I therefore wanted to check I was going the right way. When I passed a side road and checked the name on the road sign I felt slightly more confident, but I was only totally sure of myself once I reached the larger road and saw the name on the road sign there.*

This continual checking continued throughout the walk, with the exception of long, straight stretches with no choice of direction. In particular,

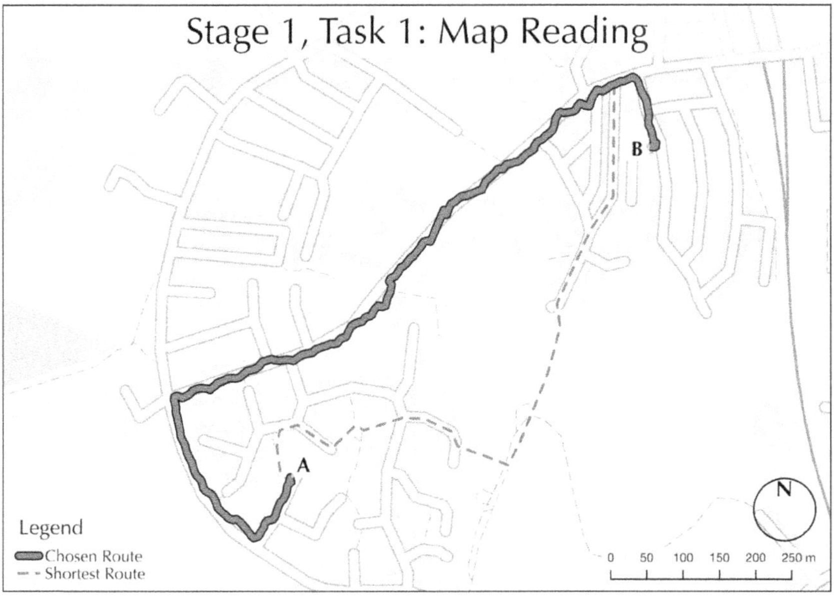

FIGURE 3.1 *A map showing a GPS trace of the route taken by the author in the Stage 1, Task 1, map-reading task, alongside the 'optimal' route, which was shorter, though complex to navigate.* Contains OS data © Crown copyright and database right (2015). Contains OpenStreetMap data © OpenStreetMap contributors (2015), licensed under the Open Database License.

checks were made when approaching a junction to confirm where a turn should be made.

> *This is something that I often do when route finding and using maps*

Overall the task was achieved without any problems.

> *Although I was continually checking my progress, for most of the journey I felt I knew where I was. But the confidence came from the map and the road signs and the fact that they matched, and matched my own idea of where I had travelled.*

The chosen route for this task is illustrated in Figure 3.1.

Task 2: Route tracing with no map

The task began with a stop at a roundabout (A) followed by a car journey to a school (B) and a request to find the way back.

> *I found myself paying particular attention to landmarks and visible signs that I would be able to use to re-orient myself. For example, noting*

a school on the left that should be on the right on the return journey, and a distinctive red railing along part of the route.

At point B, I had an idea that the point A was in a particular direction because of the turns that had been taken, but I did not feel confident enough to set out that way – my direction frame was not developed enough to have a clear idea of my exact relative position. I also wasn't sure if I would recognise point A from a different direction. Instead, I traced the route that had been taken.

The route back was navigated fairly successfully, noting landmarks such as the red fence and the school, though it was clear that this was not necessarily the shortest route.

At one point, I saw the beginning of a pathway that I was fairly confident led up to the road with the red railing. But I could not see the other end of the path and decided to take the 'safe' route that I remembered via the road. Walking past the red railing, I did indeed encounter the other end of the path – it would have been a shorter route had I decided to take it.

Orientation more generally was difficult, until a vantage point was reached which brought in sight a local landmark, the Ashton Memorial.

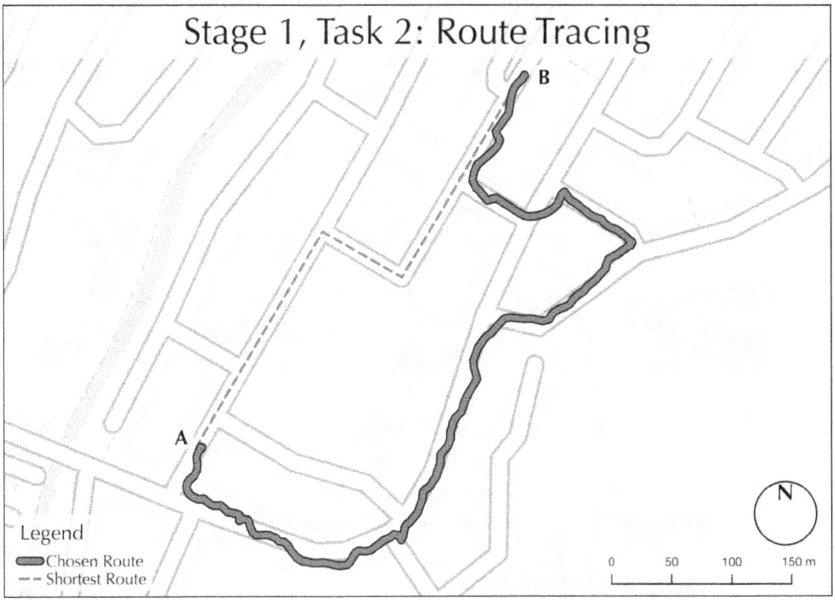

FIGURE 3.2 *A map showing a GPS trace of the route taken by the author in the Stage 1, Task 2, route-tracing task, alongside the 'optimal' route.* Contains OS data © Crown copyright and database right (2015). Contains OpenStreetMap data © OpenStreetMap contributors (2015), licensed under the Open Database License.

> *Suddenly, I found myself orienting my position in relation to the larger city I was in, realising where I was in relation to other landmarks. I still wasn't sure exactly where I was until I looked in the other direction, saw the castle and millennium bridge and then was able to place myself to one particular side of the city. This was an interesting moment of realisation because up until that point I could have been 'anywhere' and I wasn't really paying attention to my wider geographic orientation or location beyond how to get back to the origin/destination point.*

While the route was successfully navigated, it was revealed afterwards that Point B was on a connected road to Point A, and the route could have been completed in a loop.

> *That I could have taken a much shorter route was very surprising: I had no instinctive feeling that the two places linked up in a different way than via the route I had taken, they did not feel 'close together'.*

The chosen route for this task is illustrated in Figure 3.2.

Task 3: Route finding with no map

> *This task felt more challenging. I started out trying to pay attention to the direction we walked and the turns that we took, but at some point I thought that I was very unsure where we were in relation to the original starting point. My internal navigational sense, such as it was, had failed.*

After being walked from Point A to Point B the task was to find a more direct route back.

> *I didn't really have any idea of how to return to the original starting point, but I decided to follow the road in the direction that felt like the one we had 'come from' and hope that there would be some clues further in that direction that would help me establish the way to the original starting point.*

The first major moment of uncertainty was a fork in the road – one that very clearly went up the hill, and the other down.

> *I recalled that on the original route we had taken a sharp upward turn at one point, so I decided to follow the downwards route. I held with this plan at the next fork in the road, continuing the downwards trend though I wasn't sure at this point whether it was taking me closer to or further away from the goal.*

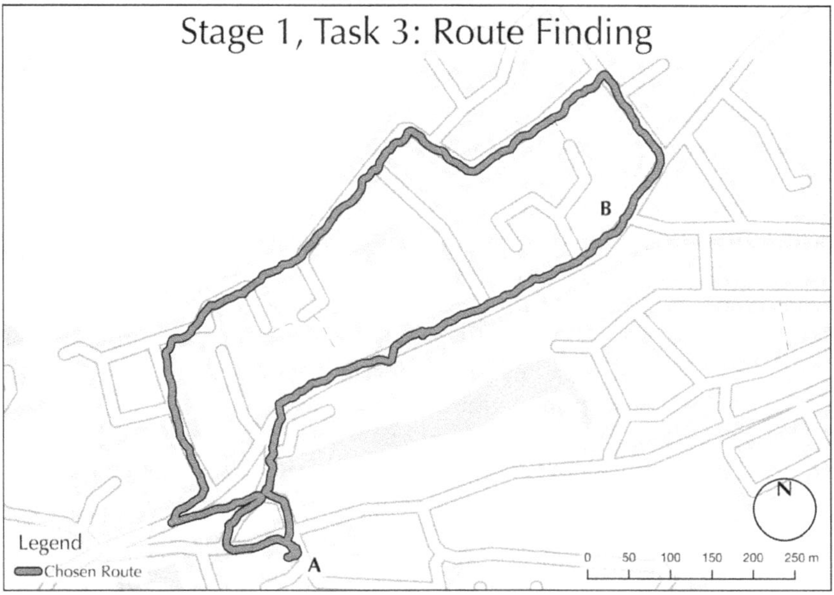

FIGURE 3.3 *A map showing a GPS trace of the route taken by the author in the Stage 1, Task 3, route-finding task, alongside the 'optimal' route.* Contains OS data © Crown copyright and database right (2015). Contains OpenStreetMap data © OpenStreetMap contributors (2015), licensed under the Open Database License.

Approaching a turn, still with no clear sense of location relative to the start point, the destination was suddenly revealed.

> *I was most surprised to find when I reached the crossroads, the marker for the original start point! I had reached the destination while still thinking I was some distance away and that I was to some extent lost, worried that I wouldn't know which way to turn at the next junction.*

Despite this lack of conscious knowledge, the shortest route back was taken.

The chosen route for this task is illustrated in Figure 3.3.

Experimental Intervention: Stage 2 (Northpaw)

The technology used to implement magnetoreception was the NorthPaw, developed by a company called Sensebridge. In many ways this may be considered a prototype device although it is sold commercially. The NorthPaw arrives as a kit which needs to be soldered together by the user and consists of an ankle bracelet with padding, eight pager motors, a battery pack and a control unit circuit board. The operation is fairly straightforward: the pager motors are spaced equally around the ankle, and the one that is positioned towards magnetic north vibrates due to commands from the magnetometer (digital compass) built into the control unit.

Several issues were experienced with the Northpaw device that meant that it was not easy to wear for long periods of time. Some of these were related to practical design issues: the anklet was very difficult to securely affix so that it did not slip down, thus causing the motors to lose contact with the leg. The motors did not function reliably, perhaps because of jostling against clothing and the ankle, and on a number of occasions the contact wires broke and required re-soldering. Additionally, contact with clothing and the small radius of the device meant that it was difficult to discern the exact direction of vibration.

The device was worn for a total of one week, but intermittently because of the issues described above. Overall, the experience was not conducive to integration.

> *It did not feel like a part of 'me' but rather an inconvenience. There was no sense that the anklet gave a true idea of where north lay at any particular time.*

The experience did not improve over the time it was working and it was concluded that it was an ineffective intervention for the purposes of giving a 'sense' of north – in this case, the technology was not 'invisible' enough (to quote Donald Norman) for the purposes of this study. With this in mind, rather than continue with this form of the intervention, a decision was made to develop the device into a form that would more closely mimic the sensory integration used by other studies with visually impaired subjects – a belt that could be worn around the waist, therefore giving a more integrated 'feeling' of directionality, since the vibration would be felt around the core of the body rather than just on one side as was the case with the ankle bracelet.

Experimental Intervention: Stage 3 (Bespoke Device)

For this intervention, the pager motors and control unit from the NorthPaw were removed from the anklet and installed into a fabric belt that could be fastened around the waist (Figure 3.4). The general operation was otherwise identical.

The belt was worn over a period of one month, with much longer periods of continuous use. In fact it was worn for the majority of days during this period, with the exception of some periods of international travel where it could not be taken through airport security.

> *Although I did not feel like the 'sense' of direction was incorporated into my awareness of the environment, I did become used to considering*

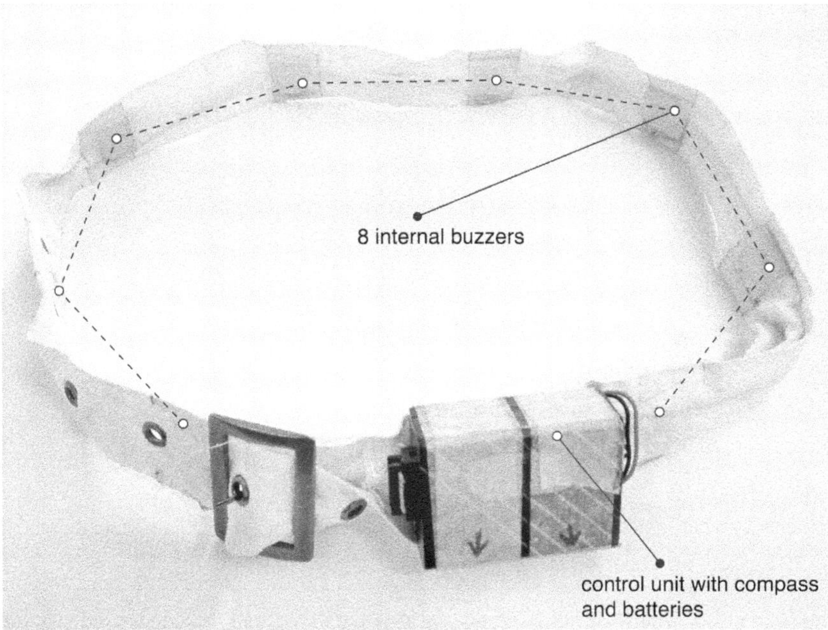

FIGURE 3.4 *The bespoke directional belt device* © Naomi Jacobs and Jonny Huck.

> *where north was and being able to tell immediately from the direction of vibration. What was intriguing was how often this corresponded to knowledge I already possessed about my location.*

A key observation from wearing the belt was becoming aware of how seldom in daily life we don't know exactly where we are.

> *I found myself retracing the same routes almost every day – walking around my house, around my office, and on simple routes around the university campus. For all of these routes, I quickly became aware of the directionality of each route – not just from the knowledge imparted by the belt but also by how they connected together, reinforced by thinking 'where is north from here?' and being able to answer that question with input from the device. Did I 'know' where north was along these routes? Yes, because they were the same ones I took every day.*

At the end of the month, the three tasks were repeated.

Task 1: Map reading

As previously, the map navigation task (finding a route from point A to point B using a map) did not pose a large challenge and was completed

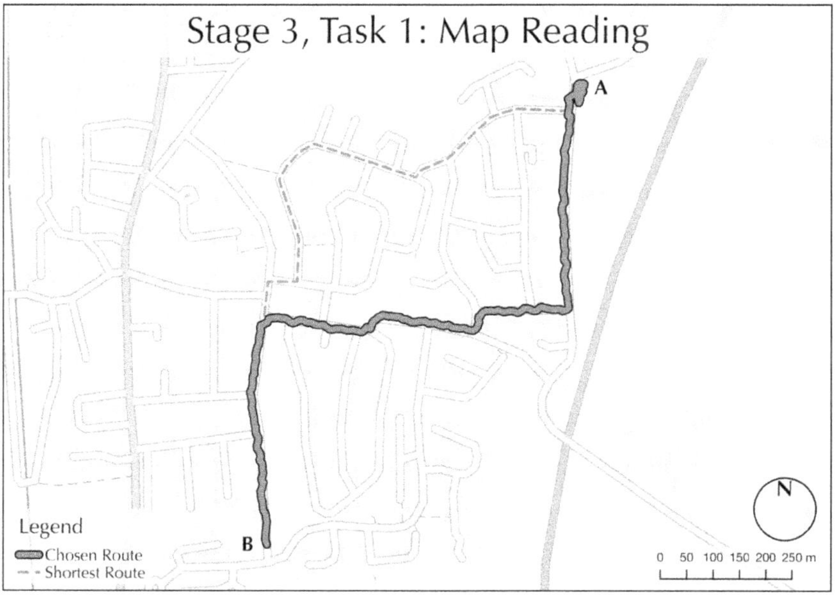

FIGURE 3.5 *A map showing a GPS trace of the route taken by the author in the Stage 3, Task 1, map-reading task, alongside the 'optimal' route.* Contains OS data © Crown copyright and database right (2015). Contains OpenStreetMap data © OpenStreetMap contributors (2015), licensed under the Open Database License.

easily. The one aspect that was noticeably affected by the belt was the initial orientation of position in relation to the map.

> *Although I was not totally confident in the knowledge imparted by the belt, I oriented myself both in terms of landmarks on the map (e.g. junction shape), backed up this information with the fact that the vibrations on the belt indicated that I was facing the right direction.*

After using road features to confirm location, the remainder of the task was completed navigating based on landmarks and road features as in the baseline task.

The chosen route for this task is illustrated in Figure 3.5.

Task 2: Route tracing with no map

The second task, retracing a driven route on foot, was experienced as being more difficult initially than it had in the baseline condition. This was possibly a factor of the particular location chosen, which was a complex estate with many similar houses, and no immediately prominent landmarks like the red fence used previously. Interestingly, it was not a shortage of potential

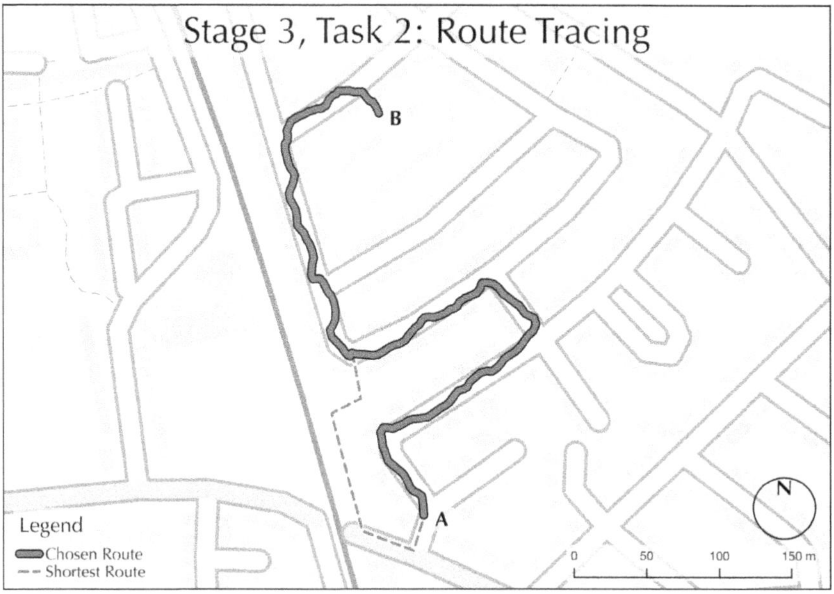

FIGURE 3.6 *A map showing a GPS trace of the route taken by the author in the Stage 3, Task 2, route-tracing task, alongside the 'optimal' route.* Contains OS data © Crown copyright and database right (2015). Contains OpenStreetMap data © OpenStreetMap contributors (2015), licensed under the Open Database License.

landmarks but an overabundance of them that caused the issues: although similar, every house was unique and had different objects in the gardens, and it felt like a long and complex route was driven.

> *I chose an initial direction based to some extent on what the belt was telling me, and from a general feeling of where I had come from, though I quickly felt disoriented.*

In spite of this, the route was re-traced exactly, though as experienced in some of the previous tasks, reaching the destination came as a surprise.

> *Although I felt 'lost' throughout the journey, I had in fact had accurately taken the shortest route to the destination with little hesitation.*

The chosen route for this task is illustrated in Figure 3.6.

Task 3: Route finding with no map

This task, to find a direct route back to the starting point having walked a less direct route, took place not in an urban area but in a woodland. This did not particularly affect the experience though the nature of the landmarks and locations were very different.

> *As in the baseline test, I quickly felt disoriented and 'lost' without a clear sense of where I had come from.*

However, extra information was available from the belt: that the route began with walking in one particular direction, apparently towards the south, given that it was in the opposite direction to the vibrating motor.

> *When asked to make my way back to the start point, there were several times I had to make a choice between two or more different paths. At the first of these, a T-junction with two paths leading in opposite direction, I did not have any clear idea which was correct, so in the absence of any other information I took the one that led towards the north – the opposite to my initial direction of travel, to retrace my steps. I did initially consider taking the other path (southwards) because although the route had travelled both up and downhill, it seemed that we had gone 'more' uphill and thus the downhill (southwards) path might be better.*

The directional information turned out to be correct. This is not information that would have been available without sensation from the belt,

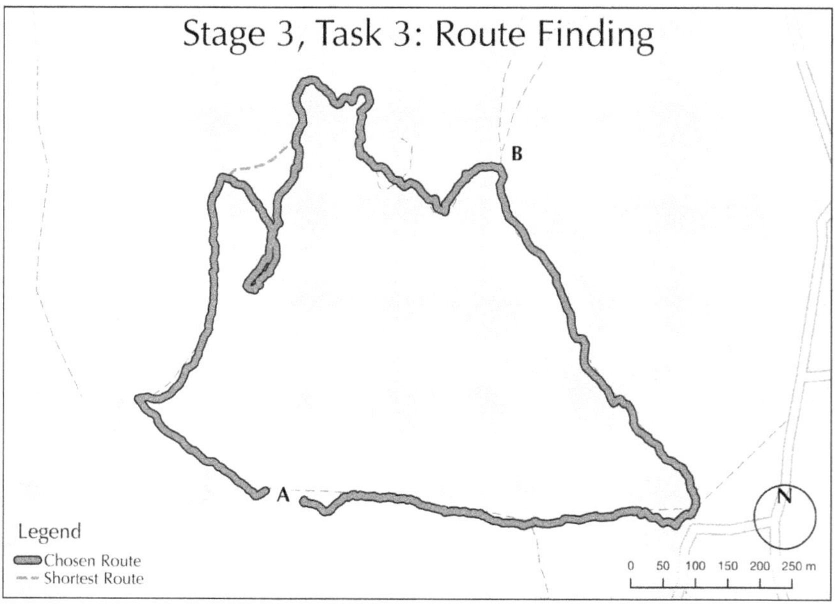

FIGURE 3.7 *A map showing a GPS trace of the route taken by the author in the Stage 3, Task 3, map-reading task, alongside the 'optimal' route. Contains OS data © Crown copyright and database right (2015).* Contains OpenStreetMap data © OpenStreetMap contributors (2015), licensed under the Open Database License.

indicating the directionality of both the initial walk and the split pathway, and it is likely the other (incorrect) path would have been taken. The task was successfully completed, returning to the start point, with the only diversion to the most direct route being at point B, where it was found that the footpath could not be followed due to a locked gate, and a small detour had to be taken. However it is interesting to note that the initial direction walked was not southwards, but in fact to the east. The information from the sensor was reliable, but not accurate.

The chosen route for this task is illustrated in Figure 3.7.

Conclusions

The result of the work here does not give conclusive answers as to whether new sensory abilities can be incorporated seamlessly into everyday consciousness. The belt technology was crude, and worn only for a limited period. However, there were some indications that being aware of the directionality became familiar and increased the feeling of 'knowing' where you were – at least in terms of improving the 'sense of direction', which appears to be highly variable between individuals. The main effect seen here appears to be in terms of mindfulness, a heightened awareness of both sensory input and specifically directionality as a result of being constantly reminded that it is a factor. Changing sensations and senses can therefore be said to affect our experience of the world, even in this limited capacity.

It is also interesting that navigational ability was seen both without the intervention, and during it, although it was not conscious. In each case the tasks were successfully completed despite a feeling of 'lostness'. It seems that directional 'sense' is something that we do have even when we are not aware of it, and it is relating this to map locations that may be a cognitive hurdle.

The urge to use digital maps to locate oneself might be a sign that direction finding cognition is offloaded to external maps, which are missed when not accessible (either as in this case through choice, or where the technology fails). This fits with observations of authors such as Willis et al. (2009) who have written about spatial knowledge acquisition with and without the aid of GPS guides. Some cognition may also be offloaded to paper maps, indicated by the constant checking to reinforce knowledge of location. Digital maps move a step beyond what can be achieved by fixed paper maps because they can be centred on the individual rather than the location, on the person rather than the journey.

Jonsson (2002) proposes that direction finding and dead reckoning are things that all can attain, but that they are skills not possessed by 'modern' peoples who have no need for them. It may be that this is because of 'cognitive unloading', at least in a modern urban setting. This outsourcing of cognitive load has the potential downside that without this technology backing us up we might be more likely to get lost, something inconceivable to someone with perfect dead reckoning and spatial awareness of everywhere they have been. However, it means we can navigate somewhere we have never been before, plan routes before we have physically seen a locale, and perhaps have an awareness of much larger areas of space. Our sense of place is extended beyond the limits our own sensory apparatus, and we are making use of shared 'knowledge' that has been collected by others.

Through our access to this pool of information it may be said that we are inhabiting a new 'digital public space' where anyone, anywhere, anytime can explore and interact with digital information.[5] This digital public space exists above and around normal 'space', in a way acting as an extra dimension to extend the familiar three. We are surrounded by a sea of information that can be accessed at multiple physical locations by many people at once. By these means we are augmenting our sense of self with a constant flow of information that can be incorporated into our experience. As the example of the expectation of Google Maps availability shows, we are becoming used to being able to access digital content wherever we are.

It may be that there are other new aspects of sensing that can be accessed through this digital public space, from the 'comobility' of being able to interact with others at a distance and know where they are (Southern 2012), to the 'ambient intimacy', coined by blogger Leisa Reichelt (2007), through which seemingly banal status updates give us knowledge of our peers and of the state of the world at all times. As connected technology and digital public spaces move inevitably into our physical world in the form of augmented technology and embedded digital–physical objects, interactions with products will involve more of our senses and interactions with products must be increasingly intuitive if we are to enable ambient computing – that seamlessly embeds into our daily lives and takes over tasks for us.

In order to achieve this, such technologies, especially those that sit on our bodies, must overcome barriers for use by becoming increasingly unobtrusive, so that they may effortlessly incorporate into our experience. The Northpaw anklet did not do this, though the belt did approach integration.

The validity of the data being fed to new senses is also important. Although the input from the belt seemed consistent, it was not always clear whether it was accurately pointing north, and in some cases did not appear to be, as in Task 3. The sensors typically used in devices such as these are low-cost, miniaturized sensors arising from emergent fields such as the 'Quantified Self' (QS) and the 'Internet of Things' (IoT). While beneficial in many ways, including portability, low power consumption and low cost, the limitations of these devices relating to precision and accuracy of collected data are often overlooked. This has significant implications for the so-called democratization of data that is frequently claimed as arising from the proliferation of these low-cost, miniaturized sensor technologies, and also for citizen science in general.

By using low-cost, miniaturized sensors such as those described in this chapter, citizens can be empowered to gain a greater understanding of the relationship between their bodies and the environment, augmenting their own senses in order to become more informed and conversant on a variety of issues (which could include navigation, but also, e.g., noise pollution, air quality and meteorological conditions). Such developments may also carry implications for the government, local councils and regulatory bodies, who may have to make changes to their operations in order to prepare for challenges to their 'official' measurements of noise, pollution, etcetera, from the public, and may have to increase public engagement on these issues in order to supply more detailed information to a public that is increasingly knowledgeable and conversant about local environmental issues such as traffic pollution, noise and so on.

However, in many cases (including that presented in this chapter), the sensors in question are not of sufficient quality to provide precise quantitative data, and as such should not be relied upon without an understanding of their limitations. This has important implications for potential users as, if the limitations of these sensors are not fully understood, then they may be unintentionally misused and produce data unsuitable for the purposes for which they are intended. For example, if citizens sought to influence policy relating to air quality using these sensors, perhaps from an industrial facility that they suspected was causing unacceptable emissions of pollution, then they would only be able to produce meaningful data if the sensors in question were of sufficient quality to produce replicable readings under calibration, which is often not the case.[6] Similarly, the sensors described in this chapter will only be successful and useful in the augmentation of our 'sense of direction' if users can have confidence that the data output from them, a haptic indication of the direction of magnetic North, are accurate and reliable. The use of such devices without proper understanding of their limitations could be said to be providing citizens with a 'false power', whereby they are led to believe that they are empowered, but in fact are not.

What they may provide, however, is a means to increase mindfulness: in the intervention, directionality was thought about more than ordinarily. The advantage of such devices might be simply that they bring otherwise 'invisible' phenomena to the forefront of people's minds.

Questions remain which should be considered when designing technology of this sort that augments our senses. How does the technology affect our place in the world, and in digital public space? Does it affect our interactions with the world, and does this have positive or negative impacts? If the data coming in to our senses do not accurately reflect the 'real' world, might this bias our interpretations? And even if we can augment ourselves, should we?

Notes

1 http://concettaantico.com/ (accessed 12 November 2015)
2 source: twitter.com

3 http://www.iaaf.org/news/news/oscar-pistorius-independent-scientific-stud-1 (accessed 12 November 2015)
4 http://fieldtripgb.blogs.edina.ac.uk/ (accessed 12 November 2015)
5 www.thecreativeexchange.org (accessed 12 November 2015)
6 This has been the experience of the authors, who have conducted laboratory calibrations on several such sensors.

References

Adame, M. R., J. Yu, K. Moller and E. Seemann (2013), 'A Wearable Navigation Aid for Blind People Using a Vibrotactile Information Transfer System'. *Complex Medical Engineering (CME), 2013 ICME International Conference*. New York: IEEE, pp. 13–18.

Baker, R. R. (1987), 'Human Navigation and Magnetoreception: The Manchester Experiments Do Replicate'. *Animal Behaviour* 35(3): 691–704.

Carr, N. (2011), *The Shallows: What the Internet is Doing to Our Brains*. London: W. W. Norton & Company.

Churchland, P. S., V. S. Ramachandran and T. J. Sejnowski (1994), 'A Critique of Pure Vision'. In C. Koch and J. L. Davis (eds), *Large-Scale Neuronal Theories of the Brain*. Cambridge, MA: MIT Press, pp. 23–60.

Clark, A. (1997), *Being There: Putting Brain, Body, and World Together Again*. Cambridge, MA: MIT Press.

Cochrane, P. (1999), *Tips for Time Travellers*. London: Orion Business.

Degenaar, J. (2014), 'Through the Inverting Glass: First-Person Observations on Spatial Vision and Imagery'. *Phenomenology and the Cognitive Sciences* 13(2): 373–393.

Jonsson, E. (2002), *Inner Navigation: Why We Get Lost and How We Find Our Way*. New York: Simon and Schuster.

Kiss, J. (2015), 'What If a Bionic Leg Is So Good That Someone Chooses to Amputate?' *The Guardian*, available at http://www.theguardian.com/technology/2015/apr/09/disability-amputees-bionics-hugh-herr-super-prostheses (accessed on 9 April 2016).

Li, S. (2015), 'The Wearable Device That Could Unlock a New Human Sense'. *The Atlantic*, available at http://www.theatlantic.com/technology/archive/2015/04/the-wearable-device-that-could-unlock-a-new-human-sense/390273/ (accessed on 14 April 2016).

Maguire, E. A., D. G. Gadian, I. S. Johnsrude, C. D. Good, J. Ashburner, R. S. Frackowiak and C. D. Frith (2000), 'Navigation-Related Structural Change in the Hippocampi of Taxi Drivers'. *Proceedings of the National Academy of Sciences* 97(8): 4398–4403.

O'Regan, J. K. (1992), 'Solving the "Real" Mysteries of Visual Perception: The World as an Outside Memory'. *Canadian Journal of Psychology/Revue canadienne de psychologie* 46(3): 461.

Reichelt, L. (2007), 'Ambient Intimacy', available at http://www.disambiguity.com/ambient-intimacy/ (accessed 1 March 2016).

Santani Teng, D. W. (2011), 'The Acuity of Echolocation: Spatial Resolution in the Sighted Compared to Expert Performance'. *Journal of Visual Impairment & Blindness* 105(1): 20–32.

Sofge, E. (2015), 'Brain-Controlled Bionic Legs Are Finally Here'. *Popular Science*, available at http://www.popsci.com/brain-controlled-bionic-legs-are-here-no-really (accessed 20 May 2016).

Southern, J. (2012), 'Comobility: How Proximity and Distance Travel Together in Locative Media'. *Canadian Journal of Communication* 37(1): 75–91.

Thompson, C. (2013), *Smarter Than You Think: How Technology Is Changing Our Minds for the Better.* New York: Penguin.

Willis, K. S., C. Hölscher, G. Wilbertz and C. Li (2009), 'A Comparison of Spatial Knowledge Acquisition with Maps and Mobile Maps'. *Computers, Environment and Urban Systems* 33(2): 100–110.

Wilson, M. (2002), 'Six Views of Embodied Cognition'. *Psychonomic Bulletin & Review* 9(4): 625–636.

Wiltschko, W. and R. Wiltschko (2005), 'Magnetic Orientation and Magnetoreception in Birds and Other Animals'. *Journal of Comparative Physiology A* 191(8): 675–693.

Yu, F., Q. J. Jiang, X. Y. Sun and R. W. Zhang (2014), 'A New Case of Complete Primary Cerebellar Agenesis: Clinical and Imaging Findings in a Living Patient'. *Brain*, awu239.

4

Sonifying Memory: Creative Approaches to Representing Socially Constructed Soundscapes

Linda O'Keeffe

Sonic Sensory Divides

While living in Chicago in 2009 I was confronted with a space both racially and sonically divided. The city, which includes a large African American population, is divided by a motorway, which splits the north from the south side of the city. On first moving to Chicago I lived on the south, predominantly Black, side, and after several months I moved to the north side. The difference in urban design, housing, paths and roadways, parks and businesses, was quite startling. Large parts of the north side contained small streets with artisanal shops, bakeries, wholefood stores and street cafes, while the south side consisted of large roadways, block-built stores and workspaces, large tracts of abandoned land, where presumably a construction project had died, with poorly built housing complexes. While recording the soundscape of Chicago what emerged was how much spatial design and architecture shaped the production of community sounds. Not only did the architecture alter the sounds of a space, it shaped how people sounded – as in produced sound – in public spaces. While this type of sonic segregation was very visible and audible, it was while attending another event in the city that I was struck by less obvious forms of sonic segregation.

The annual Chicago American Indian Powwow is held at the United Centre in Chicago, a sports stadium. This event is a response to the Indian relocation act of the 1950s, a concerted effort by governments to terminate tribal status in America and thus vacate people from their lands. The Powwow allows the first peoples to have a common social and cultural ground where they can celebrate their history. This gathering consists of a series of processional events, which are accompanied by the sounds of a number of large drums played by various community groups (see Figure 4.1). The sounds surrounded and vibrated through the space; they were both harmonic and disharmonic as each drum group shifted between rhythms. All of these sounds were contained within the dome of this vast sports centre. From the outside you could not hear any of the dances, drum beats or voices of song taking place within. This sociocultural sonic celebration was enclosed and removed from the Chicago community.

On returning to Ireland I began to interrogate the idea of sound as an important sociocultural experience, exploring spaces within Dublin city that were losing or had already lost their traditional soundscape as a result of urban planning and design. That research began with a simple premise: to define what part sound plays in the experience of everyday life in Dublin city. The original emphasis was on the urban soundscape in general. However, the research evolved substantially throughout its examination of the urban, to include interior and exterior spaces as well as mediated soundscapes. Moreover, in light of a lack of empirical qualitative data on subjective soundscape experiences, it became necessary to design a new method in which to engage with this question. The methods involved extending the reach of the discipline by using an interdisciplinary approach. It required integrating ideas from the fields of sound

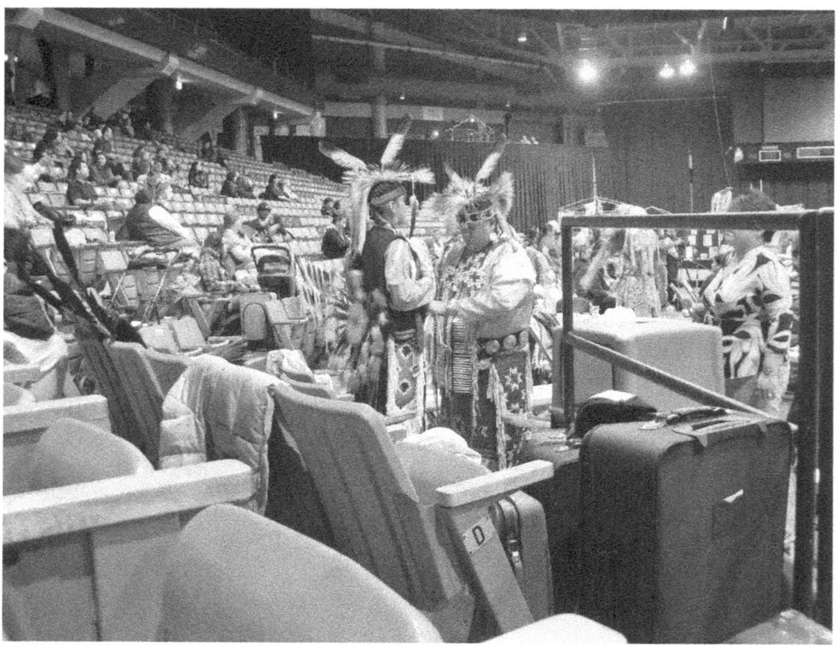

FIGURE 4.1 *Chicago Powwow, 2009*. Photo by Linda O'Keeffe.

art, acoustic ecology, psychoacoustics as well as traditional social science methods. It is only in recent studies that sound is emerging as critical to understanding social practices; however, there is still a significant gap in the area of sound as an embodied experience with the power to shape and reconstruct social spaces and social practices.

Embodying the Soundscape

The experience of listening to one's environment though common is not often acknowledged in conversation. One walks through space seeing and hearing, smelling, tasting and touching. Yet the predominant discourse of our spatial experiences is situated within the visible domain. To talk about other sensory connections means reflecting on the body and the body's awareness of space (Merleau-Ponty 1948; Ihde 2007), a sensual experience which seems private, not for public discussion. Our connections and ties to place rely on an overall embodiment and recognition of the sensory: we hear the cries of children, traffic, people shouting, birds and air, the sounds of familiar productive practices; we smell the bakers, butchers, fish markets, body odours, engine fumes; we brush against people, walls, pillars and posts; we taste the variety of food available in our culture. All of this happens simultaneously, we are contained within and embody the sensory, yet vision, the great remover and objectifier of space, is where many fields and disciplines situate the human experience (de Certeau 1988; Synnott 1992). The atomizing of the senses is a process of isolating 'one sense from the others' (Ihde 2007: 43) so that we may 'build up' or 'synthesize an object out of 'sense data' or some other form of 'sensory atom'. These beliefs lie deeply imbedded in recent times with the 'sense atomism' (Ihde 2007) that infects even the sciences at their metaphysical level.

This distanciation of the body's senses, the sensual, is part of the Western obsession with the visible as an objective view of the world, a concept which is documented as emerging during the Enlightenment, but is not restricted to that period (Schwartz 2011). The Enlightenment is said to have revealed, through the natural sciences, that which was traditionally hidden by layers of mysticism. With the natural sciences, knowledge was measured as the ability to reveal through sight the meaning of things, a move away from the mysticism of religion (Sterne 2003). Sight, therefore, became the dominant sense connected to the sciences, almost at the expense of the other senses and their abilities to reveal truths amid other sense observations. This rearranging of meaning, through language, places the experiential or empirical information at a distance. This chapter does not argue for an elevation of one sense over another but rather a consideration of a more holistic approach to sensing or representing spatialities.

Historically, sight has been significantly overestimated in its ability to reveal the accuracy of things, including the experience of things; 'seeing is believing'. Sight is said to be how we assess the spatiality of space. We see how large a space is, the tallness of structures and the skyline tell us about the possible activities economic or social that may take place there (Harvey 2001, 2011). Sounds 'are first experienced as sounds of things' (Ihde 2007: 60) – cars equal traffic sounds, factories produce the sounds of production. Experiential listening, for example, is rarely taken into consideration in the construction of objects – groups and individuals come to have an association or link between an object and the sounds it makes and this can affect our engagement with that object (Degen 2008). It is our ability to discern minute details within the listening experience that is taken for granted, yet

> this common ability of listening contains within it an extraordinary richness of distinction and the capacity to discern minute differences of auditory texture, and by it we know to what and often to where it is our listening refers. (Ihde 2007: 60)

Ihde suggests that when we first encounter sounds, we listen naively; the sound is heard on the surface, identified with a cause or a source and then meaning is applied. On next hearing that sound, even without sourcing the cause, we now have the ability to identify the sound. But Ihde goes further. Within the location of sounding experiences, the phenomenon of listening is paired with spatial awareness, a possible awareness of the *shape* of a sound, though this is significantly different to the visual seeing of shapes. Ihde proposes an extensive revision of how hearing occurs as a sensory and phenomenological event, highlighting as other authors have (Thibaud 1998), the limited understanding of the link between our auditory and visual perception of the world.

Creative Methods of Researching Sound and the Senses

The methods adopted for the collection of sonic data, and the design and construction of the art installation, placed the body at the centre of spatio-sensory experience. The sounds within the exhibition described below were designed to explore themes that had emerged during the methodological stage of my research, but they were positioned and placed in ways to transform the audience's engagement with the gallery space.

The qualitative methods were designed to engage a group of participants (eighty-four teenagers aged fifteen to sixteen, five older adults aged fifty-five to seventy) in a sensory and sonic mapping of public spaces within Dublin city between 2010 and 2013. The key space at the centre of the research was the Smithfield Square and environs, a former market area with private and public housing projects. This space has experienced significant urban regeneration projects since the mid 1990s (Peillon and Corcoran 2004). The methods included a series of sound walks, deep listening workshops, sound mapping and pyramid mapping (see Figures 4.2 and 4.3). These methods required an integration of ideas from the fields of sound art, acoustic ecology, psychoacoustics as well as traditional social science methods, focus groups and interviews. The older adults were interviewed about their memories of the Dublin city soundscape during their teenage years as well as exploring how the city soundscape has changed over the past fifty years.

During this same period I began to bring people on silent sound walks through Dublin, and in 2013 co-founded the Dublin Phonographers Union. This process was part of a global phenomenon of collecting soundscapes, generated by the growing field of acoustic ecology.

However, my study did not exclude other forms of sensory engagement with space. Sound should not be collected or studied in isolation to other sensory experiences, but be emplaced within the study of the senses and the urban environment. In examining sound as a social construct I was seeking to challenge long-standing notions that sound is ephemeral and therefore not open to interpretation 'despite the fact they are made, heard, imagined, and thought by humans' (Kahn 2001: 4). It was this data including the autoethnographic walks that shaped the proposed project at the Limerick Sculpture Centre.

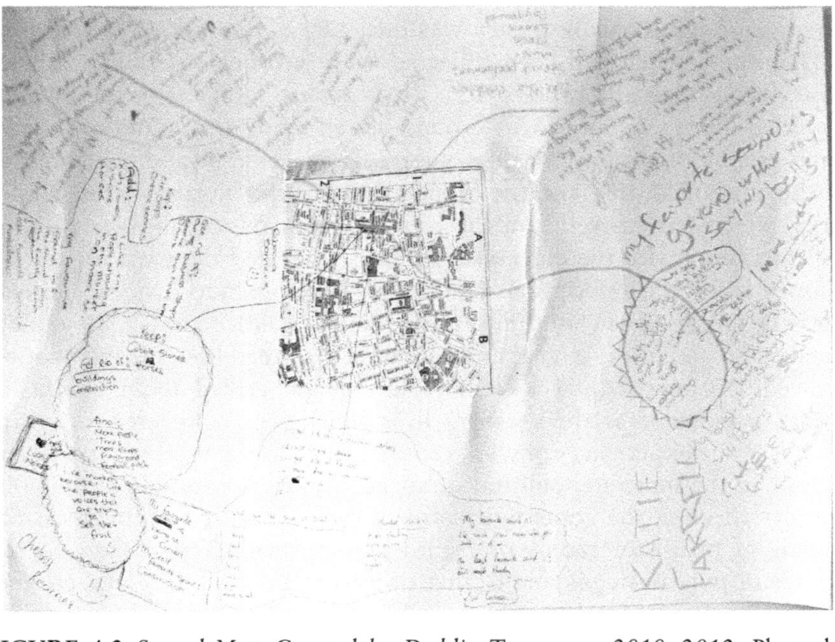

FIGURE 4.2 *Sound Map Created by Dublin Teenagers, 2010–2012*. Photo by Linda O'Keeffe.

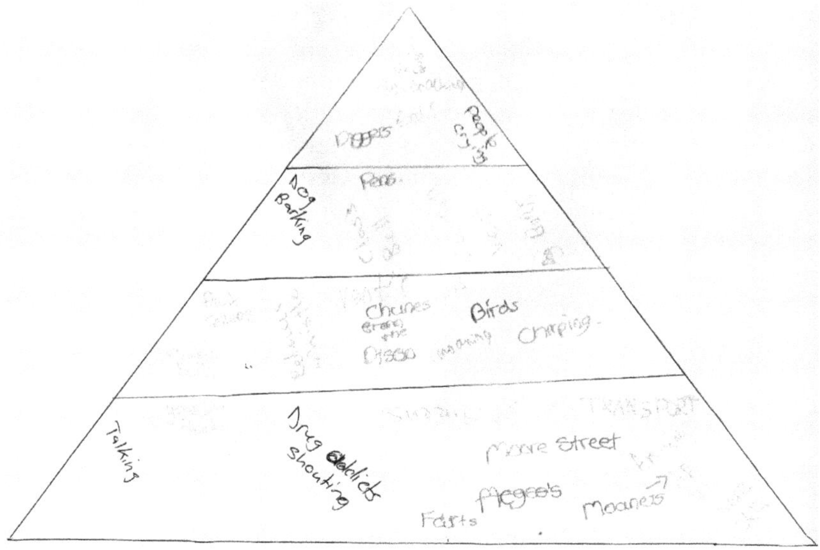

FIGURE 4.3 *Sound Pyramid Created by Dublin Teenagers, 2010–2012*. Photo by Linda O'Keeffe.

Methodology for Creating a Sonic Installation

The beginning of this residency was difficult, as the task of reconceptualizing data, which had been collected for a particular sociological purpose, seemed initially problematic. Most of this data was in the form of recorded interviews and focus groups, sound maps and sound pyramids, photographs of sound emitting objects or spaces and audio recordings of the Smithfield area and the broader area of the North side of Dublin city, collected by myself and the teenage participants. However, it was the interviews with the older adults which generated the most impressive sensory and sonic descriptions of a particular place in its historic context. Their memories of the Smithfield area from the 1940s to today, its sounds, smells, and activities – social and economic – shaped how the installation evolved. During the interviews, the older people talked about significant events or moments in their teenage lives which were connected to certain sounds: daily experiences of work routines, such as the market soundscape at four in the morning; cultural or social rituals; the sounds of religious parades through the community streets; new or older technologies; the sounds of transistor radios or record players coming from flats, or the sounds of pop music playing from a transistor amid a group of teenagers on a street corner. Sounds were described as either centripetal or centrifugal, that is, sounds that draw people towards them or push people away. In some circumstances, certain sounds were both, for example, the sounds of the delivery trucks and horses and carts bringing fresh fruit and vegetables to the markets in the morning would be defined as centripetal; 'it attracts and unifies the community in a social sense' (Schafer 1977: 54). These sounds were a familiar part of the everyday, something that allowed people to identify themselves to a unique work practice within Dublin city (Twomey 2005).

The soundscape of this space was also a reminder of the poverty and deprivation that most of the community experienced in tenement housing in Dublin at this time, a centrifugal soundscape that pushed people away from the space. From the 1960s on there was a series of mass economic emigrations from this and most other parts of Dublin city. In designing the installation, a key goal was to explore these centrifugal and centripetal sounds, as the community understood them. It was also important to interrogate how sound was defined as ephemeral, permanent, historical and modern.

Most of my art practice has involved a re-conceptualization or reimagining of a sonic event. Previous works have included interactive and immersive installations that allow the listener to experience an interpretation of other places, memories or moments in time. In 2007 the Amersfoort city council commissioned a public art installation to create a work that celebrated the five-hundredth anniversary of the town of Amersfoort in Holland. Three months were spent documenting the sounds and history of the town. This involved recording the street sounds, interviewing various people and visits to archaeological sites and museums, in an effort to try and extract the sonic past of this urban space. This also included examining how one could understand the sonic history of a space through an examination of the changes in architecture and cultural practices as well as the influences of different periods throughout history, from the Renaissance to modernity. Schafer (1993), Schwarz (2011) and Smith (1999, 2004, 2011) suggest that one can understand the soundscape of place through historical archives as well as through shifts in cultural and architectural design. The materials of construction, how the landscape was used and creative activities such as theatre, music and the arts in general, leave remnants of information that can be sonically informative. In reading a city's past we can infer a type of sonic culture. Through this process of archaeological digging it was possible to conceptualize and map a type of sonic geography. The role of the artist within the Amersfoort project was to find a way to represent the sonic history of this space and locate this within the contemporary soundscape. The link between the historical soundscape and the contemporary was further united by the art installation being constructed within a particular public space which connected these histories (see Figure 4.4). However, the installation constructed for the Leitrim Gallery space was removed from the original soundscape study. This was the white cube, a space often defined as a blank canvas, more suited to the visual than the audible, primarily because they are rarely constructed to deal with proper acoustic propagation.

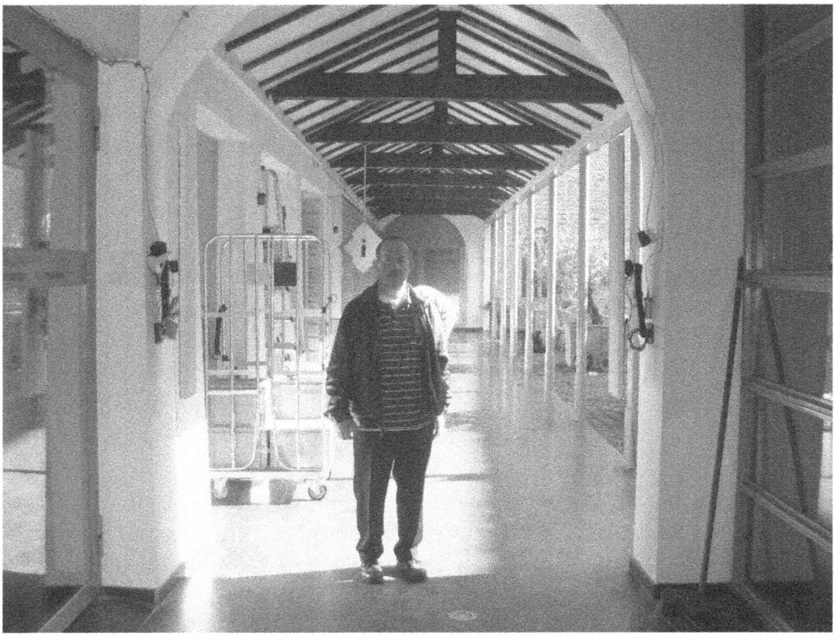

FIGURE 4.4 *Artefiction, Tourist Office, Amersfoort, Holland, 2007.* This is an outdoor space, a tourist office in Amersfoot, Holland. The participant is standing between two sound shower speakers and listening to the audio work. Photo by Linda O'Keeffe.

Practice after Research: Notes on Standing at the Precipice of a New Body of Work

Standing in the centre of the installation I am confronted by the dichotomy of sounds, sonic experiences, soundscapes, sound memories and abstracted audio that have emerged from the six-week residency at the Leitrim Sculpture centre.[1] This work represents four years of research in which a small part of Dublin city was methodologically and ethnographically examined. This interrogation of a soundscape was shaped by sociological theory, guided by writings on sound studies in all their varied forms from perception to ecology, and the mediatization of the urban (Couldry 2008). What emerged from that research highlighted key processes involved in the shaping of urban spaces, which continue to ignore the significance of sound in the experience of place (O Keeffe 2014, 2015). Translating those findings into an immersive sonic installation required a rethinking of what constitutes representation. For example, how can one narrate a soundscape memory, in what way can a gallery space represent the social shaping of community sounds, and how can a work of art reflect the loss of what is already an ephemeral experience?

Though elements of the methods incorporated techniques developed within sound art practice and acoustic ecology, such as soundwalking (Westerkamp 2007), Deep Listening (Oliveros 2005) and sound mapping (Alarcón 2013), the trans-disciplinary approach involved incorporating these methods into traditional sociological methodological enquiry. Transforming these findings into an installation required a rethinking of the model of research as art practice. Often practice-based or led research involves developing a research strategy whose end goal is the construction of some artifact (Rust, Mottram and Till 2007). The process of engaging with theory and methods is often merged with creative processes. However, this art project involved the translation of theoretical findings into a three dimensional or immersive experience. One of the key issues when working on this project was how to represent the sonic experience of the researcher and the research participants. A CD of sounds accompanied the thesis, but it was not considered necessary to understanding the text or the methods. Instead, the study had to use language as a way to describe and define the subjective and embodied experience of sound, both the internal and external, the felt and the imagined, the remembered and the lost. The installation was a way in which to engage the audience with sonic memory or psychogeography (Coverley 2010), but also a retelling through the researcher's interpretation, cuts and edits of other remembered sound stories.

When examining how the research could inform an installation I had to reflect on some of the key theoretical findings: first, sound, as an embodied experience has the power to shape and reconstruct space, and second, sound, according to both the older and younger participants, was site specific. It embodied and informed us about a place's purpose or even purposelessness. History, community, media technologies, music and community informed the participant's definition of certain sonic experiences. In order to take these elements and transform them into a work of art all of these things had to be considered, including how to create an immersive experience for the listener or viewer in the gallery which allowed them to experience and embody the soundscape memories of others. Listening back to the interviews and looking at the maps created by the teenagers offered 'new insights' when thinking about embodied auditory experiences (Rust et al. 2007: 12). Experimenting with the sounds and text from the research led to an interrogation of how one could represent sonic memories, what were the possible ethical implications of using the same data in an exhibition, and how literal or explicative should the work be? In other words, should it try to represent the findings or say something different about sonic memories? The space of the gallery would inform the placement and engagement with the sound works created for this show.

Residency

The residency allowed me the time to interrogate materials, sounds and space in which to explore what could be represented as an embodied moment of sound that someone could walk, sit and stand within. The first stage of investigation was based on a statement made by one of the older participants. During the interview, he talked about how he and a group of friends would run outside and place a transistor radio against a metal street-light pole. This would act as an antenna, picking up radio signals from other countries, particularly music stations from the United Kingdom. The teenagers would stand around these poles accessing music, news and other mediated information not broadcast or controlled by Irish media, which during the 1950s through to the 1970s was heavily controlled by the Church and state. For a moment, these spaces would become autonomous soundscapes, or as Blesser and Salter (2009) called them, acoustic bubbles. Another interviewee remembered placing his transistor radio up against 'a piece of steel so it earthed and gave you an aerial system so to pick up the signal, and you put it to the thing, right inside it, . . . the coil was picking up the metal and was extending the signal'.

This image of teenagers 'extending the signal' was very important as a concept as it highlighted the possibilities of sound as something that both transformed and liberated space. This capturing of sound allowed them a sense of autonomy over their listening spaces; it also created what Lefebvre (1974) calls a representational space. Representational space is the space that 'imagination seeks to change and appropriate' (1974: 39). It is a representational and symbolic space that is necessary for the cohesion and continuity of space. If a space is only defined by its productive practices, and given legitimacy through concrete ontological and binary codes, what is lost is the potential for a continuous discourse of space, the representational space; a space with a 'multitude of intersection(s)' (1974: 33). This image of the lamp post became part of a symbolic representation of imagined soundscapes. The installation therefore began with a search for a lamp post that could site the stories in a particular historical framework, and during the residency such a lamp post was found (see Figure 4.5).

It was this piece which became the central focus of the installation because it lead to an analysis of how the sounds within the gallery could be spaced differently, creating symbolic places within the exhibition. Sound, by its very nature, leaks and spreads, diffuses and crosses over. As a sensory experience it rarely happens in isolation to other sensory events, and I did not want to create an exhibition that was arguing for the supremacy of the auditory experience. Rather that sound was embodied, physical, tangible and intangible, it created as much as it diffused through space, but more importantly it was part of the overall experience of the gallery space, the walls, arches, walkways and objects placed within were as much a part of the experience as the sonic.

A residency is in part a period of experimentation, particularly as a lot of installations become site specific, they tend to reference the place you are within and the space you exhibit within. This particular residency offered a very different acoustic environment to the original research area, yet there were similarities to how space was defined by both participant groups. Each described this particular city space (Smithfield) as one falling into

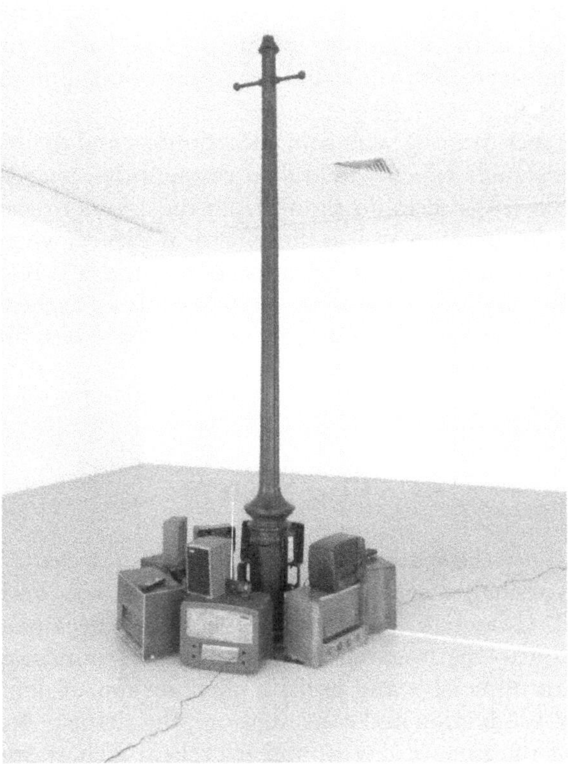

FIGURE 4.5 *Sound Radio Spaces Exhibition, Leitrim Sculpture Centre, 2014.* Photo by Linda O'Keeffe.

silence. Silence did not mean an absence of sound, but rather the absence of significant or meaningful sounds. This notion of what was considered positive and negative sound started to emerge as a key point during the residency. I began exploring how during the interviews the older participants and some of the younger participants would describe sounds heard through vocalizing a sound type or even singing sounds. Some of the younger participants often defined sound as evoking movement or music.

> Group: (Participant 1) It's not too loud, it's kind of peaceful. (Participant 2) It's like a wave. A bus is (vocalises a loud growling sound). (Participant 1) Yeah it's quiet (The Luas). Like a ballet. (Group 14a: Female)

The older participants remembered the songs sung in public spaces, the rhythm of space, its fluctuations throughout the day, connected to work and social practices.

> [S]inging, singing was a big part of it, because of a Sunday morning, Sunday around noon, you had the street singers coming around oh yes,

> they came through the streets, . . . and sing their way from Summerhill down through Sean McDermott Street down, and all through where the blocks of flats were, and you could hear their voices (2nd male aged 63).

This lead to experimenting with sonic descriptions and their voices to create music-like sounds which would float through the space, including the sounds of radio (clips of radio shows from the 1930s to the 1970s were played within the space), as well as dips into near silence, where the discreet sounds of voices floated into the main space from the next room. This time of experimentation allowed me to play with sound as a cyclical event, using stories, music, noise and silence to separate the space into different timed events of acoustic moments.

The Space

Within the gallery the space was divided into three areas, a main central space and two smaller spaces (see Figure 4.4). It was decided to treat each space as distinctive soundscapes, where one became immersed in ways significant to the research participants. The soundscape by definition is both an immersive and holistic phenomenon, it defines activities (the sounds of production and consumption), the shape of space (through acoustics) and the time of day (sound is cyclical). These sounds are not just heard where they are produced. Rather sound, because of diffusion, spreads beyond its source. Holding on to this concept meant deciding that the sounds in the space could not be closed off from other sounds, for example, all sounds restricted to headphone listening. Instead, sound would filter through each of the spaces but only one sound would be continuous.

In the second smaller space, a rectangular room, two sound showers were hung at opposite corners to each other.[2] Each speaker faced the corner of the wall, meaning that the sound reflected off that surface and moved out into the space. The listener would have to walk around the space to find the position that produced the clearest sound. The levels were quite low so one had to listen with the intent to hear what was being said. These sounds were clips taken from the interviews with the older participants, clips which stated in some way how places were transformed through the introduction of sounds, such as a radio, animals brought in to the Smithfield Square during markets days, the trucks, horses or lorries appearing in the very early hours of the morning to deliver goods. Each description was of a temporal soundscape; a soundscape that only a local would understand.

The main space had at the centre a live audio piece, which was a selection of old radio recordings from Radio Eireann as well as audio recordings from radio programs from the United Kingdom dating back to the early 1940s through to the late 1960s.[3] These clips would play for a period of time then drop to silence for approximately two minutes. Three small transistor radios were placed within the old radios that were situated around the base of the light pole. They were set to play (at a very low volume undetected until the radio sounds went off) white noise or cosmic static; this would change over time with the influence of disturbances in the atmosphere or with the other radios crossing over of signals. This would allow a listener in the next space hear the details of the vocal recordings undisturbed, which would be disrupted when the radio sounds came back on.

There were two headphone pieces also situated within the centre light pole work. Each work played a sound piece, which was a mix of voices and sounds that looped around a central theme, an important sound remembered and described by two participants.

The final piece was placed in the corner of the main space and consisted of an old record player with a headphone work. This work stemmed from the interviews and workshops with the teenagers. Making this piece required thinking a lot about the ethics of using the sounds of children and the ownership they have over their stories. The end work is a distortion of their voices, but this was not a direct response to ethics. Instead, the work was concerned with the overall experience of childhood in the twentieth and twenty-first century which has not dramatically changed since the emergence of media technologies.

Conclusion

This residency allowed for the abstracting and reconceptualizing of sonic and other sensory data as a way to explore the memories of space. It also raised questions about how to work within the white cube and all its acoustic issues. New media artists often have to engage with this traditional space, accommodating and sometimes altering the work to facilitate an appropriate engagement with non-visual-based works. The research had examined how one engages with the sonic within open and public spaces. The artwork intended to recreate this engagement through a filtered and altered representation of that experience. However, when examining the large interior spaces of the gallery it was clear that the original sonic ideas would have to be altered. The transformation, which took place in response to the gallery's architecture did in fact allow for an in-depth engagement with elements of the sound previously ignored or not considered. This included the adjustment of the amplification of certain signals or frequency ranges; the placing of certain sounds in headphones rather than in loudspeakers; the difference in the design of these sounds that would be either intimate or shared; and analyzing whether a sound would be a whole-body experience, engaging most of the senses, or a private one. This meant returning to the meaning and contexts of materials collected and considering what should or should not be amplified within all of the space. Because language played a key role in shaping sonic memories, there was a return to a deeper listening of the work and a real consideration as to what should be concealed and revealed. Each auditory description given by the interviewees defined larger social and cultural as well as spatial moments in time. In contrast, some memories triggered connections and meanings that they had not expected, one sound descriptor defining other sounds. Some of these sensory memories were private, explicated moments of terror or exclusion, others were public and involved a sensory description of a space in its entirety, smells, tastes and touch as well as sound. The installation was designed to reflect the more specific and personal elements of sensory sonic memories and how these sensory moments can trigger vast reflective memories.

Sound is not experienced in isolation to other sensory information, though it is often ignored or peripherally engaged with within urban studies. Although there has been what Howes (2006) calls a 'sensory revolution' within the social sciences, the focus on all of the senses excludes discreet examinations of how one sense, the auditory, shapes specific urban experiences. The exhibition was designed to focus the audience's attention on the sonic; each space constructed to engage them in a sensory event removed from visible information. The objects that were placed in the space were direct responses to sounding memories, and were directly linked to the production or shaping of sonic moments and memories.

Notes

1 For a virtual tour of the installation, visit https://vimeo.com/123495287 (accessed 17 October 2016).

2 A sound shower speaker is a directional speaker; it plays sound in a narrow frequency band, so vocal sounds work best.

3 Radio Eireann was the national broadcasting station of Ireland.

References

Alarcon, X. (2013), 'Creating Sounding Underground'. *Digital Creativity* 24(3): 252–258.

Blesser, B. and L. Salter (2009), *Spaces Speak, Are You Listening?* Cambridge, MA: MIT Press.

Certeau, M., L. Giard, P. Mayol and T. Tomasik (1998), *The Practice of Everyday Life*. Translated by S. Rendall. Minneapolis: University of Minnesota Press.

Corcoran, M. and M. Peillon (2004), *Place and Non-place: The Reconfiguration of Ireland*. Dublin: Institute of Public Administration.

Couldry, N. (2008), 'Mediatization or Mediation? Alternative Understandings of the Emergent Space of Digital Storytelling'. *New Media & Society* 10(3): 373–391.

Coverley, M. (2010), *Psychogeography*. Harpenden, Herts: Pocket Essentials.

Degen, M. (2008), *Sensing Cities*. London: Routledge.
Harvey, D. (2001), *Spaces of Capital*. New York: Routledge.
Harvey, D. (2011), 'Contested Cities: Social Process and Spatial Form'. In R. LeGates and F. Stout (eds), *The City Reader*, 5th edition. London: Routledge.
Howes, D. (2006), 'Charting the Sensorial Revolution'. *Senses and Society* 1(1): 113–128.
Ihde, D. (2007), *Listening and Voice*. Albany: State University of New York Press.
Kahn, D. (2001), *Noise, Water, Meat*. Cambridge, MA: MIT Press.
Lefebvre, H. (1991), *The Production of Space*. Oxford: Blackwell.
Merleau-Ponty, M. (2004), *The World of Perception*. Translated by O. Davies. London: Routledge.
O'Keeffe, L. (2014), '(Sound)Walking through Smithfield Square in Dublin' (Blog). *Sounding Out!* Available at http://soundstudiesblog.com/2014/02/10/soundwalking-through-smithfield-square-in-dublin/ (accessed 9 December 2015).
O'Keeffe, L. (2015), 'Thinking Through New Methodologies: Sounding Out the City With Teenagers'. *Qualitative Sociological Review* 11(1):6–32.
Oliveros, P. (2005), *Deep Listening*. New York: iUniverse Inc.
Rust, C., J. Mottram and J. Till (2007), *AHRC Research Review*. Bristol: Arts and Humanities Research Council.
Schafer, R. (1993), *The Soundscape*. Rochester: Destiny Books.
Schwartz, H. (2011), *Making Noise*. Brooklyn, NY: Zone Books.
Smith, B. (1999), *The Acoustic World of Early Modern England*. Chicago: University of Chicago Press.
Smith, B. (2004), 'Tuning into London c. 1600'. In L. Back and M. Bull (eds), *The Auditory Culture Reader*. Oxford: Berg Publishers, pp. 127–136.
Smith, M. (2011), 'The Garden in the Machine: Listening to Early American Industrialization'. In K. Bijsterveld and T. Pinch (eds), *The Oxford Handbook of Sound Studies*. Oxford: Oxford University Press.
Sterne, J. (2003), *The Audible Past*. Durham: Duke University Press.
Synnott, A. (1992), 'The Eye and I: A Sociology of Sight'. *International Journal of Politics, Culture and Society* 5(4): 617–636.
Thibaud, J. (1998), 'The Acoustic Embodiment of Social Practice: Towards a Praxiology of the Sound Environment'. In *Stockholm: Hey Listen*! Conference, Proceedings of the Royal Swedish Academy of Music, pp. 17–22.
Twomey, B. (2005), *Smithfield and the Parish of St Paul, Dublin, 1698–1750*. Dublin, Ireland: Four Courts Press.
Westerkamp, H. (2007). 'Soundwalking'. In A. Carlyle (ed.), *Autumn Leaves, Sound and the Environment in Artistic Practice*. Paris: Double Entendre.

Part 2

The Range of Sensory Arts and Design: Extensions, Realizations and Capacities

5

Scented Colours: The Role of Olfaction in Futurism and Olfactory (Re-)constructions

Caro Verbeek

Scented Colours: The Role of Olfaction in Futurism

> The so-called sweet perfumes of flowers prove insufficient to our nostrils that demand more violent olfactory sensations. . . . Hence we begin a new field of investigation and artistic creation.
>
> (Azari 1924)

This quote could come from one of the many contemporary olfactory artists, such as Sissel Tolaas, Peter de Cupere or Clara Ursitti, who are interested in olfactory taboos, like body odours, and in the more unpleasant side of the dichotomy of foul–fragrant, as opposed to perfumery. Instead it was formulated by the Italian Futurist artist Fedele Azari (1894–1970) in 1924. The elaborate manifesto entitled *La Flora Futurista ed equivalent plastici di odori artificiali* (The Futurist Flora and Plastic Equivalents of Artificial Odours) is the first Futurist manifesto that discusses smell as a direct medium.[1] It contains all the Futurist bullet points: the typical bold and expressive use of language, the role of education, the claim of originality, the shock element, and the interest in the bodily or lower senses. A manifesto on touch had already appeared (Marinetti 1921) and one on taste would soon follow (Marinetti and Fillia 1930).

Futurism provides many more examples: texts that refer to smell, or directly address the sense of smell in performances, artists' books, and even toys with an aromatic dimension.[2] Some of the texts recording these events were in fact published, although it is not always clear if the events actually took place. Founded by the fascist poet F. T. Marinetti (1876–1944), Futurism was born as a literary movement, and there are numerous textual sources that enable us to study and analyse not just which substances the artists may have used, but also what role olfaction played within the movement. In the following paragraphs I will discuss several of these manifestos, including '*La Flora futurista*' and conclude by discussing the value and meaning of sensory reconstructions. How should we present and interpret historical scents? To answer this question, the chapter will deal first with concrete Futurist case studies, and second open a more general debate on sensory and olfactory reconstructions.

The Painting of Sounds, Noises and Smells

On the eve of World War I, Carlo Carrá published 'The Painting of Sounds, Noises and Smells' encompassing three senses: sight, hearing and olfaction. It should be noted in passing that the Futurists make a clear distinction between sounds and noise, noise being classified as chaotic sound. He stated that 'sounds, noises and smells are nothing but different forms and intensity of vibration' (Carrá 1913a).

This is one of the most important lines in the text, because it tells us something about a widespread contemporary belief concerning perception. The correspondence between the senses – and consequently the possibility of moving from one sense to another – was explained by this very notion of vibrational theories. On this premise, all sensory input, no matter from which realm, could be manifested visually. He further explains:

> We Futurist painters maintain that sounds, noises and smells are incorporated in the expression of lines, volumes and colors, just as lines, volumes and colors are incorporated in the architecture of a musical work. Our canvases will therefore express the plastic equivalents of the sounds, noises and smells found in theatres, music-halls, cinemas, brothels, railway stations, ports, garages, hospitals, workshops, etc. etc. (Carrá 1913a)

Since Futurists tried to merge art and daily life, it comes as no surprise that Carrá involves all of the institutions that played a pivotal role in society. More interestingly, the artist presents the relation between painting and music as completely obvious. It is important to realize that what we now refer to as 'synesthesia' was a highly popular idea from the 1850s onwards.[3] It didn't just appeal to painters, such as Vassily Kandinsky, but also to writers and composers. The French Symbolist Charles Baudelaire wrote the sensual poem 'Correspondances' as early as 1857, containing the lines 'Vast as the dark of night and as the light of day/ Perfumes, sounds, and colors correspond' (1954). At this time the condition was described as *audition coloree* (coloured hearing).[4] Claude Debussy composed music exceeding the auditory realm and even stretching to odours in *Iberia, Les parfums de la nuit* (*Spain: The Fragrance of the Night*, 1905–1908). This title was intended to be more than just metaphorical. These are not isolated examples.

Although he does not literally refer to it in his manifesto, it is certain that Carrá was well acquainted with Kandinsky's synesthetic endeavours. The *Blaue Reiter* artist sought visual equivalents to Schoenberg's music. Carrá mentions having seen Kandinsky's *Una composizione musicale* in 1912 (1945). In his essay 'On the Spiritual in Art' Kandinsky extensively described the merging of the senses, devoting only a one sentence to smell:

> The expression 'scented colours' is also frequently used. Finally, the sound of colour is so precise that it would be difficult to locate anyone who would attempt to express the impression of bright yellow in the bass notes of the piano, or rose-madder as a soprano voice. (Kandinsky 1912: 42)

Carrá, maybe in his effort to create something original and innovative in relation to the work of Kandinsky, then well known as an artist and Bauhaus professor, dedicated considerable attention to olfaction, making his text about cross-modality in art quite unique.

> We do not exaggerate in claiming that smell alone is enough to create in our minds arabesques of form and color which constitute the motive and justify the necessity of a painting. In fact, if we are shut in a dark room (so that our sense of sight no longer functions) with flowers, petrol or other strong-smelling things, our plastic spirit gradually eliminates the memory sensations and constructs particular plastic wholes whose quality of weight and movement corresponds perfectly to the smells found in the room. These smells, through an obscure process, have become an environment-force, determining that state of mind which for us Futurist painters constitutes a pure plastic whole. (Carrá 1913a)

The remark about eliminating memory sensations is meaningful. The subjectivity of odour-perception and olfactorily evoked memories was and still is a main point of critique when smells are used in a public artistic context. When music critic John F. Runciman discusses Scriabin's idea of combining music, colour and perfume in 1915, he elaborates on these 'inevitable' problems.[5]

> The perfume of tar is not, I should think, in great favour with fashionable ladies, nor for the thing itself have I any mighty fancy. Yet it reminds me of the banks of the Tyne on sweet evenings, an old-fashioned seaport before iron ships had entirely ousted the old sailing ships, and sailors used to tar their wooden craft while the tide was out, and the litter of ropes, chains, canvas and timber suggested only romance to a boy's

> imagination. My case is not rare. Everyone to whom I have ever spoken on this subject had his or her particular association with a particular odour or smell; but the visions evoked were never alike and each person had a favourite smell [. . .] The message sent through the nostril to the brain or the thoughts and emotions aroused in the brain by any one odour, are not the same in two cases. (Runciman 1915: 157)

Runciman (falsely) presumes the experience of odours is solely related to idiosyncratic or episodical memory and could therefore never address a wider audience and evoke the same sensations or associations.[6] But by treating smell as (additionally) possessing abstract qualities, in this case equivalents of weight and movement, this problem could be avoided. In fact, every scent, besides being linked to an episode, can be judged on its distinctive aromatic character. Lavender might remind us of a holiday spent in France, but we can also recognize its sweet yet fresh aroma, at a second glance or 'sniff' though, because associations always come first.[7]

Now what would these 'arabesques of form' ignited by scent have *looked* like? Luckily Carrá provides us with examples, some of which can still be seen in museums and on the World Wide Web. Unfortunately digital smells, which we can perceive with a few mouse clicks, still elude us. By visually analyzing and comparing these visual manifestations or representations of smells, noises and sounds, we get a glimpse of what the often used Futurist term 'environment-force' might mean.

> This bubbling and whirling of forms and lights composed of sounds, noises and smells has been partly rendered by me in my *Anarchist's Funeral* and *Jolts of a Taxi-cab*, by Boccioni in *States of Mind* and *Forces of a Street*, by Russolo in *Revolt* and Severini in *Pan Pan*. (Carrá 1913a)

What all of these canvases have in common is the use of diagonal lines, sharp angles, dramatic contrasts and fragmented, colourful and overlapping planes that lack any clear contours or borders, enhancing a strong sense of chaos and movement. It is impossible to focus on one part, because our eye is confused and led in every possible direction. This represents the dynamic character of light, sounds and perfumes, which expand over space and time and cannot be captured in a static image. So it is not just the aroma of the perfume that is portrayed, but also its inherent dynamic nature.[8]

Carrá makes more concrete and less abstract assertions with the following: 'While the sounds, noises and smells of animals are yellow and blue, those of a woman are green, blue and purple' (Carrá 1913a).

Does this mean that every time a Futurist soaks his brush in blue paint, he is trying to express something animalistic or feminine? It is unclear how the artist drew these conclusions. Was it from experiment, intuition or an obscure theory, now lost?

La Pittura dei Suoni, Rumori, Odori received a fair amount of attention from important European newspapers. Some journalists found the idea of 'vomiting sounds and smells' on a canvas despicable and ridiculous. And even worse, an Austrian critic contradicted Carrá's claim of originality, one of the Futurists' most important assertions. The journalist argued that painters had already experimented with conveying other senses. Yet Carrá remained rather confident in justifying his claims:

> In their bold revolution, the Impressionists made some confused, hesitant attempts at sounds and noises in their pictures. Before them nothing, absolutely nothing! (Carrá 1913a)

One of the 'Impressionists', or rather post-Impressionists, he was probably referring to was the French master Paul Cézanne. Cézanne seems to have assumed that all objects were present for all the senses at once, through the modality of sight. Phenomenologist Maurice Merleau-Ponty discusses this presumption in 'Cézanne's Doubt': 'We see the depth, the smoothness, the softness, the hardness of objects. Cézanne even claimed that we see their odor' (Merleau-Ponty 1964: 15). According to Martin Jay, in his series *Monte Sainte Victoire*, Cézanne tried to 'capture reality before it was broken down into isolated senses, and the hegemonic autonomy of sight' through bodily and multi-sensory act of painting' (Jay 1994: 159).

The Futurists were interested in a completely different approach to reality, one they considered more objective. In an article published in the Futurist magazine *Lacerba*, Carrá explains how Cézanne's figurative representations of a specific moment in time and his mimetic use of colour (a blue sky, a green field) cannot possibly be considered translations of universal (objective) sensations (Carrá 1913a: 99). The Futurists were depicting our multisensory reality as a whole, manifested through synaesthesia. And these 'universal sensations' could only be expressed abstractly, through contrast, movement, direction and volume (99).

Still, the problematic aspect of this kind of representation is that the result, crystallized in a painting, remains merely visual, and does not consequently communicate to or necessarily address other senses. These visual creations might seem merely to affirm the dominance of the eye than to challenge it.

The Futurist Flora and Plastic Equivalents of Artificial Odours

In the manifesto *La Flora Futurista ed equivalenti plastici di odori artificiali*, 1924, Fedele Azari discusses the possibility of translating contemporary synthetic perfumes into plastic (three-dimensional) objects, such as giant, wooden, brightly coloured flowers and subsequently adding to these an olfactory layer (Azari 1924). Like all Futurists, Azari believed in the supremacy of mankind and the machine over nature, and of the artificial (or synthetic) over the natural. Azari elaborates on some of Carrá's ideas. He speaks about smell–colour synesthesia in a similar manner: 'I state that, beyond such affinity caused by habituation of two simultaneous sensations, there is a connection between form–colour and perfume like there is between music and colour' (1924).

By this, he means that one might associate the colour of a rose with the smell of a rose because of its mutual source, a habituation of two simultaneous sensations, but there are more abstract connections between the two sensory modalities, such as intensity, sharpness or volume.[9] Interestingly, in addition, Azari introduces new concepts related to odour and perfume beyond Carrá's olfactory gaze as a more autonomous means of expression. At least that is what some of his claims indicate:

> Ascertained by this time that the flowers provided to us by nature do not interest us any more, we futurists, in order to brighten, animate and decorate our paintings and our environments, have started the creation of a plastic flower.
>
> Most original
>
> Absolutely invented
>
> Most colorful
>
> Most aromatic (Azari 1924)

And

> We keep plastically constructing our flower and violently colouring and perfuming her with the most intense perfumes. (Azari 1924)

Excitingly he mentions some of these by name. The first two have been reproduced, which makes it possible to study their cultural backgrounds and inherent aroma: 'I have realised a few plastic coloured interpretations of synthetic perfumes that are most in vogue' (*Origan*, *C[h]ypre*, *Contessa Azzurra*, etc.) (Azari 1924).

Chypre (1917), now a famous composition created by French perfumer François Coty, is often described as the first step to abstract perfumery. It consisted of synthetic ingredients, substances that 'amplify' or highlight other ingredients, generating extreme contrasts between top, heart and base notes (Stamelman 2006: 186).[10] Furthermore, Coty was one of the few contemporary perfumers to use raw materials without waxes. As a result, his compositions were much stronger or 'loud', as if someone turned up the volume. Naturally this appealed to the Futurists who glorified noise and speed expressed by bright colours, fragmented planes and dramatic contrasts.

Strikingly, or maybe rather logically, the most famous perfumer and perfume theoretician of all time, Edmond Roudnitska, also sees correspondences between visual and olfactory art: he describes l'Origan (1905) – the other Coty perfume mentioned by Azari – as 'a translation of fauvist sensibility' borrowing all its 'vividness, violence and audacity' (Stamelman 2006: 186). Perfumers are often aware of art and art history. But besides knowing which perfumes were fashionable, there is little indication that Futurists knew about perfume theory or history.

We cannot be sure if the scents Fedele Azari mentioned were actually used to add an olfactory layer to the many, mostly wooden, constructed flowers the Futurists created to substitute for the natural ones they detested. No one has ever taken a headspace sample of the still remaining specimens by Balla and Depero.[11] But it is almost certain that Azari experimented with the actual perfumes, as proven by a letter, sent to his friend Depero just a few days prior to his first presentation of his text during a Futurist conference. In the post scriptum we read:

> I need to remind you to bring me: one bottle of the perfume '*dans la nuit*' by Worth (the flat one, not the spherical one, 12 cm in height, costing appr. 100 fr.) and a bottle of '*tabac blond*' by Caron (the perfume, not the eau de toilette). Don't forget!!![12] (Azari 1924)

Tabac blond (1919) was one of those revolutionary post-war perfumes designed to appeal to those independent European women wearing trousers and smoking cigarettes. The powdery leathery aroma would blend in with the smell of tobacco, now part of their unusual and new olfactory identity. It was the first in a class of masculine non-floral perfumes (Stamelman 2006: 226, 234).

The Meaning of Sensory and Olfactory Reconstructions: Producing Sense

In his critical and influential essay 'Producing, Sense, Consuming Sense, Making Sense: Perils and Prospects for Sensory History', Mark Smith states that sensory history only becomes history when a particular sense is analysed and put in the right historical context (Smith 2007: 841–58). Scents are neither universal nor trans-historical, he argues, emphasizing the role of both perceived object and perceiving subject. Smith grants language the power to overcome such subjective interpretation. Since language and olfaction are poorly connected, though, there being very few words in the Western language to describe smells, this appears somewhat problematic. Furthermore, even if there was a satisfactory lexicon, unlike visualizing, 'olfactorizing' or imagining scents by verbal cues is only possibly for 30 per cent of the Western population (Köster 2002: 33).[13] Olfactory memory – unlike our visual memory – is passive and incidental. Smell memories occur when one *re-encounters* a scent from the past, not when we try to *imagine* a scent from the past, at least for most subjects.

In a famous episode from the novel cycle *Á la recherché du temps perdu*, Proust strikingly identifies this passive aspect of the olfactorily triggered memory. The novel's protagonist, Marcel, is suddenly and involuntarily transported back in time, vividly remembering the days he spent in Combray years ago, while consuming his tea in the exact same way he did during that specific period, soaking a madeleine in lime tea. He considered it to be an aesthetic experience:

> weary after a dull day with the prospect of a depressing morrow, I raised to my lips a spoonful of the tea in which I had soaked a morsel of the cake. No sooner had the warm liquid, and the crumbs with it, touched my palate than a shudder ran through my whole body. (Proust 1913, in Van Campen 2014: 9)

The author expresses the huge emotional impact of the memory, for he had completely forgotten about the episode it revealed. He starts contemplating: neither the word 'madeleine' nor the sight of the cake was capable of granting him access to these 'things lost'. Only the unmediated experience was able to do so.

Even if we can imagine a scent we are familiar with, it will not have the effect of the actual scent. In *The Multi-sensory Museum*, neurologist Richard Stevenson explains that olfaction seems to be phenomenologically more proximinal than vision.

> That is we feel as if an odor is actually in contact with us, directly acting upon us, making us feel ill, disgusted, fearful (or perhaps happy), in a way that we do not feel with most forms of visual or auditory sensation. First, imagine just smelling an imitation fecal odor (one you know to be an imitation) versus its visual equivalent, looking at a picture of a piece of feces. Both experiences would be unpleasant, but I suspect that the visceral nature of your response to smell would more rapidly impel you to move away from it than from the picture. (Stevenson 2014: 157)

This doesn't just count for stench, but also for scents we encountered in the past in general.

What Proust researched artistically is now scientifically proven: memories evoked by the chemical senses, taste and smell, are involuntary, most vivid and emotional, and cannot be substituted by images or language (Herz 1992, 2002, 2004, 2007). In case we encounter smells we never perceived before, their physical presence can still convey knowledge. As Annick Le Guerer puts it eloquently:

> [J]ust because the sense of smell is coined as anti-intellectual, does not mean we cannot benefit from its information intellectually. Smell is revelatory not just of substances, but also of moods, climates, and even existential states. Olfaction is a subtle tool of knowledge that allows for

> an intuitive and prelinguistic understanding, It enables us to have a profound relationship with our environment. Hippocrates recommended that a doctor be 'a man with an open nose'. (Le Guerer 2014: 11)

Another argument for the unmediated use of smell as methodological tool in addition to language is expressed by sensory anthropologist David Howes:

> Rudolf Arnheim argues that 'visual perception is visual thinking'. As for smell and taste: 'one can indulge in smells and tastes but one can hardly think in them'. (Howes 2014: 67)

Howes argues that one is not aware of this huge difference in smelling and seeing related to thinking and language. A personal experience with a student can illustrate this 'problematic' approach to smell. The student was critical of the assumption that olfaction is a stronger inducer of memory than sight, because when he thought about his home country, Japan, only images and sounds came to his mind. As explained before, thinking about a smell is not the same as triggering a memory by means of smell (Howes 2002: 67).

While I have already argued that historiographer Mark Smith discusses sensory stimuli effectively in his influential article on sensory reconstructions (2007), specifically the case of olfaction and fragrant substances, he seems to leave out these particular characteristics of the *sense of smell* as a faculty.

Consuming Sense

Many of the conditions in a museum are designed to enhance our sense of sight and to preserve the visual aspect of objects for future generations. Smells, being volatile, invisible and uncontrollable, defy many museum norms. What makes them so intriguing, so unique and elusive, makes them equally 'unexhibitable'.

The exhibition *Something in the Air – Scent in Art* which took place at the German museum Villa Rot, dealt with the role of smell in both contemporary and classic modern art and featured about fifteen installations by artists from eleven different nations. It took on the challenge of staging dozens of scents across fifteen spaces. The works on view, designed to be sniffed, were selected to represent the most frequently occurring themes within olfactory art from the beginning of the twentieth century until the present day (Verbeek 2015: 10–20).[14]

The curators of the show installed an olfacto-visual room because most of the avant-garde's volatile heritage is now long gone. Photographs of Surrealist and Futurist exhibitions, catalogues, original manifestos and other texts adorned the walls and filled the showcases. Glass laboratory vials containing scents provided the onlookers and smellers with olfactory cues of fragrant events that took place almost a century ago. The use of headspace (aromatized air) instead of liquids prevented scents from blending and 'bleeding' into spaces they weren't supposed to go.[15]

One of the scents on display was Chypre. We have already learned that it was considered modern and revolutionary when it was conceived in 1917, which was exactly the reason Carrá judged it to be an equivalent to Futurist paintings. It was so popular that the accord patchouli-oakmoss-bergamot became a new category within perfumery, which means that similar perfumes are still marketed as such.[16] This emphasizes the peril Smith has pointed out: we will not understand what made it so innovative by just smelling it. Its prevalence even today might evoke memories linked to our grandmothers. Not until we realize what perfumes were like before this creation came to light can we value the impact Chypre once had. This means that in addition to reading about the aroma of contemporary and older perfumes, we should use our nose and compare perfumes *aromatically*. It does not take a trained nose to notice the difference between the less voluminous, more innocent and floral bouquets that were previously *en vogue*. Only in relation to other compositions does it become possible to judge a perfume for its inherent aromatic qualities and ascertain what made it unique. These qualities were what made perfumes so interesting for artists.

Another smellable invisible object was the previously discussed, *Tabac Blond*, the name referring to its smoky character. Although associations have changed – the sight or smell of a smoking woman won't be perceived as shocking anymore – we instantly understand how its leathery misty aroma would have blended with the smell of a burning cigarette, even though they were more woody and opiate at the time. Again, both olfactory context combined with background information can play a role in gaining deeper understanding of our olfactory past.

Making Sense

Photographs, lacking actual plasticity and conveying only one sensory dimension, are rarely questioned as a means of representation of the multisensory three-dimensional world of the past. They do not just document, but additionally *shape* collective visual memory. Perfumes could be treated the same way and fulfill that task: when we are confronted with important historical smells from our formative years, these scents will become part of a memory that is collective, beyond the idiosyncratic and individual, ideally leading to a so called *period nose*, that is capable of putting aromas in a historical context by the faculty of smell. Sounds and images are already accepted as methodological tools. Musical scores allow musicologists, historians and a wider interested audience to listen to Bach and Wagner. Centuries-old paintings and sculptures are an inexhaustible source of knowledge for which no text could ever substitute. The chiaroscuro of Rembrandt's *Nightwatch* can be described extensively, but even now it takes only a glance to fully understand and live its dramatic effects. In the same way a single inhalation of an odour, when put in the right context, can transmit knowledge. The *Nightwatch*, also known as *The Shooting Company of Frans Banning Cocq and Willem van Ruytenburchor*, once adorned one of the walls of the Kloveniersdoelen – the meeting place for this militia company, and later the Town Hall. Both are quite different environments from the artificiality of the contemporary museum. Like visual artefacts, smells too will always be perceived differently in new contexts.

If we can somehow secure these fleeting art historical objects, by documenting and replicating our volatile heritage, in the future it will be up to perceiving subjects to interpret them and put them in the right context. When technology allows us to conserve and diffuse the smells that once played essential roles in artworks, nothing will stand in our way of using our noses to create a more profound connection to our sensory past and to start developing a *period nose*, equivalent to the period eye. The pages of olfactory history of art may one day transcend their aura of electronics or ink and paper, with texts being accompanied by both visual and olfactory illustrations, for future generations to (re)contextualize and interpret, both academically and for a wider 'audience'.

Notes

1 The posthumously found manifesto 'Arte degli Odori' (Art of Scents) was written by the Italian Futurist Ennio Valentinelli around 1916. It was discovered in the drawer of fellow artist Giacomo Balla. It is unclear why it was not published.

2 This text is the first out of two on the role of smell in Futurism. Whereas this is based on written sources, the second one will focus on actual aromatic works of art. It will appear in *Designing with Smell: Practices, Techniques and Challenges*, compiled by Victoria Henshaw and published by Routledge in 2016.

3 Synaesthesia is a neurological condition in which a stimulus usually perceived by one sense is simultaneously experienced by another.

4 The symbolist poet René Ghil coined the term in his *Traité du Verbe*. See Piet Devos (2013).

5 Runciman treats Scriabin as a member of the Futurists, although in a strict sense, he is not.

6 The idea of subjectivity/objectivity of perception was subject to heated debate during modernism (1880–1950). The insight into the role of culture in perception and intersubjective differences made some artists even more eager to visualize (and in this case make perceivable through other senses) the (invisible) universal and the objective. The famous contemporary perfumer Jean-Claude Ellena, like many of his colleagues, states that his appreciation of scents has nothing to do with their hedonic qualities, but with absolute (or abstract)

qualities, confirming the ideas of Carlo Carrá: 'Whether odors are good or bad doesn't matter. My nose is nothing more than a measuring instrument. I use it to test, to compare, and to evaluate in order to mark, correct, repeat the work in progress.'

7 This process can be facilitated by comparing two different odours: one is always relatively fresher, sweeter, sharper, warmer, colder, smoother, more powdery in relation to the other.

8 This idea of the dynamism of odours is expressed in some texts. In Marinetti's poem *Ritratto olfattivo di una donna* (1932), for example, there are numerous descriptions of movements and shapes of odours, such as '*tre spiragli di odore di sigaretta*' (three spirals of cigarette smoke) and '*archi mobili di odore*' (mobile arches of smell).

9 Avery Gilbert et al. (1996) conducted research among non-synaesthetes that indicates that there are common abstract correlations between colours and smells, such as between red and cinnamon, green and galbanum.

10 Perfumes are composed according to the principle of variation in volatility. We first smell the most volatile molecules in the so-called top notes. Heart notes and base notes consist of heavier molecules and are perceived later, sometimes after a couple of hours. Together these three layers form a *fragrant accord*.

11 Headspace is the gas emitted by solid objects. Gas chromatography enables researchers to determine the molecular structure of volatile substances. Since only a few molecules suffice, perfumes that cannot be perceived any more by human noses are still detectable by these machines.

12 Originally in Italian: "*Ti raccomando vivamente di portarmi: un flacone di profumo "dans la nuit" da Worth (piatto e non sferico, alto circa 12 cent. e costa circa 100 fr.) e uno di: tabac blond da Caron (profumo, non acqua di toilette). Non ti dimenticare!!*" Letter by Fedele Azari to Fortunato Depero.

13 Köster uses the word 'olfactorise' as meaning 'the capacity to imagine smells'.

14 *Something in the Air – Scent in Art* was curated by Stefanie Dathe and Caro Verbeek. The themes were listed in the accompanying catalogue as follows: synaesthesia, olfactory mapping, bodily or non-intellectual knowledge, the taboo on body odours and olfactory identity, olfactory storytelling, mood setting and memory evocation.

15 This didn't always work out. Job Koelewijn's baby-powder room was sometimes overtaken by the scent of synthetic sperm by Clara Ursitti's installation 'Bill'. Ironically, sperm cells can detect the womb because it emits a smell similar to lily-of-the valley, the main ingredient of the baby powder in question.

16 The terms used in perfumery, such as notes and scales, are mostly borrowed from music. An intentional blend with different notes is called an 'accord'. An accord is part of a larger composition, which would be the perfume.

References

Azari, F. (1924), *La flora futurista ed equivalent plastici di odori artificiali.* Presented during the annual Futurist Congress in November 1924.

Baudelaire, C. (1954), *Les Fleurs du Mal.* Translated by William Aggeler. Freso, CA: Academy Library Guild.

Carrá, C. (1913a), 'La pittura dei suoni, rumori, odori'. Available at http://www.futurismo.altervista.org/manifesti/pitturaSuoni.htm (accessed on 17 November 2015).
Carrá, C. (1913b), 'Da Cèzanne a noi futuristi'. In *Lacerba*, 15 May (nr. 10), p. 99.
Carrá, C. (1945), *La mia vita*. New York: Rizzoli.
Devos, Piet (2013), *Talend Lichaam*. Groningen: University of Groningen.
Gilbert, Avery N., Robyn Martin and Sarah E. Kemp (1996), 'Cross-Modal Correspondence between Vision and Olfaction: The Color of Smells'. *The American Journal of Psychology* 109(3): 335–351.
Guerer, A. Le (2002), 'Olfaction and Cognition, A Philosophical and Psychoanalytic View'. In C. Rouby, B. Schaal, D. Dubois, R. Gervais and A. Holly (eds), *Olfaction, Taste, and Cognition*. Cambridge: Cambridge University Press.
Herz, R. S. (2007), *The Scent of Desire: Discovering our Enigmatic Sense of Smell*. New York: HarperCollins.
Herz, R. S. and G. C. Cupchik (1992), 'An Experimental Characterization of Odor-evoked Memories in Humans'. *Chemical Senses* 17: 519–28.
Herz, R. S. and J. W. Schooler (2002), 'A Naturalistic Study of Autobiographical Memories Evoked by Olfactory and Visual Cues: Testing the Proustian Hypothesis'. *American Journal of Psychology* 115(1): 21–32.
Herz, R. S., J. Eliassen, S. Beland and T. Souza (2004), 'Neuroimaging Evidence for the Emotional Potency of Odor-evoked Memory'. *Neuropsychologia* 42: 371–378.
Howes, D. (2002), 'Nose-wise: Olfactory Metaphors in Mind'. In C. Rouby, B. Schaal, D. Dubois, R. Gervais and A. Holly (eds), *Olfaction, Taste, and Cognition*. Cambridge: Cambridge University Press.
Jay, M. (1994), *Downcast Eyes – The Denigration of Vision in Twentieth-Century French Thought*. Berkeley: University of California Press.
Kandinsky, W. (1912), *Über das Geistige in der Kunst* (On the Spiritual in Art). Munich: R. Piper & Co. Verlag.
Köster, E. P. (2002), 'The Specific Characteristics of the Sense of Smell'. In C. Rouby, B. Schaal, D. Dubois, R. Gervais and A. Holly (eds), *Olfaction, Taste, and Cognition*. Cambridge: Cambridge University Press.
Marinetti, F. T. (1921), *Il Tattilismo*. Futurismo Italiano. Available at http://www.futurismo.altervista.org/manifesti/tattilismo.htm (accessed 1 June, 2009).
Marinetti, F. T. (1930), *The Futurist Cookbook*. Edited by L. Chamberlain. (1989). San Francisco, CA: Bedford Arts Publishers.
Runciman, J. F. (1915), 'Noises, Smells and Colours'. *The Musical Quarterly* 1(2): 157.
Smith, M. (2007), 'Producing, Sense, Consuming Sense, Making Sense: Perils and Prospects for Sensory History'. *Journal of Social History* 40(4): 841–858.
Stamelman, R. (2006), *Perfume: Joy, Scandal, Sin: A Cultural History of Fragrance from 1750 to the Present*. New York: Rizzoli.
Stevenson, R. J. (2014), 'The Forgotten Sense'. In N. Levent and A. Pascual-Leone (eds), *The Multi-Sensory Museum*, Plymouth: Rowman & Littlefield.
van Campen, C. (2014), *The Proust Effect*. Oxford: Oxford University Press.
Verbeek, C. (2015), *Something in the Air – Scent in Art*. Exhibition catalogue. Villa Rot: Burgrieden.

6

Museums of Good Taste, Artworks of Good Taste: Gastronomic Contemporary Art

Mark Clintberg

Introduction: Good Taste

The sense of taste has long been used as a convenient metaphor for aesthetic acuity in the fields of art history, connoisseurship, philosophy and other cultural practices. However, in the twentieth century, museum visitors have generally been required to appreciate exhibitions primarily through the sense of sight, with emphasis on the *aesthetic* sense of taste, leaving the literal, *gustatory* sense of taste at the museum entrance.[1] Judgements about both art and food are often summarized with the Latin phrase *de gustibus non disputandum est*: there is no disputing about taste. At the core of this aphorism are links between what it means to eat, to perceive and to judge. The core similarity between these two varieties of taste – gustatory taste and aesthetic taste – seems to be that they both involve internal and subjective judgements that are shaped by and influential upon basic notions of 'good' and 'bad'. This commonality may have engendered the homograph of 'taste' itself, as well as a profusion of analogies and similes between these two types of taste in philosophy, art history and popular culture. However, in many art exhibitions taste has taken on much more than metaphoric significance. Many of today's art museums are going through a radical sensory shift, whereby the non-visual senses and taste in particular are increasingly stimulated in the gallery.

A growing number of museum exhibitions and programs in North America and Europe are designed to profile and stimulate the non-visual senses, including the sense of taste. Although this tendency to invite audiences to have a range of sensory contact with artworks – by allowing visitors to touch museum collections, for instance, as is the case with many tours for blind and partially sighted visitors – might seem new to Western museum practices, the trend marks a return to European attitudes and practices from the pre-Victorian era. Prior to the nineteenth century, members of upper social classes were admitted to and toured museums freely; during their visits, these guests were given the opportunity to encounter objects from collections through several sensory modes (Classen 2007: 897; Candlin 2010). Englishman John Evelyn's diaries from the seventeenth century reveal that he was given license to handle, to smell and even to shake artifacts in European collections (Evelyn, cited in Howes and Classen 2014: 18). Constance Classen notes the account of a German tourist, Sophie de la Roche, who visited the British Museum in the eighteenth century. De la Roche handled various Greek and Roman artifacts – and was particularly captivated by an urn filled with cremated remains of a woman. In rapt phrases this tourist describes that she touched the object and the dust that covered it 'tenderly, just as her best friend might once have grasped her hand' (2005: 278). In this case a proximal sense provides the visitor with an opportunity to imagine a physical and emotional proximity to a woman from antiquity. This account reveals the potentially intimate and socially evocative nature of non-visual contact with collections. If in the seventeenth and eighteenth centuries to invite visitors to touch was a mark of good hospitality to elite visitors, in the twentieth- and twenty-first-century Canadian museum it would appear that the same invitation is offered to include ostensibly marginalized visitors but also to heighten a sense of social connection between museum-goers and the cultures represented in collections.

There are several registers at which these recent changes in attitude and policy have occurred. Contributing to this shift, many contemporary artists create pieces that are designed to stimulate multisensorial experiences involving edible materials. This chapter responds to the increasing number of gastronomic art practices making their way into museum galleries, and explores the changing philosophical terrain first used to block such gastronomic experiences from the museum, and the reasons why taste is being increasingly celebrated as a mode for experiencing artwork. For instance, Rirkrit Tiravanija's ongoing food service artworks, such as *Untitled (Free)* (1992), offer free food to gallery visitors, including Thai 'national dishes', such as curry and pad thai. In many cases, the dirty dishes and cooking equipment used during the service of these meals are left on display as a record of the event. This practice will be used as an example to animate a larger discussion of the dynamic between aesthetic taste and gustatory taste with a focus on the broader implications for museum collections and exhibitions.

Taste and Multisensory Experience in the Gallery

It can be argued that entry into any museum collection or exhibition automatically involves the non-visual senses, since visitors will smell the building's air quality, for example, regardless of whether the chosen theme of the exhibition is 'scent'. Indeed, as Tony Bennett points out, a museum visit can be equally considered a kinetic action, not simply a visual one (1995: 36–45), and Classen reminds us that 'the first galleries in private houses were employed precisely for walking. Paintings were added to these galleries in order to give people something at which to look as they walked' (2007: 897). The museum is a decidedly multisensorial environment regardless of its curatorial program. However, in the past decade there have been museum exhibitions that accent particular senses, including the exhibition *Odor Limits* at the Esther M. Klein Art Gallery (2008, Philadelphia) curated by DisplayCult (Jim Drobnick and Jennifer Fisher), which featured four artists whose work was scent-based. *The Art of Scent* at the Museum of Arts and Design (2012, New York) was a detailed study of olfactory design surveying twelve perfumes. *Sound Art: Sound as a Media of Art* opened at the Zentrum für Kunst und Medientechnologie in Karlsruhe, Germany in 2012. The Museum of Modern Art's *Soundings: A Contemporary Score* (2013) was the institution's first major survey of sound-based artworks. Other, earlier group exhibitions dedicated to audio-based artworks include Rene Block's *Für Augen und Ohren* (1980), and Robert Smith and Bob Wilhite's *Sound* (1979) at the Los Angeles Institute of Contemporary Art (Cluett 2014).[2] What these exhibitions have in common is that they implicitly legitimate the value of sound and smell *specifically* as artistic forms, or they address the apparent neglect of these senses in daily life.

Certain exhibitions have been designed to give sensory access to specific demographics. In these cases, the perceived or actual needs of a particular public determine the content delivered. Some museums have gradually broadened the spectrum of the sensory modes permitted in their spaces, as with the Royal Ontario Museum's and the National Gallery of Canada's (NGC) multisensory exhibition components (Clintberg 2014a, 2014b) and the British Museum's touch tour program (Hetherington 2003). The NGC, for instance, offers tactile tours featuring selected objects from collections, which registered visitors are allowed to touch while wearing protective gloves. Other exhibitions have focused on particular senses in order to bring attention to avant-garde and contemporary art practices. In these cases, artistic practices themselves may determine the starting point for the exhibition, and the positive outcomes for the public (accessibility for many learning styles and types of sensory engagement) are a welcome byproduct. For example, in her text 'Walking with Janet Cardiff, Sitting with Massimo Guerrera, and Eating Apples with R. Murray Schafer', Elizabeth Sweeney draws from the public programs at the National Gallery of Canada to describe examples of artworks that have distinct aesthetic meaning and provide sensory access for both blind and partially sighted visitors, and visitors who are not visually impaired. Although a Cardiff audio walk artwork may not be designed specifically for visitors who are vision impaired, such a practice offers public program departments the opportunity to develop unique sensorial programs centred on her artwork (2009).

The programming of multisensory museum experiences has been influenced by many factors, but noteworthy force has been exerted by official legislation requiring cultural institutions to be accessible to a wide variety of citizens. In Canada, key legislation that has had an impact on sensorial components of museum programming is related to prohibition of discrimination including the Canadian Charter of Rights and Freedoms (1982), the Canadian Human Rights Act (1985) and the Ontarians with Disabilities Act (2005). Similar legislation and policies have shaped museum design and collections programming internationally, including the Americans with Disabilities Act (1990). Accompanying these regulations are attitudes suggesting that when more sensory registers are highlighted through programs at museums, more audiences will be included in and attracted to programs, further expanding attendance and anchoring public institutions into their surrounding communities. In brief, such thinking holds that sensory engagement can be alluring and satisfying for visitors, but these attitudes frequently involve a connection between multisensory engagement and democracy, especially in cases where the non-visual senses are activated by artworks. In their co-authored writing, Nina Levent and D. Lynn McRainey present examples of exhibitions and artworks that have claimed to use touch because it is a 'democratic medium' (2014: 65). Offering one example, artist Felix Gonzalez-Torres's beaded curtains, which are installed in an orientation that invites visitors to touch their strands of beads and walk through them in order to progress through the gallery space, have been praised for their democratic nature because they allow tactile engagement. The contemporary art curator Jen Mergel refers to one of these beaded curtains as a 'living piece, an experience as opposed to the object' (see Levent and McRainey: 65–66). Touch not only enlivens Gonzalez-Torres's inanimate object, but in this case also encourages an experience that is assumed to be more approachable, genuine and democratic than it would be if the audience were not allowed to touch the artwork. Such ideas about the broad appeal of his artworks, in part sparked by the fact that some of them can be touched by the public, have likely been further encouraged by the artist's remarks linking his own practice to the functions of democracy.[3] Yet, if something has broad sensory appeal and offers multisensory access, is the object itself democratic in quality? This is a question I will return to momentarily in light of Tiravanija's practice.

Fiona Candlin, focusing on the role of touch in museums, points out that there has been a change in the perceived uses and roles of museums, whereby 'museums are now being characterized as resources for informal learning and social inclusion . . . so they simply cannot *afford* to alienate their visitors. On the contrary, museum staff need to make sure that the displays are appealing to a wide range of age and class groups, including non-traditional museum goers' (2007: 90). The non-visual senses are important sensory factors in such inclusive programming. This sensory turn represents a cultural shift towards proximal sensory contact because these seem to be inclusive, non-alienating senses by which visitors can engage with collections and exhibitions in a democratic fashion.

Philosophies of Taste

These discussions of sensorial access operate within a larger, Western philosophical debate about the nature of the human senses. Although the volume of literature dealing with such questions is far too extensive to grapple with here, I will introduce selected episodes in this ongoing debate. Martin Jay's *Downcast Eyes* (1993) presents evidence that the ancient Greeks had a higher estimation of sight than the non-visual senses: the use of visual verbs in the Homeric period, the appearance of the Greek gods in physical form, the advanced use of theatre in Greece and, especially, discussions of vision in Greek philosophy (1993: 22, 23). But Jay points out that the Greeks also expressed a 'a certain anxiety about vision's malevolent power' in several of their myths (1993: 28), which warn that looking can be a dangerous act. Complicating any claims that ancient Greek culture was scopophilic, the German philosopher Friedrich Nietzsche's *The Birth of Tragedy* (1872) presents a different view of the Apollonian (or visual) and the Dionysian (or bodily and sensual) aspects of Greek theatre. In Nietzsche's view, sight and mind, and the non-visual senses and the body, continually do battle for supremacy in the theatre of ancient Greece. While philosophies of the senses in classical Greek thought are certainly more complex, these two authors present narratives of vision as a potentially ordering and rational principle for knowledge of the world.

Taste, by contrast, has often been described as an inherently disordered sense. The philosopher Kevin W. Sweeney points out that some aesthetic philosophers have claimed that gustatory taste is incapable of delivering 'ordered aesthetic structures' (1999: 21) meaning that food and drink resist description and reflection because our experience of them takes place in a disordered fashion and internally, unlike vision, which experiences its object at a distance and organizes it in spatial, temporal terms. Perhaps more gravely, comestibles are said to have the potential to disorder thought itself. A significant source guiding my research in this matter is philosopher Carolyn Korsmeyer's book *Making Sense of Taste: Food and Philosophy*, which grapples in detail with the philosophical, scientific, symbolic and artistic potential of gustatory taste. Author of *A History of Cooks and Cooking* Michael Symons presents that for Plato, food and its pleasures figure as clear examples of the 'transient, inadequate, inferior, material world of the senses, bodily pleasures, and humdrum, non-philosophical activities' (2007: 24). The sense of taste is not the only problem when it comes to food, in Plato's view. Plato also critiques cooking itself with even more vitriol, describing it as a 'kind of knack gained by experience . . . a knack of . . . producing gratification and pleasure', that is at its core 'pandering' (24). Cooking is an ignoble art for Plato. Aristotle has a similar bias against taste, and considers sight to be the most valuable and noble sense of them all. He writes,

> All men by nature desire to know. An indication of this is the delight we take in our senses; for even apart from their usefulness they are loved for themselves; and above all others the sense of sight . . . The reason is that this, most of all the senses, makes us know and brings to light many differences between things. (Quoted in Korsmeyer 1999: 18–19)

This passage describes the human sensorium as a system that delivers knowledge to us, with vision being the strongest signal received by the sensorial system because its transmission allows us to differentiate between things. Aristotle has other reasons for praising sight as superior and for diminishing taste and touch: he believes that the proximal senses, which involve being in physical contact with the thing sensed (touch, smell and taste), are inferior to the distal senses, which hold their sensed objects at a distance (sight and hearing) (Korsmeyer 1999: 21). The risk of the proximal senses, for both Plato and Aristotle, is that they can be easily indulged to excess and cause an immoral life. Korsmeyer notes that according to these two philosophers, the distal senses of 'vision and hearing actually appear to be senses that cannot be overindulged' (Korsmeyer 1999: 22). These philosophies suggest that vision's ability to keep its subject at a physical distance allows for stronger objective judgements than could ever be possible with the senses of taste and touch. As Korsmeyer has effectively demonstrated,

> in virtually all analyses of the senses in Western philosophy the distance between object and perceiver has been seen as a cognitive, moral and aesthetic advantage. The bodily senses are 'lower' in part because of the necessary closeness of the object of perception to the physical body of the percipient. (1999: 12)

According to philosophies put forward in the eighteenth century by figures such as Immanuel Kant, the so-called lower senses cannot succeed in critical judgements because they too easily yield to sensory pleasure. Kant's requirement for 'disinterestedness' in critical judgements of beauty will not allow for senses such as taste and touch. In short, when food is 'beautiful' we want more of it, meaning that it can never be truly beautiful in the sense that Kant means. As he puts it,

> everyone must allow that a judgment on the beautiful which is tinged with the slightest interest, is very partial and not a pure judgment of taste. One must not be in the least prepossessed in favour of the existence of the thing, but must preserve complete indifference in this respect, in order to play the part of judge in matters of taste. (Kant 2007 [1790]: 38)

Appetite and gustatory taste are obstacles for pure judgements of aesthetic taste by Kant's evaluation, and the other proximal senses similarly cloud judgement. Nonetheless, in everyday speech it is common to discuss the quality and even aesthetics of foodstuffs. To this extent, gustatory taste is for Kant merely a 'vehicle of conversation', and Kant holds such conversations around food in very low esteem. Kant proposes that true beauty has to be unclouded by personal interest. He argues that true critical judgements of taste cannot involve any personal interest, a difficult criterion to realize when it comes to edible goods because a diner has an inherent stake in the nutritional content and flavour of the food. Based on this idea, Kant is quick to disqualify the rites of the table and food itself as possible sources of beauty worthy of aesthetic contemplation. Appetite can only attain limited registers of affect and these are instinctual rather than rational in Kant's view, since 'the senses of taste and smell are both more subjective than objective' (2005 [1798]: 210). Smell and taste provide 'enjoyment, rather than the cognition of the external object' (210). Enjoyment stands in the way of cognitive reflection on objects that are tasted and smelled.

Some philosophers in the Western tradition have examined the philosophical potential of gustatory taste and have even valorized the sense of taste. Taking a position distinct from that of Aristotle and Plato, Epicurus (308–270 BCE) enjoys simultaneous and contradictory reputations as a hedonistic thinker and an ascetic cult leader of antiquity. Being the namesake for the term epicurean, Epicurus is sometimes misunderstood as a philosopher who argues for the blind pursuit of sensual pleasures through food and alcohol.[4] His ideas are much more complex, however. A core aphorism of Epicurus is: 'The beginning and root of all good is the pleasure of the stomach; even wisdom and culture must be referred to this' (Symons 2007: 19). Perhaps in keeping with this quote, Symons somewhat erroneously describes Epicurus's reputation in antiquity as 'the belly-centered philosopher' (2007: 17). As discussed by David Sedley, the belly is just one organ of interest to Epicurus, who in truth was interested in bodily pleasure as well as what people's predispositions are with respect to belief, desire and so on (2011: 38). Elizabeth Asmis investigates how Epicurus argues that pleasure should be pursued and pain avoided, but he makes allowances for tolerating periods of pain that lead to eventual pleasure, meaning that he encourages a rational rather than hedonistic approach to pleasure (2011: 164). His philosophy involves much more than blind abandon to hedonism, but rather presents a moral view of the pleasures that the body does allow. He writes, 'For I at least cannot conceive the good if I take away the pleasures due to tastes, the pleasures due to sex, the pleasures due to sounds, and the pleasant visual motions due to shape' (quoted in Purinton 1993: 281). Epicurus calls these varieties of pleasure 'kinetic', or pleasures of motion, distinguished from 'static' pleasures. Kinetic sensory pleasures, including gustatory taste, are intrinsically part of the good in Epicurus's view.

Another advocate of gustatory taste is philosopher David Hume. His essay 'Of the Standard of Taste' predates Kant's text, and raises some of the same paradoxes of taste: taste is entirely subjective, yet people frequently hold that their taste is superior to that of others and that there is such a thing as 'bad taste'. Hume writes,

> To seek the real beauty, or real deformity, is as fruitless an enquiry, as to pretend to ascertain the real sweet or real bitter. According to the disposition of the organs, the same object may be both sweet and bitter; and the proverb has justly determined it to be fruitless to dispute concerning tastes. It is very natural, and even quite necessary, to extend this axiom to mental, as well as bodily taste. (Hume 1898 [1757]: 1:269)

Hume believes that the subtle differences of taste can be overlooked in favour of a general human proclivity towards pleasure when encountering certain tastes. Hume also identifies a special class of individuals – those of 'delicate taste' – who have cultivated a sensitivity enabling them to identify things of fine taste, including works of art. To illustrate this delicate taste, Hume refers to the well-known oenological episode of Spanish novelist Miguel de Cervantes's *Don Quixote* (1605). During a wine-tasting contest, two characters remark that a certain vintage is quite good but each of them senses a mild undertone discoloring the bouquet of the wine. The first character senses a whiff of metal, the second the aroma of leather. Their audience laughs in disbelief, considering their oral reports on gustatory taste as the products of affectation; these naysayers are silenced when a metal key on a leather strap is discovered at the bottom of the wine vat. Hume's account of this story is meant to suggest that even those sources of sensation that are out of view – much like the hidden key and leather strap – can be apperceived *through taste* by those who are sensitive enough, and those who cannot detect these subtleties should listen to those of delicate taste, who are authorities on a world that is out of view for most people (Hume 1898: 202). Hume does believe that a rule of beauty can be developed – something Kant denies – and also holds that exposure to 'a particular art, and the frequent survey or contemplation of a particular species of beauty' can increase one's acuity and 'delicacy' of taste (203). In other words, to desire more of a thing or increased exposure to it does not necessarily prevent the possibility of experiencing aesthetic feeling. According to Hume, gustatory taste and aesthetic taste are both highly discerning senses.

Adding further detail to this discussion, a final advocate of gustatory taste is philosopher Anthony Savile, who adds to the discussion of food's ability to affect both mind and body by further expanding on Kant's view of gustatory taste and beauty. Kant meant to frame beauty, Savile argues, as the philosophical analogue of food because of its capacity to 'feed' and 'nourish' the human faculties (Savile 2003: 91). Savile's argument hints that foodstuffs can lead to aesthetic experience, and thus become an art form. He writes, 'Just as it is of the essence of food to strengthen the body and promote its growth, so too with beauty; with the difference that what it strengthens and promotes the growth of is the mind or the spirit, not the body' (91). The crucial difference, as Savile is aware, is that Kant's so-called true judgements of beauty should not involve personal interests, and food's stimulation of appetites automatically negates the possibility of disinterestedness.

Rirkrit Tiravanija

As part of his art practice Thai artist Rirkrit Tiravanija has cooked and served food in teahouses, supermarkets, street stalls, gallery offices, museum galleries and at the side of roads. A pivotal piece for the artist in this body of work was *Untitled (Free)* (1992), for which he moved the entire contents of the offices of commercial dealer Gallery 303 into its exhibitions area, and converted the offices into a food service site. Vessels, cooking equipment and utensils used during *Untitled (Free)* were left on display in the space as a record of the dining experiences that took place there. Visitors were invited to relax, to converse, and to share in the meal made by the artist. In such exhibitions the intersection of gustatory taste and aesthetic taste is promoted as a democratic means by which to generate social cohesion and amicability – but, as I will explain, such allegedly democratic outcomes should not be taken for granted.

To a certain extent, Tiravanija repurposed the commercial setting of Gallery 303 as a free food service site that in some ways seemed to be entirely de-commoditized, serving to highlight the specially commoditized environment of galleries. Because he often presents Thai cuisine to visitors, Tiravanija's work can be understood in relationship to questions of identity and judgements of taste. Since the food served at *Untitled (Free)* was traditional Thai curry, a dish that serves as a strong marker of Thai food culture, this piece could also be considered as an artist's self-portrait,[5] which serves forth his ethnic identity.[6] During *Untitled (Free)*, Tiravanija served two kinds of green curry in the space: one was cooked by the method used by New York-based Thai restaurants, the other 'was an authentically made Thai curry', as the artist describes it. Tiravanija continues, 'I was working on the idea of food, but in a kind of anthropological and archeological way. It was a lot about, the layers of taste and otherness.'[7] Since Tiravanija is of Thai descent, if this work follows an anthropological method, it appears to be one of auto-anthropology or auto-ethnography. Clearly gustatory sensitivity and connoisseurship are at play in this case study, since it tests the visitor's ability to recognize allegedly authentic Thai cuisine.

Some authors praise Tiravanija's food service sites as being social equalizers that invite people of all backgrounds, incomes and persuasions to dine on free food. Curator Alexandre Melo claims that,

> Tiravanija's work is one of the rare examples of an intervention that effectively breaks down the barriers isolating the small audience in the

> art circuit. Tiravanija's food is available to anyone who turns up. In this way, he also dismantles the elitist model of the meal of the initiates as a form that reproduces the special social position of artists as a group. (Melo 1995: 105)

Melo's certainty that Tiravanija's work rejects elitism and is boundlessly generous to any person 'who turns up' should be interrogated according to the special relationship that museums and galleries have with the 'anyone' – 'the public' – Melo refers to. Tiravanija's practice stages an illusion of democratization, by allowing 'all people' to enjoy his free food gift. It could be said that Tiravanija's installations have been used to attempt a kind of social inoculation that will bring divergent demographics of museum visitors into harmony. Yet Gallery 303, like museums and other commercial galleries (and restaurants), is a private space where some people could be refused entry, and not a democratic abstraction. Clearly, there are filters that determine who is made aware of Tiravanija's practice (through education, media and so on) and thus determine who experiences his generous gift of food. Also, institutions that host his projects frequently charge admission; those who cannot pay admission cannot receive the 'free' meal of the artist. According to Claire Bishop's contentious analysis of this practice, it is advantageous to the artist's practice that his work appears accessible to the public in order to rationalize connections between his food service sites and the goals of the democratic project (2004: 67–68). Bishop is sceptical of just how widely accessible Tiravanija's events are and how 'fundamentally harmonious' in quality because they support benign social encounters between people of a particular demographic. However, Bishop does not address the importance of *sensorial* access in this case study. The allure of sensorial proximity described by Korsmeyer – which has been used to position taste as a morally culpable sense – seems to be the very quality of Tiravanija's piece that intrigues visitors and curators. And yet, building on Candlin's discussion, it can be said that because it *profiles* gustatory sensation, it would seem that Tiravanija's piece is inclusive with wide appeal to diverse visitors. Mary Jane Jacob introduces Tiravanija's work as 'generous art as a free commodity' (2005: 3). Her emphasis on the gift economy inherent in this art practice suggests that foodstuffs are ushered into the museum context with the rationale that these are free, nutritional, socially ameliorative gifts available to all.

Tiravanija's latest version of his piece, now titled *Untitled (Free/Still)* (2011–2012), was acquired and exhibited at the Museum of Modern Art, New York, in 2012, revealing that the artist's act of food generosity is certainly one that can be commoditized and purchased.[8] Its new title alludes both to the connection this piece has to the genre of still life and to the perennial promise of free food. Nonetheless, for most audience members there are costs involved in experiencing the piece: as of 2015 admission fees for entry into the museum are $25 USD for adults, $18 USD for seniors, and $14 USD for students. With the exception of Friday evenings between

4:00 and 8:00 p.m., when the MoMA grants free admission to visitors, Tiravanija's *Untitled (Free/Still)* will in fact *not* be free at all whenever it is exhibited there. No free gift, *Untitled (Free/Still)* is in fact an edible commodity with a price tag that admits only individuals with the ready money to pay admission.

Emma Allen describes the clientele for the piece at the MoMA when she attended in 2012:

> [I]t was a room filled with European tourists and other museum-going types, who spoke in hushed tones and photographed one another with smartphones as they downed their curry . . . All in all, it was like a sacred soup kitchen for the middle-to-upper classes. (Allen 2012: 97)

Allen's report of the demographics that attended the MoMA installation quite complicates Melo's hopeful observation that 'Tiravanija's food is available to anyone who turns up', and by extension any claim that his work is automatically democratic simply because it involves the non-visual senses. Obviously there are systemic reasons that keep many people from visiting the MoMA and therefore prevent the blend of demographics that Melo has in mind, and the democratic outcomes that such a situation implies.

Tiravanija's projects also seem to be broadly appealing because they involve multiple sensory registers, echoing some of the allegedly democratic qualities introduced in Gonzalez-Torres's work. Through Tiravanija's practice, negative critiques of the gustatory senses (all the human senses stimulated during the ingestion of food) are inverted, and the very properties of taste that have been pejoratively framed are celebrated: the disputed qualities of taste, a sense upon which no two people can entirely agree, are in parallel to the unsettled, contested qualities inherent to democracy. Yet the democratizing framework assembled around Tiravanija's practice should not be taken for granted as benevolent and limitlessly inclusive. Similarly, while the sensory turn in museum studies and exhibition design certainly can allow broader access to many demographics, such developments are only democratic to the extent that they engender and support dissent, dispute and discussion about the nature of sensorially and socially inclusive programming, as well as the public nature of institutions such as museums.

Conclusion: Sensorial Democracies

The socially ameliorative aspirations institutionally associated with Tiravanija's work suggest that taste is a socially ordering (rather than disordering) sense, a sense that coheres communities. Also, this work combines the 'delicate taste' of the connoisseur discussed by Hume with sensory, gustatory taste. Although MoMA seems to take on a positive attitude towards the sense of taste because it is considered to be a democratizing sense, it is clear that in reality Tiravanija's practice nonetheless exists in a pre-existing system of social stratification; in this case it is questionable if taste has indeed democratized the museum.

The nature of democracy – what is meant by the term in any particular historical or contemporary context – is too complex to conclusively explore here, but it is important to note that the term comes from Greek, referring to the power (*kratia*) of the people (*dēmos*). Democracy is more than a matter of access or appeal, but also a matter of power and control. To touch, to taste, to smell, to hear or to see an artwork does not necessarily guarantee control or power of that object, its presented meaning or the ideologies of the institution that exhibits it. Theories connected to interactive artworks that involve social outreach are useful in further illuminating how sensory stimulation can reveal political and ideological qualities of museum settings. In her recent critiques of theories relating to socially intervening art practices, Bishop challenges the precise nature of rhetorical evocations of the term 'democracy'. Specifically, she has questioned the value of artworks that attempt to formulate democratic scenarios through dialogue and the creation of new social relations, a way of working encapsulated by the curator Nicolas Bourriaud's term 'relational aesthetics' (Bourriaud, 1998). Tiravanija's work is an important (although briefly discussed) case study in Bourriaud's typology of relational art, and according to Bishop, '*what* Tiravanija cooks, *how* and *for whom*, are less important to Bourriaud than the fact that he gives away the results of his cooking for free' (2004: 64). This attitude coincides with Jacobs' analysis introduced earlier, which stresses the generous capacity of Tiravanija's practice and its accessibility. She writes that by virtue of such relational practices,

> all relations that permit 'dialogue' are automatically assumed to be democratic and therefore good. But what does 'democracy' really mean in this context? If relational art produces human relations, then the next logical question to ask is what *types* of relations are being produced, for whom, and why? (Bishop 2004: 37)

Similarly, practices that permit enlarged sensory access should not be taken for granted as democratic and therefore as 'good'. Bishop's observations are equally useful in critiquing other forms of artwork and museum programming that attempt to incite democracy, including multisensory programming in museums. Seeking the nature of relations produced through sensorial, allegedly democratic museum programs is a revealing undertaking. The right to touch and engage the senses through gustation in museum contexts is certainly a matter of power, as Levent and McRainey's remarks reveal. But if the public is permitted only to touch or taste certain artworks in a given collection, the institution is still clearly in control of the nature of relations that will occur between visitors, objects and one another relative to sensory engagement. Beyond this, there are endemic barriers that keep certain populations out of museums. The systems of inclusion or exclusion at play in museums will reveal just as much about the 'good taste' or 'bad taste' of the institution. The possible democratic power of the human sensorium as it is instrumentalized or activated in museums through practices like Tiravanija's should not be underestimated. The social conversations that take place during *Untitled (Free/Still)* may be utterly banal or determinedly sophisticated, but it is not the *subject* of these conversations that should serve to demonstrate whether such a practice gives evidence of any democratic quality. Rather, as Bishop's observations imply, it is the conditions under which such gustatory practices are exhibited that serves to reveal more about the 'types of relations' that are happening between either broad or narrow swaths of that amorphous body called 'the public'. What is more, when sense-specific and multisensory exhibitions are mounted, it can be said that institutions are both focused on extending but also defining and demarcating the powers of those senses and how they will be understood by publics who are in relation with one another.

Since there can be no disputing about taste, at first blush the ingestion of an edible artwork would seem to function as a social astringent, able to settle any democratic argument through 'agreement to disagree', thus uniting the gustatory and aesthetic terms of taste. If a group of diners can agree to disagree on the gustatory value of pad thai, while still permitting the pleasure or displeasure of other diners, then perhaps it is also possible to similarly defer any conflict surrounding other even more contentious religious, political or social disputes. In this way, 'good taste' is an analogue for the tremendously complex subject of what is 'good' in the world. Gustatory taste and aesthetic taste are, as Hume argues and as Tiravanija's practice implies, both discerning senses that deserve our attention because they uncover the deeply chaotic and productive qualities of dispute that are inherent to democratic pursuits: continual discussion about the relative value of what is good.

Notes

1 The Victoria & Albert Museum (London) was the first public museum to include a restaurant. Its Refreshment Rooms opened in 1856. Since then, museum cafés and restaurants are an important exception to this proscription of taste in the museum.

2 Seth Cluett gives a compelling discussion of curating sound in 'Ephemeral, Immersive, Invasive: Sound as Curatorial Theme, 1966–2013', in Nina Levent and Alvaro Pascual-Leone, eds, *The Multisensory Museum: Cross-Disciplinary Perspectives on Touch, Sound, Smell, Memory, and Space*, 109–118 (Lanham: Rowman & Littlefield, 2014).

3 His interview with Tim Rollins provides a notable example. See, in particular, page 25.

4 The popular recipe website www.epicurious.com and the American food retailer Epicure have further confused Epicurus's legacy in popular culture.

5 Another artist who has used curry as a marker of ethnic identity in her art practice is Elaine Tin Nyo. Her *Egg Curry* (1997) is a cooking and food service performance where the artist fashions a curry in the style her mother taught her while narrating events from her upbringing. See Barbara Fischer, ed. *Foodculture: Tasting Identities and Geographies in Art* (Toronto: YYZ Books, 1999).

6 For one example of this apparent connection between the cultures of South East Asia, identity and the artist's practice, see Yvane Chapuis, 'Rirkrit Tiravanija: The Space of Unconditional Action', *Parachute*, no. 101 (January–March 2001): 14–25. Weil also makes rather spurious observations about the food practices of Buddhist monks in relation to the artist's work.

7 From an audio program excerpt featuring Rirkrit Tiravanija and MoMA director Glenn Lowry. 'MoMA: The Collection: Rirkrit Tiravanija. untitled 1992/1995 (free/still)', http://www.moma.org/collection/object.php?object_id=147206 (accessed 28 February 2013).

8 In this new version of the work, MoMA employees serve Tiravanija's food – vegetarian green curry – to visitors. Strict fire regulations prohibit the service of food in the MoMA's galleries, and so when *Untitled (Free/Still)* is exhibited, curry is prepared in the kitchen of the museum's cafeteria and then brought to the gallery space.

References

Allen, E. (2012), 'Curry up!' *ArtNews* 111(3): 97.

Asmis, E. (2011), 'The Necessity of Anger in Philodemus' On Anger'. In J. Fish and Kirk R. Sanders (eds), *Epicurus and the Epicurean Tradition*. Cambridge: Cambridge University Press, pp. 152–82.

Bennett, T. (1995), *The Birth of the Museum: History, Theory, Politics*. London and New York: Routledge.

Bishop, C. (2004), 'Antagonism and Relational Aesthetics'. *October* 110: 51–79.

Bourriaud, N. (2002 [1998]), *Relational Aesthetics*. Dijon, France: Les Presse Du Réel.

Candlin, F. (2007), 'Don't Touch! Hands Off! Art, Blindness and the Conservation of Expertise'. In E. Pye (ed.), *The Power of Touch: Handling Objects in Museum and Heritage Contexts*. Walnut Creek: Left Coast Press, pp. 82–106.

Classen, C. (1993), *Worlds of Sense: Exploring the Senses in History and across Cultures*. London: Routledge.

Classen, C. (ed.) (2005), 'Touch in the Museum'. In *The Book of Touch*. Oxford; New York: Berg.

Classen, C. (2007), 'Museum Manners: The Sensory Life of the Early Museum'. *Journal of Social History* 40(4): 895–914.

Classen, C. and D. Howes (2006), 'The Museum as Sensescape: Western Sensibilities and Indigenous Artifacts'. In E. Edwards, C. Gosden and R. B. Phillips (eds), *Sensible Objects: Colonialism, Museums and Material Culture*. New York: Berg.

Clintberg, M. (2014a), 'Where Publics May Touch: Stimulating Sensory Access at the National Gallery of Canada'. *The Senses & Society* 9(3): 312–322.

Clintberg, M. (2014b), 'Multisensory Tours and Programming at the Royal Ontario Museum'. Unpublished manuscript.

Cluett, S. (2014), 'Ephemeral, Immersive, Invasive: Sound as Curatorial Theme, 1966–2013'. In N. Levent and A. Pascual-Leone (eds), *The Multisensory Museum: Cross-Disciplinary Perspectives on Touch, Sound, Smell, Memory, and Space*. Lanham: Rowman & Littlefield, pp. 109–118.

Herring, F. W. (1949), 'Touch: The Neglected Sense'. *The Journal of Aesthetics and Art Criticism* 7(3): 199–215.

Hetherington, K. (2003), 'Accountability and Disposal: Visual Impairment and the Museum'. *Museum and Society* 1(2): 104–115.

Hume, D. (1898 [1757]), 'Of the Standard of Taste'. In T. H. Green and T. H. Grose (eds), *Essays Moral, Political and Literary*. London: Longmans, Green.

Jacob, M. J. (2005), 'Reciprocal Generosity'. In T. Purves (ed.), *What We Want is Free: Generosity and Exchange in Recent Art*. Albany: State University of New York Press, pp. 3–10.

Kant, I. (2005 [1798]), 'Objective and Subjective Senses: The Sense of Taste'. In Carolyn Korsmeyer (ed.), *The Taste Culture Reader*. Oxford; New York: Berg, pp. 209–214.

Kant, I. (2007 [1790]), *The Critique of Judgement*, translated by James Creed Meredith. Oxford: Oxford University Press.

Kearney, R. (2014), 'Losing our Touch'. *The New York Times*. Available at http://opinionator.blogs.nytimes.com/2014/08/30/losing-our-touch/?hp&action=click&pgtype=Homepage&module=c-column-top-span-region&region=c-column-top-span-region&WT.nav=c-column-top-span-region (accessed 31 August 2014).

Korsmeyer, C. (1999), *Making Sense of Taste: Food and Philosophy*. Ithaca and London: Cornell University Press.

Melo, A. (1995), 'Guess Who's Coming to Dinner'. *Parkett* 44: 105.

Purinton, J. S. (1993), 'Epicurus on the Telos'. *Phronesis* 38(3): 281–320.

Rollins, T. (1993), 'Interview with Tim Rollins, April 16, June 12, 1993'. *Felix Gonzalez-Torres*. New York: A.R.T. Press.

Savile, A. (2003), 'The Idealism of Purposiveness'. In P. Guyer (ed.), *Kant's Critique of the Power of Judgment: Critical Essays*. Lanham: Rowman & Littlefield, pp. 87–99.

Sedley, D. (2011), 'Epicurus' Theological Innatism'. In J. Fish and Kirk R. Sanders (eds), *Epicurus and the Epicurean Tradition*. Cambridge: Cambridge University Press, pp. 29–52.

Smith, G. A. (2011), 'To Touch or Not to Touch: That is the Question!' *The Journal of Museum Education* 36(2): 137–146.

Sweeney, E. (2009), 'Walking with Janet Cardiff, Sitting with Massimo Guerrera, and Eating Apples with R. Murray Schafer: Meaningful Museum Experiences with Participatory Art for Visitors with and without Visual Impairments'. *The Journal of Museum Education* 34(3): 235–248.

Sweeney, K. W. (1999), 'Alice's Discriminating Palate'. *Philosophy and Literature* 23(1): 17–31.

Symons, M. (2007), 'Epicurus, the Foodies' Philosopher'. In F. Allhoff and D. Monroe (eds), *Food & Philosophy: Eat, Drink and Be Merry*. Oxford: Blackwell Publishing, pp. 13–30.

7

The 2015 Chicago Architecture Biennial: The State of Sensory Design

Joy Monice Malnar

The curators for the inaugural Chicago Architecture Biennial invited more than 120 artists and architects from thirty countries for the purpose of determining 'The State of the Art of Architecture.' Opening on 3 October 2015 with 31,000 people in attendance, this three-month event included the notable architecture of the city, exhibits, full-scale installations and new lakefront kiosks. This major event presented an opportunity to evaluate the state of contemporary architecture, and determine the extent to which multisensory experiences are being considered in its realization. Yi-Fu Tuan has noted: 'What begins as undifferentiated space becomes place as we get to know it better and endow it with value' (1977: 6). In this article, the lakefront kiosks competition winner, and the three Chicago architecture schools that collaborated with internationally renowned architects, are evaluated for their ability to contribute to a sense of place that characterizes Chicago. *Place* will be defined for this purpose as the sensed characteristics of land, water, air, sun and seasons, along with the built cultural heritage Chicagoans are proud of, and wish to continue. This will limit the exhibits discussed to those located outdoors. The historic beach houses and pavilions currently located within the twenty-eight miles of public lakefront parks have sheltered generations during the hot summer months, offering places to feel the cooling shade and wind, as well as affording protection from the sudden lightning storms. The question is: does 'The State of the Art of Architecture' indicate that global designers are taking into account the specific sensorial conditions of place? Have architects moved beyond a belief in universalism, and an ocular-centric, Cartesian view of typology?

Over a half-million people attended the inaugural Chicago Architecture Biennial (CAB), the first such in North America. For three months, Chicago, known for its historic architecture, was engaged in determining architecture's current state. As could be expected, the exhibits selected by curators Sarah Herda and Joseph Grima received comments ranging from praise to criticism to snark, but few reviewers actually evaluated the 'state of architecture'. In fact, CAB succeeded on many levels. While Biennials typically display models and drawings that test and demonstrate new ideas, here there were a remarkable number of full-scale prototypes built inside the glorious 1897 beaux-arts style Chicago Cultural Center – the main venue. As part of the event, an open international competition was run to select a kiosk that would be located along the shoreline of Lake Michigan. The competition drew interest from 420 applicants from more than forty countries. Three other kiosks were designed by local architecture schools that worked in collaboration with internationally known architectural firms. The winning competition kiosk was temporarily located along Lake Michigan, north of the Museum Campus. Of the three school submissions, one was built, another represented in Millennium Park, and the third remained on the Illinois Institute of Technology (IIT) campus. As a lasting legacy all four will eventually be relocated along the lakefront.

In the interest of complete accuracy, it should be noted at the outset that not a single finalist actually designed a kiosk at all. The definition as given in the Chicago Architecture Biennial: Lakefront Kiosk Competition was brief, 'A kiosk is a small open-fronted structure used for the sale of food or retail goods' (Herda and Grima, 2015: 14). In this regard the announcement is quite consistent:

> The Chicago Park District currently oversees over forty kiosks that punctuate the shoreline, which during the summer offer food, retail, and recreational services – ranging from beverages to clothing to surf rentals. Although these kiosks are, by necessity, modest in size, these structures are an exciting opportunity to explore creative architectural solutions. The competition calls for the design of a new kiosk that will be a fully functioning commercial space during the summer, but also asks applicants to consider how the kiosk might perform as an architectural intervention on the lakefront when its commercial functions are inactive. When open, how does the kiosk engage with both visitors and the surrounding environment? When closed, how does the kiosk maintain an active presence on the lakefront and attract visitors year-round? How can its design adapt to changing programs, as well as different locations on the lakefront? (Herda and Grima 2015: 4)

Every Chicagoan is familiar with such structures from practical experience; but this set of parameters was ignored in virtually every particular. In fact the designer of one of the kiosks, Paul Preissner, said the market-based program 'bothered us a little bit' (Raskin and Sitz 2015: 104). On the other hand, a pavilion is defined as 'an ornamental building, usually of light construction and designed for temporary shelter, refreshment, etc.' (Oxford English Dictionary). Using this definition, the winning entries were somewhat more successful, although it is disappointing to see designers disengage from aspects of a program they obviously felt limiting. Nor were the proffered rationalizations for missing functions any real help. It thus becomes necessary for this analysis to rely on other existing Chicago pavilions – rather than any actual kiosks – for the purpose of design comparison.

One of the least physically engaging stretches of Chicago's lakefront is the one-mile-long, straight concrete sidewalk used in the introductory photograph of the Lakefront Kiosk Competition announcement.[1] This sidewalk sits between the sheet piling holding back the lake and the traffic of Lake Shore Drive. The concrete path connects the sands of Oak Street Beach with the sands of the Ohio Street beach. This harsh photo may have confused many of those not familiar with the true identity of the 'iconic shoreline of Lake Michigan'. The Chicago Architectural Biennial Trailer announcing the event also focused entirely on the rectilinear street and building grids of the city to the exclusion of the nodal gathering of radial streets and the curvilinear shoreline (Chicago Architecture Biennial Trailer 2015). This reveals a particular vision of the city held by the organizers of the Chicago Architecture Biennial. One of the dangers of an international competition is the limited understanding of a place that results from not having the knowledge that can only occur from long-term accumulation of observation, and such a photo does not help.

The Lakefront Kiosk announcement stated: 'Though the winning kiosk will be a small structure – a work of micro-architecture – it will reinforce the city's broader commitment to forward-thinking design. The competition is a challenge to demonstrate how small-scale architectural design can transform public space' (Herda and Grima 2015: 4). The programmatic requirements were that it must accommodate a commercial function on the lakefront during the summer (May–August) and also be 'an iconic work of architecture that will attract visitors and enliven the lakefront year round – including the off-season months (September–April), when its retail services will be suspended' (Herda and Grima 2015: 5). This therefore requires an understanding of the weather conditions of Chicago and their sensorial effect on people. And as a final reminder of this elementary fact, the competition announcement provides the basic yearly temperatures and notes that summers are hot and humid with periods of rainstorms and high winds. The rainstorms are actually often sudden downpours with lightning, during which lifeguards must clear the beaches and encourage people to find shelter. Many of Chicago's older lakefront beach houses did provide such shelter. Fine precedents, such as at the 63rd Street and the North Avenue Beach Houses, were also designed to provide 'cool' zones. A central aperture allows for the *venturi* effect to take place, where air movement accelerates through a constricted opening. The breeze helps with the stultifying humidity and, when coupled with the shade, offers a place to retreat from the hot sun. The more recent beach houses have picked up on this building-type opening, but treat it as a formalist technique rather than actually understanding the sensory mitigation it provides. In fact, being in direct sunlight makes the air feel 10 to 15 degrees Fahrenheit warmer, while a breeze will make it feel 4 to 5 degrees Fahrenheit cooler.

A clear outline of 'Criteria for Evaluation' focused entrants' attention on *originality* and *feasibility*. Originality was defined as being an 'original and inventive contribution to the field', encompassing 'creative use of materials and technology'. Also listed were 'innovative fabrication', a 'thoughtful engagement of the lakefront landscape', and 'sustainability'. Feasibility required that the kiosk be 'realizable within the budget', constitute 'ease of on-site installation', be 'transportable', be a 'weather sustainable design', and that the designers have a 'demonstrated capacity to complete the project'. None of the criteria called for an explicit consideration of human sensory capacity, although a 'thoughtful engagement of the lakefront landscape', could be expected to bring this about.

The kiosk design, titled *Chicago Horizon*, by the firm Ultramoderne was selected as the winner of the BP Prize in the Chicago Lakefront Kiosk Competition to stand as a lasting legacy of the inaugural Chicago Architecture Biennial (Figure 7.1). The principals, Rhode Island designers Yasmin Vobis and Aaron Forrest, explain on their website that they are committed to designing projects 'that are at once modern, playful, and generous' (Ultramodern.net 2015). Thus these will serve as my evaluative terms. The name of the firm indicates a clear aspiration to be 'more than modern'. The kiosk was constructed in the Museum Campus lakefront area and opened to the public on 1 October 2015. It displays a number of the Modern Movement's edicts such as the belief that decoration must be eliminated, roofs must be flat, with the building's structure clearly expressed; and this is referred to as 'honesty'. This ideological indoctrination, taught in architecture schools everywhere, stands in sharp contrast to local knowledge. The designers explain that they were 'Inspired by two

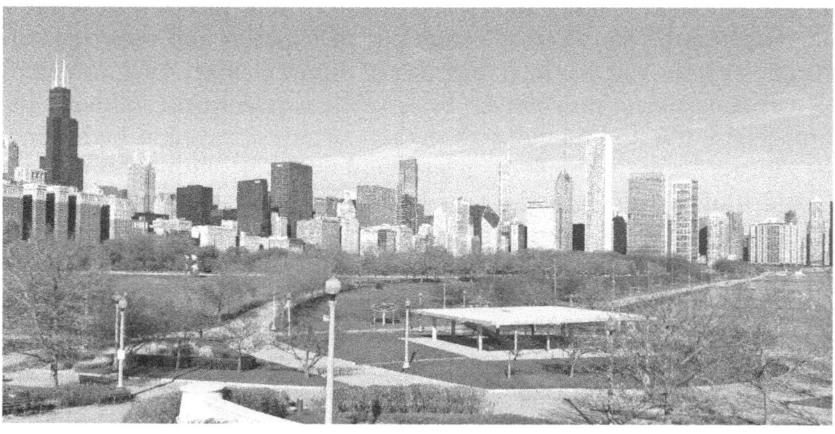

FIGURE 7.1 *Chicago Horizon*, Ultramoderne, 2015. Photo by Joy Monice Malnar.

Chicago prototypes – Mies van der Rohe's experiments in flatness and the Eames' explorations of scale in Powers of Ten' (Ultramodern.net, 2015).

A major problem in architectural education remains its deeply embedded belief in (Western) universal design. The Cree ethicist Willie Ermine describes this condition that occurs in many areas of education as a 'dissemination of a singular world consciousness, a monoculture with a claim to one model of humanity and one model of society' (2007: 198). Ermine is describing what indigenous scholars refer to as 'cognitive imperialism' and points out that it 'remains simmering, unchecked, enfolded as it is, in the subconscious of the masses and recreated from the archives of knowledge and systems, rules and values of colonialism that in turn will into being the intellectual, political, economic, cultural, and social systems and institutions of this country' (2007: 198). This is an even more difficult problem in Chicago where Mies van der Rohe, who promoted the universal model, remains a major architectural figure of abiding significance.

The catalogue copy explains: '*Chicago Horizon* seeks to build the largest flat wooden roof possible with the available budget' (Grima et al. 2015: 110). The driving premise is cognitive, one surely appreciated by structural engineers; whether others find it similarly scintillating is questionable. This 'quest' resulted in a 'generous 56' ft. (17m) square' (110) that would 'demarcate a zone of the city for all to enjoy' (Ultramodern.net 2015). Aside from providing a place of shade, it is difficult to imagine what makes this a place 'for all to enjoy'. It is difficult to imagine someone walking over and saying, 'Wow, that is the largest wood roof possible that the budget allows'. In any case, without a sign posted who would be aware of this particular virtue? The designers express the more romantic notion of creating 'an abstract floating plane', but the reality is that it is nothing more than a flat roof with a slight cantilever beyond the columns. This brings to mind Juhani Pallasmaa's observation: 'The flatness of today's architecture extends to temporal experience; we live in a world of flattened time' (2001: 52).

Quite the opposite occurs at the 1957 *Chess Pavilion* designed by architect Maurice Webster with free-standing figures and incised decoration sculpted out of local limestone by Boris Gilbertson (Figure 7.2). Its dramatic cantilevered roof comes closer to actually providing a floating roof. Robert McCarter and Juhani Pallasmaa articulate a similar condition when they point out: 'Architecture takes place under the laws of physics, and it usually deliberately expresses these constitutive physical forces . . . All physical structures are bound to recognize the force of gravity . . . As structural forces are inescapable physical facts, they provide the ground for a heightened sense of reality; an architectural approach that aims at precise structural articulation and expression turns into a form of poetic realism' (2012: 117). For over fifty years, the Chess Pavilion, located south of the North Avenue Beach has been a popular summer gathering place for hundreds of chess players. The thin concrete roof dramatically tilts upward toward the lake while it shelters built-in chess tables located at varying

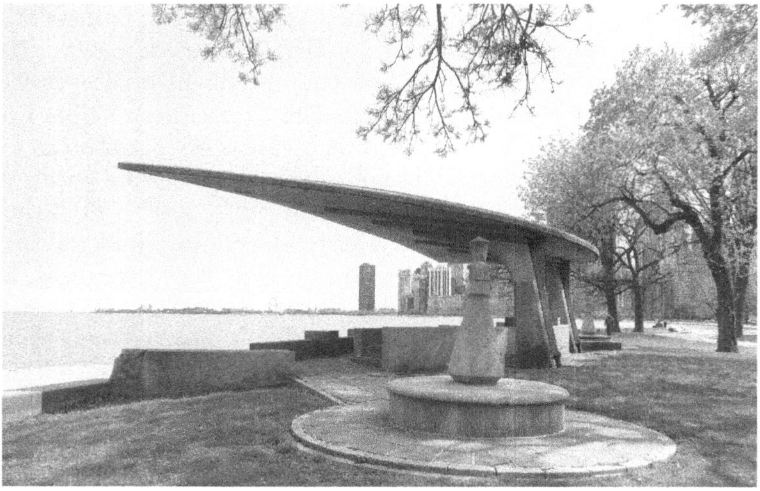

FIGURE 7.2 *Chess Pavilion*, Maurice Webster, 1957. Photo by Joy Monice Malnar.

heights. The delightful almost human-scale king and queen chess figures flank the pavilion.

Continuing the analysis of the *Chicago Horizon* kiosk, attention is shifted to the stairs to the roof opening (Figure 7.3). These stairs invite people to walk up with the intent of providing a different view of the city. If they are meant to establish a sense of prospect through a peephole it does not work, because the roof plane disrupts the continuity of view for too short a time. It does not frame views or refocus attention on any specific building. Here there are no surprises. Once one pops up beyond the opening there is nothing more than what was seen below, except for a large flat rubber membrane roof sure to become progressively dirty. (It is worth noting that one of the advantages of a pitched roof is that rainwater washes it down.) This roof in the summer will be radiating heat adding to the heat island effect and negatively impacting the microclimate. This is contrary to the direction the city has taken toward encouraging the greening of every inch of roof. And given that the kiosk is located in the lakefront park, a green roof would replace natural ground cover. Rather than establishing relationships between people and the water, the stairs' orientation cause people to turn their back to the lake horizon. Shortly after the *Chicago Horizon* kiosk opened, people climbed not only up the stairs but onto the roof, causing the Chicago Park District to wrap the stairs with a chain-link fence – thus making them predictably inaccessible. There was an obvious safety concern that without a railing people could fall off the edge of the roof. The result is that what was designed as the main experience is now not accessible – not only to those in wheelchairs – but to everyone.

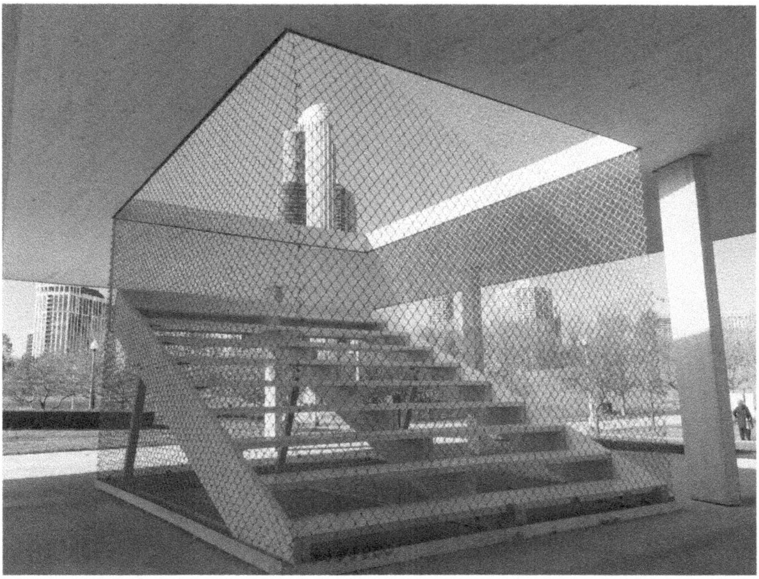

FIGURE 7.3 *Chicago Horizon Stair*, Ultramoderne, 2015. Photo by Joy Monice Malnar.

Charles and Ray Eames describe their marvelous film *Powers of Ten* as one, 'dealing with the relative size of things in the universe and the effect of adding another zero' (1977). The film begins with an overhead view of a couple lying on a one-meter square picnic blanket on Chicago's lakefront. From that location it zooms out to 10^2 meters and then back in to 10^{-16} meters. The designers of the *Chicago Horizon* provide only one frame of the movie, so to understand the reference one must have previously seen the Eames movie. It reminds one of Italo Calvino's complaint about a student interpreter, who 'condenses whole stories into one sentence that is comprehensible but lacking in emotional appeal' (1984; 2013: 181). The scale shift in the movie reminds us of our place within the universe and that when designing things it should not be done in isolation. This requires an intimate understanding of context and that relationships matter.

Summer Vault was designed by students at the University of Illinois at Chicago with Colorado architect Paul Andersen and Chicago's Paul Preissner (Figure 7.4). Placed in close proximity to Anish Kapoor's highly engaging *Cloudgate*, it simply could not compete; passers-by for the most part passed it by. Blair Kamin found children having fun swinging on the metal gate. But soon after being placed in the park, the Chicago Park District realized this 'kinesthetic action' needed to be prevented and locked the gate in place. Many questions arise when comparing the designers' description with the built kiosk. First and foremost is determining the 'thoughtful engagement of the lakefront landscape'. The drawings illustrate an oval ground disengaged

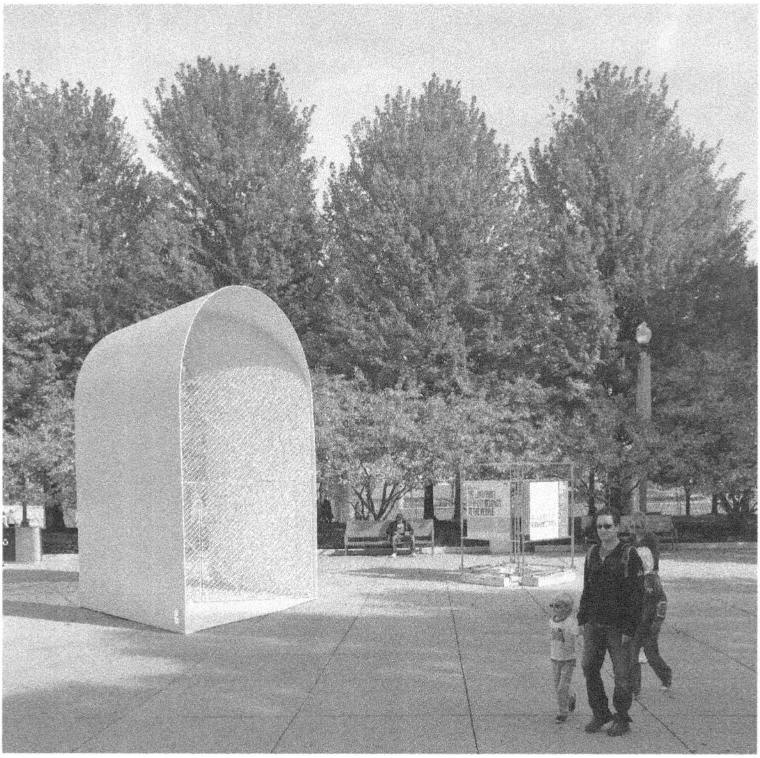

FIGURE 7.4 *Summer Vault*, Andersen and Preissner, 2015. Photo by Joy Monice Malnar.

from any context. The kiosk appears in both the drawing and built structure like an isolated, slightly more elaborate Quonset hut that can be deployed and erected anywhere needed. It is intended to reflect the 'kiosk's Persian origins as a 13th-century garden pavilion' (Chicagoarchitecturebiennial.org 2015). Native American buildings of the Great Lakes region, such as the Algonquian bark house or Midewiwin lodge, would have been more appropriate (and more appealing as well). The designers said: 'It consists of basic geometric shapes – a 12-foot-diameter barrel vault, a parallelogram, triangles – combined to create a curious, freestanding hangout within the park' (Chicagoarchitecturebiennial.org 2015). In its present state, it is not likely to become a hangout.

'The interior of the skewed vault is divided into two triangular spaces – one enclosed by expanded metal screens and doors, and one open to the air but still within the vaulting' (Grima et al. 2015: 111). In short, the kiosk is an object that is all about itself; there is no description as to how it connects to the sun, wind or edge of the lakefront. In their rush toward the new they give no thought to the careful, time-honored watching of the sky. Christopher Tilley's words are instructive as he discusses the coast as a place where the sun rises to 'be reborn from a watery underworld' and that there are 'auspicious days of the year, such as midsummer, the equinoxes, and midwinter [which can also be an important feature for a site's lived geography]' (2012: 462). Ancient civilizations would mark the equinox and solstice with celebrations; when architects take the sun into account today it is more often as an energy or light source, not for 'a site's lived geography' or its perception. What should have been of concern to the designers of the lakefront kiosks is described in Robert McCarter and Juhani Pallasmaa's book *Understanding Architecture*. When analyzing Glenn Murcutt's Simpson-Lee house, they found it, 'Open to the movement of the sun and the change of the seasons, the details and materials are kept intentionally quiet and reserved to enable the subtle dramas of the natural setting to become the foreground, rather than the background of daily life' (McCarter and Pallasmaa 2012: 248). The design of structures as landmarks, on the other hand, places them in the foreground.

It is hard to imagine, given its small footprint that 'this two-part plan allows for commerce and community to occur simultaneously' (Chicagoar chitecturebiennial.org 2015), as it simply is not large enough and is too open. The size is likely limited by the budget, but then that was one of the original criteria. The designers believed "its openness allows year-round use, so that it remains active even in its retail slumber during the Chicago winter' (Chicagoarchitecturebiennial.org 2015). This is a quasi-romantic notion that indicates they did not actually check Chicago's winter temperatures and wind patterns, as the open, thin, steel structure offers no protection at all. The aspirations in terms of programming sound good, but again are not related in any specific way to the lakefront.

Cent Pavilion (Figure 7.5), designed by Mauricio Pezo and Sofia von Ellrichshausen with IIT students, was 'meant to convey silent and convoluted simplicity. It repeats the same angled design over and over, resulting in an opaque monolith' (Chicagoarchitecturebiennial.org 2015). The forty-foot structural frame was built in front of Ludwig Mies van der Rohe's iconic, horizontal IIT Crown Hall. It was roped off with signs posted saying it was a temporary structure and warned that 'Climbing the structure is expressly prohibited'. Of course, these stacked, progressively smaller layers are begging to be climbed. Perhaps the Chilean architects did not realize the interactive character of Chicagoans. When placed on the lake it will be clad with a surface material, which they believe will prevent the climbing – or perhaps add to the challenge. 'When its commercial function ceases at the summer's end, the kiosk will complement the verticality of Chicago's iconic skyline year-round' (Chicagoarchitecturebiennial.org 2015). This hardly addresses one of the criteria: 'When open, how does the kiosk engage with both visitors and the surrounding environment? When closed, how does the kiosk maintain an active presence on the lakefront and attract visitors year-round?' (Herda and Grima 2015: 4). This formal play is satisfying to cognitive designers, but a strictly visual tower offers no winter shelter for joggers.

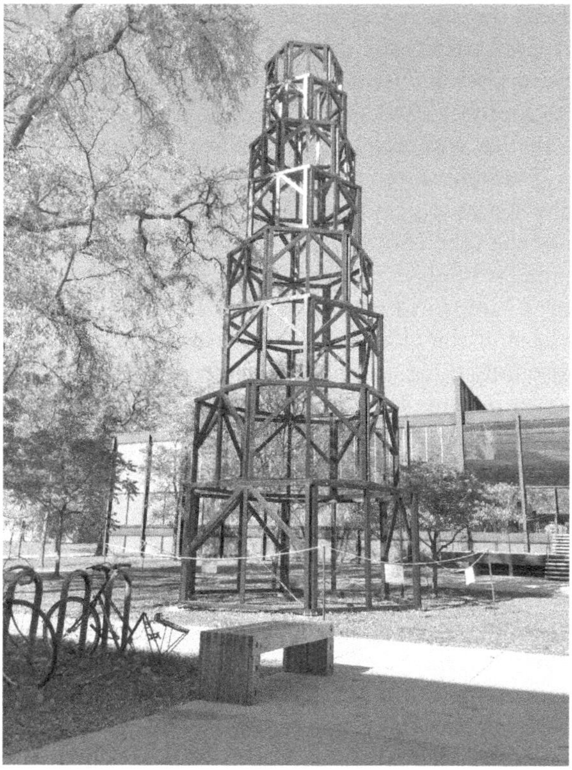

FIGURE 7.5 *Cent Pavilion*, Pezo and Ellrichshausen, 2015. Photo by Joy Monice Malnar.

Also problematic is its derivative nature – a kind of New World Tatlin – which would appear to argue against originality.[2]

With all of the recent interest in integrating buildings with the landscape it is surprising to see that only one kiosk did so. *Rock*, designed by Nigerian architect Kunle Adeyemi in association with the School of the Art Institute of Chicago, designed a kiosk 'composed from the raw and historic limestone blocks that once protected the city's shoreline' (Nleworks.com 2015). Unfortunately, due to the cost involved in moving the kiosk from Millennium Park to its final location at Montrose Beach – completely ignoring the portability requirement – it was decided to place only a few representative rocks in Millennium Park. Therefore there is not sufficient development for evaluation, aside from observing the fun children had in climbing onto the individual rocks.

The point of immersing people within an environment is to activate the full range of the senses. Chicago is a hands-on, feet-on-the-ground city. Their embrace of public sculptures can be seen as urbanites walk through Calder's *Flamingo*, children slide down the *Picasso*, and everyone engages in touching and waving at their image in *Cloudgate*. Interestingly, these sculptures are all made of steel. Chicago is a city where steel mills emerged, and steel rails converge. It knows steel's durability. Signs saying 'Do not touch' posted at sculpture parks such as Seattle Art Museum to protect the steel sculptures are silly, merely reducing interaction. It is unnecessary to treat steel in a pristine manner. No Chicagoan would dare say 'Do not touch.' One immediately knows the human desire to interact was not taken into account when a sign needs to be posted or a barrier placed.

Thousands of people flock to the thirty miles of lakefront. There is still hope that the patterns of nature and behaviour of people will be studied and the new kiosks will be appropriately placed to serve as gathering nodes. But of course this requires the designers to want to connect people with the sun, wind, sand and water. Perhaps it is the confusion of wind and the seeming unpredictability of drifting sand that causes architects to run toward the clarity of basic geometry. When reading Italo Calvino's essay 'Collection of Sand' the unique place-oriented aspect of sand is brought to our attention. Fascinated by 'an exhibition of bizarre collections', it was the jars of sand taken from all over the world that 'was the least showy but also the most mysterious, the one that seemed to have most things to say, even through the opaque silence imprisoned behind the glass of the jars' (1984; 2013: 5). Calvino first notices the differences in colour, then looking closer the texture. This material made of thousands of years of erosion; its existence is dependent on the interaction of water, wind and sun. So it is with indigenous cultures. Melissa K. Nelson points out that, 'A Cahuilla coiled basket, for example, is a beautiful piece of art with unique elements of design, colour, symmetry, and texture. But the knowledge it took to make it includes an understanding of plant lifecycles, seasonal variation, moisture and tensile strength, and weaving pattern – all things encompassed by our modern sciences of botany, climatology, engineering, and mathematics' (2015: 198). The designers of the kiosks have focused on the engineering and mathematics of the equation to the exclusion of botany and climatology that connect people to nature.

Chicago is a great city in large part because it is located on one of the Great Lakes. It has thirty miles of shoreline sculpted, not by natural erosion, but entirely by geo-engineering. Even given that this urban shoreline is entirely man-made its purpose remains to provide people with a place where they can directly sense and enjoy the natural conditions created by the interaction of water, wind, sand and sun. Typically earth and water engage each other in a give and take motion that has been altered in many of Chicago's miles of shoreline where a defensive concrete edge sits behind corrugated steel. This dialogue has been altered in order to maintain an unyielding edge protecting the land from erosion. In some ways, this illustrates Peter Buchanan's observation when discussing 'sensitive relationships with context', that 'a major consequence of modernity's undervaluing of relationship is the creation of an alienating built environment and a general disenchanting of the world. A necessary step to

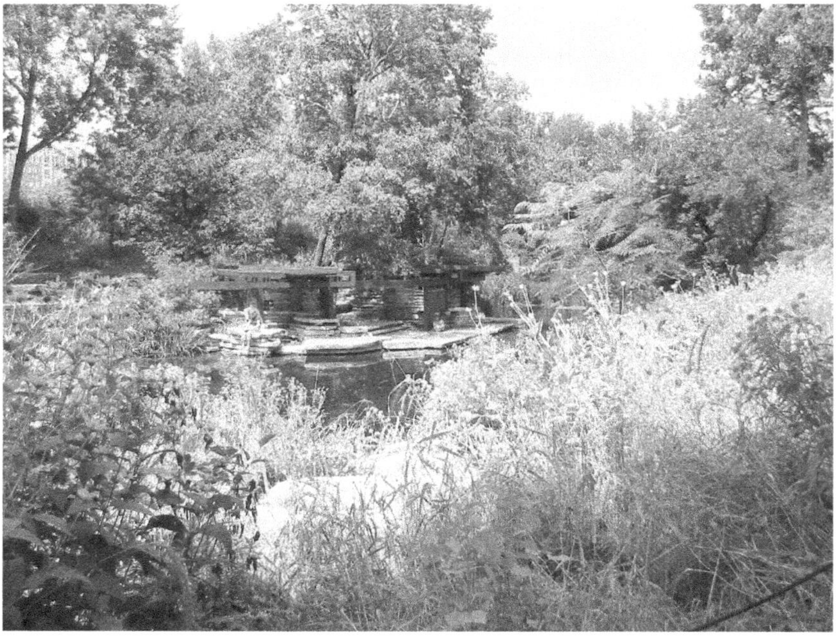

FIGURE 7.6 *Caldwell Lily Pond*, Alfred Caldwell, 1937. Photo by Joy Monice Malnar.

sustainability is to re-enchant the world and evoke reverence and connection with it' (2012: 83).

This occurs at the Caldwell Lily Pond, a magical, hidden refuge for birds and people (Figure 7.6). It offers a quiet place where people can meander along the edge of the pond on a path flanked by stratified limestone ledges while listening to bird songs, a melodic waterfall and wind rustling through the trees. The moist scent of earth, moss and stone prevails. The film critic Roger Ebert said he would come here after his rehab to 'walk around [the pond] and affirm my continuing existence' (2010). Designed in 1936 by the Prairie School landscape architect Alfred Caldwell, the concept was based on his observation that 'water has cut deep into prairie soil' revealing a unique glaciated terrain of the great lake region (1942; 1997: 158). The eroded limestone speaks of the geologic forces that formed the land. The success of Caldwell's pavilion arises from its ability to integrate itself into the landscape. The architecture is composed of scraped rock surfaces and dark stained wood that works with the essence of the land. Sitting on the cool limestone or lying on the warm, wood bench one is literally in touch with nature. The pavilion is divided, with each part turned in a slightly different direction, subtly allowing people to indulge in private moments of quiet contemplation as well as provide options to sit in the sun or shade. The deeper recesses of the pavilion provide places of refuge with additional privacy. Children enjoy games of hide and seek, popping up above the ledges and behind screens. It confirms that a pavilion can unite with place, establishing a memorable experience for people of all ages.

When Robin Wall Kimmerer writes from her Anishinabekwe and plant ecologist perspectives, she points out that '*Becoming indigenous to place*' requires people to 'redefine their evolving relationship with nature . . . [As] It is born of long intimacy and attentiveness to a homeland and can arise wherever people are materially and spiritually integrated with their landscape' (2000: 9). This is something that is sadly difficult to achieve in a fast-paced competition, located in an area that the entrants might not have ever visited. This reveals itself in many ways, but in particular the sensorial aspects of the glorious lakefront being completely ignored. While some might argue this is merely a competition for a small kiosk, it begins to reveal the current 'state of the art of architecture'. In the pursuit of something new, in trying to create an object that will stand out, the time necessary to pause and understand the life forces of Lake Michigan is eliminated. In the words of Wendell Berry there is a need for a 'complex knowledge of one's place' and 'faithfulness to one's place on which such knowledge depends' (2007: 39).

Thoughtful engagement requires both an understanding of why people gravitate to waterfronts and local knowledge that recognizes how the weather cycles of the region effect the life forces of Lake Michigan. In *The Great Lakes Water Wars*, Peter Annin calls water the 'foundation of life' (2006: 256). Lake Michigan is the source of drinking water for Chicagoans and creates a microclimate along its shores, often referred to as 'cooler by the lake'. Aside from haptic comfort levels, it provides a restorative experience. In the *1909 Plan of Chicago*, Daniel Burnham wrote, 'The lakefront by right belongs to the people. It affords their one great unobstructed view, stretching away to the horizon where water and clouds seem to meet' (1909; 1993: 50). His rationale for giving this valuable land to the people was: 'These views of a broad expanse are helpful alike to mind and body. They beget calm thoughts and feelings, and afford escape from the petty things of life' (1909; 1993: 50). Research has confirmed the stress-reducing properties of being in nature. Peter F. Smith in *The Syntax of Cities* points out: 'Psychologists have for long recognized the existence of a "rhythm-demand." It has been plausibly suggested that, through rhythm, man becomes incorporated into the wider system of nature which can be conceived as a marvelously complex symphony of rhythms' (1977: 66). Unfortunately, as Ralph L. Knowles explains, 'Architects have generally ignored the temporal dimension that nature adds to our perceptions of architectural space. Of course most designers acknowledge that buildings may be transformed or deteriorate over time. But on the whole their artistic idea of space is compositional complete and static, the end product of many imaginative design decisions' (1998).

At the lakefront, people experience both its rhythmic, wind-dependent waves and sunrises over its expansive horizon. It is a place where we can, as described by John O'Donohue in *Eternal Echoes*, 'rediscover ascetical tranquility and come home to the temple of our senses . . . Our bodies know that they belong; it is our minds that make our lives so homeless . . . An increasing majority of people feel no belonging. We have fallen out of rhythm with life. The art of belonging is the recovery of the wisdom of rhythm' (1999: 3). The attraction people feel toward Lake Michigan might be due to a need to reestablish the fluctuating rhythmic features of breath, heartbeat, circadian rhythms, and brainwave activity. This connection requires more than visual rhythm that is typically displayed in buildings by the spacing of parts, such as windows, columns and ornament. Equally importantly architects should create places where rhythmic connections can occur to achieve harmony between people and nature.

The heartbeat of Lake Michigan is unique. Unlike the continual roar of the ocean and its salty sea air there is quietude to the lake with some describing its smell as fresh rain on stone. Lake Michigan waves tend to be smaller and gentler than ocean waves offering a contemplative tranquility. And unlike the ocean tides, Lake Michigan's water level changes six feet gradually over periods of years. The *Monument to the Partisan Woman* in Venice by sculptor Augusto Murer and architect Carlo Scarpa is an excellent example of how to design to make apparent the changing water levels. A platform supports the bronze sculpture that the rising and falling of the tide exposes and conceals, thus, 'producing a continuous, silent interference by the water of the lagoon. By design, the movement is not perceptible, both because it develops within the time arc of the cycle of the tide and because the entire elevation mechanism is conceived to follow the inclination of the energy of the water rather than express something stagy or obvious. This is the meaning of dialogue with context achieved in Scarpa's handling of an extremely difficult theme' (Codello 2009).

To design a structure that provides a place where 'thoughtful engagement of the lakefront landscape' occurs requires a place that orients people so they can better sense these natural rhythms. Creating an intimate relationship between the rhythms of the place and actual embodied experiences of people would bring about this thoughtful engagement. Indigenous understanding of places provide instruction on how this can occur, as Melissa K. Nelson explains:

> Native sciences are local knowledges of specific places, geographies, and homelands. They are site-specific, place-based, *in situ* knowledges. Local knowledge is about persistence in place and orientation. This orientation operates on a spatial level with both vertical and horizontal dimensions, among others. In my Ojibwe tradition, for example, the number 7 is considered very sacred and significant, because it orients us to the four cardinal directions horizontally, and the two major vertical dimensions: the sky above and the Earth below. The seventh direction is the inner or spiritual direction of where we are individually located; it is also sometimes referred to the dimension of Mystery or the Unknowable space. (2015: 198)

How does this relate to the biennial? It is not that these 'kiosks' are bad, just dull, not engaging our human sensorial systems, nor taking into consideration the unique character of the lakefront. The pavilions are designed by and as a result of the rational, cognitive mind that sees the world as static. The British writer Norman Douglas realized, 'How hard it is, sometimes, to trust the evidence of one's senses! How reluctantly the mind consents to reality' (1928; 1982: 82). If the designers drew on their own personal experience of being on a waterfront, it is not evident in their work. While there have been great inventions providing comfort for the human body the human body has not evolved much. We still sense our environment with the same sensory systems.

Historic Chicago architecture has some truly beautiful light wells, such as architect Daniel Burnham's *Motorola Building* with its sun-reflecting, white brick and the *Rookery*'s sparkling light court of white marble and gold leaf by Frank Lloyd Wright. The Chicago Cultural Center's central light well has always been merely functional, dutifully bringing in daylight and air from the center of the building. Yoshiharu Tsukamoto and Momoyo Kaijima of Atelier Bow-Wow were, as might be expected of Tokyo designers, intrigued by this large, empty outdoor space and selected it for their *Piranesi Circus* installation (Figure 7.7). Piranesi, the eccentric artist with an unfulfilled desire to be an architect, has influenced many with his whimsical series of labyrinthine prints. Within this exterior space, the designers placed ramps, stairs, ladders, balconies, bridges and a swing, all beckoning one to enter. The proposed model indicates the initial intention was to draw people in at the ground level, up a series of ramps that lead to one of the first-floor arched windows, where people could reenter the building. Unfortunately, as the architect of record, Woodhouse Tinucci Architects, pointed out, due to claims of 'security, safety, and facility management' concerns, the intent was not realized (2015). As visitors journeyed through the over one hundred CAB exhibits they were continually confronted with the inaccessibility of the central lightwell. Eventually it becomes clear that the *Piranesi Circus* is imprisoned and unusable. The exhibit becomes frustratingly inaccessible while visible from all levels and sides of the rectangular building. Anyone approaching *Piranesi Circus* begins a search for the entry point. Since people were prevented from entering the exterior, the exterior ramps and balconies could have been brought into the interior by means of extensions. Where the circulation elements meet the windows they could have had a beginning platform on the inside of the building forming a relationship between the inside and outside. This would have moved the exhibit beyond its purely ocular-centric stance to one with progressively thwarted thresholds.

The Atelier Bow-Wow designers consider themselves behaviourologists who 'study the functional relations between behavior and its independent variables in the behavior-determining environment' (2010, cover). But in this case everything has been reduced to the visual. ' "It's about the possibility, and the impossibility, of architecture," the co-artistic director, Sarah

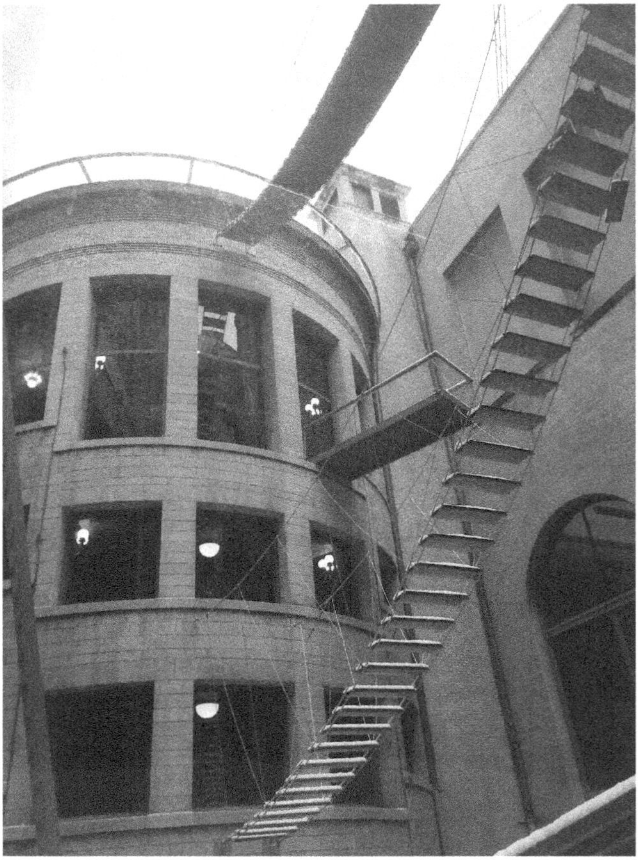

FIGURE 7.7 *Piranesi Circus*, Atelier Bow-Wow, 2015. Photo by Joy Monice Malnar.

Herda, said of the display, which the public will be able to see but not use. The design, she said, will hint at the question: "What if?"' (Kamin 2015). This positive spin is not due to intent, but rather supposed 'security and safety' concerns by facility managers' overreaction to possible litigation. While there are the ever-present concerns of slip-and-fall accidents, the less tangible cost is the sensory neutralizing of the built environment.

Patrick Lynch found the Biennial 'makes for a lively romp through the gamut of the many different things the word "architecture" is now applied to, but the sheer breadth of approaches, combined with a distinct lack of any central idea, can make it a frustrating experience' (2015). Many critics commented on a lack of a central idea, and it is perhaps too easy to use the *Piranesi Circus* as a metaphor for what we are circling but cannot access. 'Unfortunately, and some would say tragically, the metaphoric part of our minds has generally atrophied in modern Eurocentric societies, especially since the Industrial Revolution when so much emphasis was placed on the machine as the metaphor to live by. Supreme emphasis was placed on quantitative analysis, reductionistic science and technology in education, industry, and media' (Nelson 2015: 198).

So, where are we? What is the current state of the art? Sadly, the current research on multisensory environments appearing in journals such as *The Senses & Society* does not appear to be impacting the artists and architects participating in the Chicago Biennial. Nor are the discoveries in neuroscience offering new information about how the brain relates to the physical environment. In *Functional Connections of Cortical Areas: A New View from the Thalamus* by S. Murray Sherman and R. W. Guillery, leading authorities in neurobiology argue: 'Each cortical area depends on the messages linking it to body and world' (2013, Overview). It becomes the role of architects to facilitate this link between people and the world. 'We need to have these conversations anyway', Herda said about Chicago's need to keep on innovating. 'I think if we're having them with the world, it's a much richer possibility' (Kamin 2015). But unless the conversation is broadened beyond those embedded within the ocular-centric world, architects will not innovate.

As Grima puts it, the Biennial is 'a platform through which theory and practice can converge', adding that they were keen 'not to make disciplinary distinctions' (Wainwright 2015). But in not doing so, we no longer know what the distinction between art and architecture actually is. The connection between people and the lakefront was also avoided in favour of cognitive theoretical positions. The designers of the full-scale outdoor kiosks and exhibits designed for the mind. The conversation needs to include Merleau-Ponty's voice, 'rather than a mind *and* a body, man is a mind *with* a body' (1948, 2004: 56).

When evaluating the full-scale installations, the conclusion is that architecture is still working mainly in the sphere of obscure universal cognition. The kiosks are perhaps visually intriguing but they have left the body behind, and nature out of the equation. There is a separation in Chicago architecture between those who build and those who exhibit. The best architecture is coming from those who do both, such as Jeanne Gang. There is a risk that architects begin to think collectively that the exhibit is more important than the real thing, just as some academics today stake their credentials on the mistaken claim that Piranesi's desire to be an architect made him one.

The anthropologist Edmund Carpenter notes, 'All peoples have the same senses, though not all use them alike . . . Any sensory experience is partly a skill and any skill can be cultivated' (1973: 20). The belief in universalism hampers architects in cultivating their sensory skills thus trapping them within the limited ocular-centric expression. The question presented in my book *Sensory Design* remains: what would our built environment be like if sensory response, sentiment and memory were critical design factors, more vital even than structure and program? (2004: xi). Judging by the Biennial, we still do not know.

Notes

1 A similar view of the lakefront between Oak Street Beach and the Ohio Street Beach can be seen on Google Earth V 7.1.1.1843. 41° 53' 49" N 87° 37' 7" W, Altitude 3,018 feet. DigitalGlobe © 2013. http://www.earth.google.com (accessed 25 April 2016).

2 Vladimir Tatlin was best known as the architect who designed the similar *Monument to the Third International* in 1919, a reference any architect could not fail to recognize.

References

Annin, P. (2006), *The Great Lakes Water Wars*. Washington, DC: Island Press.

Atelier Bow-Wow and T. Fujimori (2010), *The Architecture of Atelier Bow-Wow: Behaviorology*. New York: Rizzoli International Publications.

Berry, W. (2007), 'The Regional Motive'. In V. B. Canizaro (ed.), *Architectural Regionalism: Collected Writings on Place, Identity, Modernity*. New York: Princeton Architectural Press, pp. 37–41.

Buchanan, P. (2012), 'The Big Rethink Part 8: Lessons from Peter Zumthor and Other Living Masters'. *The Architectural Review*, 28 August. Available at http://www.architectural-review.com/essays/the-big-rethink-part-8-l...rom-peter-zumthor-and-other-living-masters/8634689.article#comments (accessed 4 January 2015).

Burnham, D. and E. Bennett (1909, 1993), *Plan of Chicago*. New York: Princeton Architectural Press.

Caldwell, A. (1942), 'The Lily Pool, Lincoln Park'. In D. D. Domer (1997), *Alfred Caldwell: The Life and Work of a Prairie School Landscape Architect*. Baltimore: The Johns Hopkins University Press, p. 158.

Calvino, I. (1984), *Collection of Sand*, translated by M. McLaughlin (2013). Boston: Houghton Mifflin Harcourt.

Carpenter, E. (1973), *Oh, What a Blow That Phantom Gave Me!* New York: Holt, Rinehart and Winston.

Chicago Architecture Biennial Trailer (2015) [video], USA: Chicago Architecture Biennial. Available at https://www.youtube.com/watch?v=heOuwXh0mAQ (viewed 2 September 2015).

Chicagoarchitecturebiennial.org (2015), *Lakefront Kiosks*. Available at http://chicagoarchitecturebiennial.org/lakefront-kiosks/lakefront-kiosk-competition/ (accessed 18 November 2015).

Codello, R. (2009), 'Carlo Scarpa's Monument to the Partisan Woman'. Translated by J. Dezio, *Future Anterior* 6(1): 38–34. DOI: 10.1353/fta.0.0024 (accessed 23 March 2016).

Douglas, N. (1928, 1982), *South Wind*. New York: Dover Publications.

Eames, C. and R. Eames (1977), *Powers of Ten* [Film] USA: IBM. Available at https://www.youtube.com/watch?v=0fKBhvDjuy0 (viewed 20 March 2016).

Ebert, R. (2010), 'The London Perambulator'. *Roger Ebert's Journal*, 13 February. Available at http://www.rogerebert.com/rogers-journal/the-london-perambulator (accessed 20 March 2016).

Ermine, W. (2007), 'The Ethical Space of Engagement'. *Indigenous Law Journal* 6(1): 193–203.

Grima, J., S. Herda, A. Bagnato and I. Sunwoo (eds) (2015), *The State of the Art of Architecture Guidebook: Chicago Architecture Biennial*. Chicago: Chicago Architectural Biennial.

Herda, S. and J. Grima (2015), 'Chicago Architecture Biennial: Lakefront Kiosk Competition', 1–14. Available at https://steelandglass2015.files.wordpress.com/2015/01/150109_cablkc_pdf_final-v4.pdf (accessed 18 December 2014).

Kamin, B. (2015), 'City's Architecture Biennial will House Bold Ideas, Co-curator Says', *Redeye*, 28 August. Available at http://la2www.redeyechicago.com/news/cta/ct-chicago-architecture-biennial-sarah-herda-20150903,0,1392320.column (accessed 13 March 2016).

Kimmerer, R. W. (2000), 'Native Knowledge for Native Ecosystems'. *Journal of Forestry* 98(8): 4–9.

Knowles, R. L. (1998), 'Rhythm and Ritual: A Motive for Design'. Available at http://www-bcf.usc.edu/~rknowles/rhythm_ritual/rhy_rit.html (accessed 11 August 2014).

Lynch, P. (2015), 'Critics Take On "The State of the Art of Architecture" in Chicago'. Available at http://www.archdaily.com/774970/critical-round-up-chicago-architecture-biennial (accessed 15 October 2015).

Malnar, J. and F. Vodvarka (2004), *Sensory Design*. Minneapolis: University of Minnesota Press.

McCarter, R. and Juhani Pallasmaa (2012), *Understanding Architecture*. New York: Phaidon Press.

Merleau-Ponty, M. (1948), *The World of Perception*, translated by O. Davis (2004). New York: Routledge.

Nelson, M. K. (2015), 'Indigenous Science and Traditional Ecological Knowledge: Persistence in Place'. In R. A. Warrior (ed.), *The World of Indigenous North America*. Routledge: New York, pp. 188–214.

Nleworks.com (2015), *Rock-Chicago Lakefront Kiosk, NLÉ*. Available at http://www.nleworks.com/case/chicago-lakefront-kiosk/ (accessed 18 November 2015).

O'Donohue, J. (1999), *Eternal Echoes*. New York: HarperCollins.

Pallasmaa, J. (2001), 'Our Image Culture and Its Misguided Ideas About Freedom'. *Architectural Record* 189(1): 51–52.

Raskin, L. and Miriam Sitz (2015), 'Chicago's Next Generation'. *Architectural Record* 203(10): 102–106.

Sherman, S. M. and R. W. Guillery (2013), *Functional Connections of Cortical Areas: A New View from the Thalamus*, 'Overview'. Cambridge, MA: MIT Press. Available at https://mitpress.mit.edu/books/functional-connections-cortical-areas (accessed 13 March 2016).

Smith, P. F. (1977), *The Syntax of Cities*. London: Hutchinson & Co.

Tilley, C. (2012), *Interpreting Landscapes: Geologies, Topographies, Identities – Explorations in Landscape Phenomenology 3*. Walnut Creek, CA: Left Coast Press.

Tuan, Y. (1977), *Space and Place: The Perspective of Experience*. Minneapolis: University of Minnesota Press.

Ultramodern.net (2015), 'About'. Available at http://www.ultramoderne.net (accessed 29 November 2015).

Wainwright, O. (2015), 'Chicago Architecture Biennial Secures the City's Place as a Mecca for Building Buffs'. *The Guardian*, 5 October. Available at http://www.theguardian.com/artanddesign/architecture-design-blog/2015/oct/05/chicago-architecture-biennial-a-mecca-for-building-buffs (accessed 13 March 2016).

Woodhouse Tinucci Architects (2015), *Chicago Architecture Biennial – Piranesi Circus*. Available at http://www.woodtinarch.com/2015-cab/ (accessed 1 April 2016).

8

Music: Seeing and Feeling with the Ears

Alan Marsden and Richard Leadbeater

Introduction

Music is sound, clearly, but when listeners report their experience of listening to music, they often recount sensations of light, space and movement. Hearing music is not just a sonic experience, but also one which recruits senses other than hearing to create experiences which range from the mundane to the sublime. A listener to the music of Sibelius reported, 'All my senses are turned on, even smell and taste.' (Gabrielsson 2011: 359) In this chapter, we investigate listeners' non-sonic sensations in listening to music, in the context of four hypothesized theoretical explanations. We draw on three sources of accounts of musical experience, two from other published sources and one from our own research. We conclude with observations about the value of listening to music, and how experience of music might be fundamentally changing as a result of technological innovations.

One does not turn off senses other than hearing when listening to music, so one at least sees, smells and feels one's surroundings while listening. The degree to which these sensations can be separated from the music is uncertain, and in many situations they are clearly not separated as, for example, in the case of marching bands, or performances of John Cage's *4' 33"*, or of I Fagiolini's *The Full Monteverdi* where performers appear as members of the audience. Even in more regular situations, it is important to recognise the impact that the physical space and immediate environment has on music engagement (Krause and Hargreaves 2012; Greasley, Lamont and Sloboda 2013). We aim to focus here, however, on those sensations which are reported not as the context of listening but as *part of the experience of the music*, for example, a listener sensing dark not because the place of listening is dark but because the music is sensed *as* dark.

We also set to one side those non-sonic music experiences which arise as a result of synaesthesia. The range of phenomena which are properly described as synaesthesia are open to debate, but it is clear that some individuals have the rare experience of automatic and involuntary sensations in a sense different from the one stimulated. In the case of music, the most common synaesthetic sense associations are between pitch or harmony and colour (Marks 1975). While some famous composers are claimed to have been synaesthetes (e.g. Skryabin and Messiaen) and while synaesthesia might provide useful insights to the development and workings of the perceptual system, it seems to us, because of its rarity, to form an unpromising basis for explanation of common musical experiences. We aim instead to explore non-sonic experiences in music which do not rely on synaesthesia for their explanation.

Not every listening experience involves non-sonic sensation, but it seems sufficiently common, especially in connection with strong experiences of music, to be worthy of investigation. A middle-aged woman gave this account of hearing the electronic music of Ralph Lundsten at his studio:

> [I]nto your entire consciousness goes the most delightful, most powerful, most caressing lyrical nature music. You see the stars, you see the snow and can smell it, you enjoy the peace, you shiver in the cold, and are swept along by enormous waves. I felt as if I was transferred in time and space, as if I was in another world. (Gabrielsson 2011: 168)

This one quotation has many of the elements we will examine: memories, metaphor, a sense of movement – in the sound and in the listener, fictive objects and transportation to a different reality.

Sources

We base this chapter on three particular sources of data which we will refer to as LED (*Listening Experience Database*), SEM (*Strong Experiences with Music*) and MAM (*Magpies and Mirrors*).

The *Listening Experience Database* (LED)[1] is an online database of written accounts of listening experiences compiled in a project at the Open University and the Royal College of Music. This is a growing collection of extracts from writings which recount a particular experience of listening to or hearing music. Many are incidental accounts, where the music is not the principal subject, but many others focus on the listening in particular, whether the music is heard deliberately or accidentally. On 19 May 2015, the database was reported to include 1405 records of listening experiences. When the research on which this chapter is based was conducted, it contained 1405 records of listening experiences; on 20 April 2016, it was reported to contain 6485.

Strong Experiences of Music (SEM) (Gabrielsson 2011) is the outcome of reports from about 965 Swedes about their experiences of music, collected from the late 1980s to the present century. Respondents were asked, 'Describe in your own words the strongest (most intense, most profound) experience with music you have ever had. Try to revive it in your mind and describe your experience and reactions in as much detail as possible' (Gabrielsson 2011: 7). Most responses were written but a few were obtained by interview. The respondents were aged thirteen to ninety-one, with an even spread across this range, but a majority of women (62%) and a preponderance of musicians, amateur or professional. As the experiences reported came from any point in a respondent's life, some were from early in the twentieth century, though more than half of them occurred after 1980 (Gabrielsson 2011: 7–12). The reports were translated from Swedish by Rod Bradbury.

Our third source of data *Magpies and Mirrors* (MAM) comes from the second author's doctoral research (Leadbeater 2014) and consists of interviews conducted in 2012 with sixty-two individuals concerning their musical preferences and listening habits. As in the case of the Gabrielsson data, the respondents covered a wide age range (18 to 73), and a majority were women (61%). Their nationalities varied, but most were associated with Lancaster University, as either students or members of staff. The main purpose was to explore through heuristic semi-structured interviews the development, meaning and trajectory of music preferences across the lifespan. One's sense of identity may shift as a result of important events, such as going to university, career development, changing social friendship groups, social and cultural activities, independent travel and exposure to a variety of cultural experiences and unexpected disequilibrating events such as unemployment, illness, hospitalization and bereavement. Following the practice of Leadbeater (2014), pseudonyms are used in referring to participants with respect to the quotations from MAM below.

A key finding of this research was that music preferences evolved in response to an array of personal and social factors. The trajectory and evolution of taste took on many guises, but the accounts given by the participants broadly supported the claim that music is interpreted by many as a symbolic object of the self. For the most part music was understood to act as a powerful emotive and sensory conduit to address a wide range of functions. For our present purpose we are interested in those cases where individuals' musical engagement extended beyond pure sonic experiences. As expected, many noted that they used their music to transport themselves back in time to revisit a specific place, real or imagined, or an event in their lives, in effect to be 'there'. Yet, for others, nostalgia was only part of the experience. Some individuals experienced a sense of movement or a blurring of the boundaries of their physical presence and their immediate environment. These individuals described how the music entered or enveloped them, as if the music had become a living entity. Musical engagement was a total corporeal experience to the extent that there was no separation in body or mind between their own existence, their moods and the music. Others reported a different kind of distortion of sense of time and location. For them, engagement with music and music-related activities afforded the space to adopt and assimilate an 'exo-identity' which existed beyond their immediate socio-cultural temporal location and mundane identity.

In the following sections, we present four possible theorizations of non-sonic sensations of music, together with examples taken from our source data. We do not regard the theorizations as mutually exclusive; very likely in any particular situation more than one might be in play. Our approach to the data has been to seek and select interesting and illustrative cases. In the case of the LED data we searched using terms which were considered likely to be associated with accounts of interest (e.g. 'light', 'dark', 'wide', 'hard'). The results were trawled for suitable cases, regardless of whether or not the case reflected the kind of non-sonic sensation implied by the search term used. In the case of SEM we profited from Gabrielsson's own summaries of his data (chapters 28 and 29) to find and select noteworthy cases. The second author was of course already familiar with the MAM data. Because our approach has involved deliberate selection, with no attempt to measure the size of the pool from which we have selected, we make no claim about the prevalence of non-sonic sensations in music. Rather, our claim is that such sensations play a part in at least some cases of music-listening, and that these sensations are important because they are associated with strong experiences of music.

Memory

Music can bring a memory to mind sufficiently strongly for the listener to sense something associated with that memory. Memory of some particular earlier occasion or period when the music has been heard is often reported as a cause of strong musical experiences. Indeed, 'episodic memory' is one component of Juslin and Västfjäll's BRECVEM[2] model of music and emotion (Juslin and Västfjäll 2008), and Davies refers to this as the 'darling, they are playing our tune' phenomenon (1978).

In the book *The War Letters of a Light Infantryman*, a British soldier in France in 1917 wrote home:

> The gramophone is playing '*Un peu d'amour*,' bringing back memories of Sloley at Christmas 1914. Music is awful for reminding you of lovely times . . . This land of France is most excessively boring, and I am fed up with the war. To think that at this moment the last scene of 'Bubbly' is being played, and everyone is preparing to go and try to find a cab. Time 10.45 p.m. All the fine ladies in their fine dresses, enjoying life to

> the full, and flirting with penniless subalterns to the detriment of both. The contrast is what amazes me. (Neville 1930: 45)

Of course, this account reflects the soldier's longing to return home as much as it does his experience of the music he hears, but it is noteworthy that his account slips seamlessly from talk about music into memories of ladies in fine dresses. There is no boundary between the music as sound and the memories it evokes. The same is clear in the account of a young woman in SEM who had recently returned from Africa.

> I had never sung [*'Jesus, Du är kung'*] before in Sweden, but in Africa we often sang it. So when they start singing it here at home it is like being transported in time and space. I was back in Africa in the midst of all the missionaries who had come to mean so much to me during that year. I could even almost feel the special smell and hear the goats bleating outside. (Gabrielsson 2011: 111)

These two cases perhaps report kinds of experience which differ in their essential sensory nature. For the soldier, it is possible that the music is merely a trigger to a chain of thought and recollection, which clearly is strongly sensory – a particular song, the sight of people trying to find a cab and of ladies in fine dresses – but might operate essentially because of the associations of thought rather than of sense. In the case of the Swedish missionary, by contrast, the memory is a multi-sensory package – the felt actions of one's own singing, the interior sound of companions' singing, the exterior sound of bleating goats, and the smell. The soldier has been led into a reverie in which '*Un peu d'amour*' is no longer an essential component, but for the missionary '*Jesus, Du är kung*' is a focal part of the recollected, and re-felt, experience.

This experience of being 'taken back' or 'being there' is common. In MAM, a large proportion of participants noted that they used music to transport themselves to a specific place, a particular time or event in their lives or to remember a relationship or close family member. As TJ (male, 30, a university lecturer) commented, his music was always 'fixed in joyous nostalgia', a position echoed by Webster (male, 44), who suggested that 'music can bring you to another place . . . that's why I listen to music'. It is not just the 'joy' which is important but also the *sense* of being in a different time or place.

Significant memories associated with music were often recollected in the MAM interviews with clarity. Individuals could still remember minute details of the event, the conversations, the physical surroundings, the social context, their self-views and values of that time of their lives. For example, Ieuan (56), who considers himself to be a connoisseur of Monteverdi, can recall in detail the first time that he heard Monteverdi in the early 1980s. He openly admitted that this event was pivotal on the trajectory of his music tastes. He was visiting a friend's house for Sunday lunch when his friend put on Monteverdi's *Vespers*. With some amusement he also remembered the friend's son throwing his arms up in horror at the album, groaning aloud, 'Oh no not more Monteverdi again Dad', and stormed off. After thirty years, this event is clearly still an important event for him as a pivotal aspect in the development of his music taste palate.

Metaphor

The non-sonic sensations of music engendered by memory were originally sensed from the music's context or environment and so perhaps might be considered to have become a part of the music by association rather than being essential (though the accounts above indicate how essential they have become for the individuals concerned). This cannot apply in cases where the recounted non-sonic sensations do not depend on memory of a specific earlier experience, to which we now turn.

It is possible, in both the accounts we discuss below and in the accounts of memory discussed above, that the recourse to reports of non-sonic sensation arises because the speakers lack a vocabulary for reporting about the music as sound. In speaking about sights, smells and other sensations, perhaps the speakers mean to say things about the sound through metaphor and analogy rather than reporting real sensed experience. If this were the case, we would expect fewer non-sonic 'metaphorical' accounts from professional musicians, who have recourse to the rich vocabulary of music theory for communicating about music. There is insufficient data in the sources we have used to establish whether or not this is the case, but it is noteworthy that even the composer Aaron Copland (quoted in LED), who presumably did not lack facility in musical terminology, wrote in 'metaphorical' language: '[E]verything comes out of there in great unwashed gobs of sound that billow about you' (Copland [1943] 2013).

Even if listeners take recourse to metaphor because they have no other way of relating their experiences, the metaphors they use reveal something of the sensation of the music. Consider, for example, the words of a middle-aged woman in SEM: '[The music] was so unbelievably beautiful and [it] sort of came in waves roughly like a swell out at sea' (Gabrielsson 2011: 68). Other things could function as a metaphor for cyclic increase and decrease, a bank balance rising and falling monthly, for example, but this listener and others use a metaphor of something *sensed*, like the motion of the sea, not something of which we have perhaps more frequent or consequential experience but do not sense. Furthermore, the woman did not describe the music as becoming louder and softer, or higher and lower, language which surely must have been available to her, but sought language for a more bodily experience of 'a feeling that washed all over me'.

Indeed, perhaps we are wrong to attempt to make a distinction between 'actual' non-sonic sensations and 'metaphorical' ones. Unless we scan her brain, or use some other technique which we believe gives more direct access to her sensations, we have only the words of the woman referred to above to go on. From these, we cannot distinguish between a woman who, lacking suitable vocabulary to describe a purely sonic experience, uses words about the sea to describe her experience of music, and a woman who experiences the music *as* motion like the sea. If Lakoff and Johnson are right about the centrality of metaphor for human cognition (Lakoff and Johnson 1980), perhaps even a brain scan would show that there is no difference between 'actual' and 'metaphorical' sensation apart from the absence of the peripheral stimulus from the appropriate sense organs in the latter.

In MAM, one of the most prevalent themes to emerge was the notion that music as an object could be transformed from a sonic experience on one level to exist on another level as an engendered object, distorting the senses. Sensory perception could be transformed as the individual came to inhabit an engendered or imaginary sphere of existence within which the music could envelop the individual to the extent that they had no distinct *corpus habitus*, with no obvious separation between themselves and the emotions or identity engendered by the music. For example, one of Clay's (male, 23) favourite music styles was to listen to drone, ambient, noise death metal for its 'dark' qualities and nihilistic apocalyptic lyrical texts. Engagement with this music style often evoked a sense of physical darkness that enveloped his immediate environment. Irrespective of the brightness of the ambient light, he felt the darkness envelop him so that in effect he was 'blind'. He believed that he and the music were in unison. His physical corpus had succumbed to the power and sensory perception afforded by the music. In another example, Angela (66) described a live performance of a wind orchestra at Lancaster University that had a strong impact on her.

> And I remember physically feeling it 'there' (clenches her fist against her breastbone) the drums in particular and you don't get that from the radio. You actually get, it's not just auditory, and you actually get a corporeal experience with live music.

It is interesting to note that the clenching of the fist was for Angela a representation of both the physical and spiritual impact of the music. Similar to Clay, the music existed on two distinct but interconnected planes of existence, analogous to the 'target' and 'source' domains of linguistic metaphor. Indeed for some individuals, the amalgamation or triangulation of physical, sonic and spiritual planes of existence could cause physical movement. This action lies far beyond the minute rhythmic movements that are often associated with music engagement but may necessitate an imperative desire to move, a topic to which we now turn.

Motion Cognition

Music can 'move' its listeners, and not only in a metaphorical sense of stimulating emotions. Listeners often physically move, tapping their foot or nodding their head, often involuntarily, but we are concerned here not with such induction of movement but rather with the *sensation* of movement. Listeners commonly report either that they feel themselves to be in motion, even if in reality they are still, or that they sense the music as a moving body.

The connection between music and movement is very strong, and has been a topic of considerable recent research (Todd 1999; Godøy and Leman 2010; Larson 2012). One line of study is the phenomenon of entrainment whereby an organism – in this case a listener or performer – matches the rate of some pulsation (whether actual or immanent) with the rate of the phenomenon witnessed – in this case typically the beats of the piece of music (Clayton 2012). Entrainment is claimed to be an involuntary tendency acquired by our species because a physical or social benefit can follow from attuning to external processes. It thus explains motion in music in terms of response rather than sensation, but it might be difficult to draw a sharp distinction between automatic responses and sensations.

The other line of research on motion in music (Clarke 2005) is based on the importance of sound in the everyday environment as a carrier of information about movement. Physically, sounds can only be produced when something moves and, conversely, nothing can move without making a sound (though the sound might be one so quiet, high or low that we cannot hear it). This is not to say that for every sound we are strongly aware of the movement involved – when someone speaks our focus is not on the movement of air from their throat – but there are often cases where our focus is on the movement, such as when we hear a car approaching from behind. Many everyday sounds are thus sensed as movement, and it is not surprising that this should carry over to music also.

Aaron Copland has already been quoted above in LED where he referred to 'great unwashed gobs of sound that billow about you' (Copland [1943] 2013). LED also contains a description by Philip Larkin of a particular jazz recording, 'especially one suicidal note in the last chorus that gives me the impression of falling from an enormous height to be dashed to pieces' (Larkin 1992: 72). (It is possible that Larkin sensed himself as 'falling from an enormous height', but since it is the note which is described as 'suicidal' it seems more likely that Larkin sensed the note as falling.) The sense of sound as a moving object is conveyed particularly explicitly in an account of an ensemble performing beneath a geodesic dome.

> [The quintet] play . . . in the middle of the dome, sitting directly under the five points of the topmost pentagon, and I am very struck by how antiphonal things in the music really seem antiphonal, not experienced flatly, or on one plane as they are when you watch the players on the stage, going 'tick-tock' from side to side like a pendulum, but passing in 'deep' space from one part to another part of the dome, north-south and east-west. (Tomes 2004: 49)

Antiphony is a musical technique in which a fragment of music from one performer or group of performers is answered by another, and it is common to physically separate the groups, for example, two choirs on opposite sides of a church. For the reporter here, the three-dimensional space affords a richer experience of sound moving from place to place. In this case, the space traversed by the moving sounds was the real space under the dome, but in other cases the space is virtual, such as this from SEM:

> [A]fter some introductory downward bow movements in the accompaniment comes a soprano solo where the tone foundation of the strings becomes like a catapult for the exultant flight of the solo voice, as if lifted by invisible wings towards the heights. (Gabrielsson 2011: 329)

Sometimes music is sensed not as movement in an external space, whether real or virtual, but as music entering into or moving inside the listener, as in this account from SEM.

> Then the organ music began to fill the church. A music that I had never heard before. It was notes whirling around like snowflakes, weightless. . . . The music flooded into me, it felt as if it filled every fibre of my body and I shivered and felt frozen. (Gabrielsson 2011: 279)

A similar sense of music inside the listener is recounted in MAM by Lara (22), though this time in an unpleasant manner: 'I genuinely can't stand it [Trance / electronica music] now . . . it genuinely makes me feel like, not angry but I feel like a bubble inside me.'

Sounding Objects and Environments

Sound has two main affordances for humans: it is a carrier of messages, most often in speech but also in cases such as alarms, and it gives us information about the objects and events in our surroundings. Music hovers between, around or perhaps above these. In the twentieth century, interest grew in sound as pure sound, seen most influentially perhaps in the work of Pierre Schaeffer (1966), who originated the notion of the *objet sonore*, usually rendered in English as 'sound object', a sound as sound and not as a carrier of some message or as a sign of some object or event. To achieve the sensation of an *object sonore*, Schaeffer advocated repeated 'reduced listening' in which the listener disregards the origin of a sound and focuses purely on its sonic properties (properties which Schaeffer set out to define in his treatise). Even in the absence of reduced listening, there are good reasons for believing that sounds in hearing are more object-like than images in vision (Marsden 2014). However, the very fact that Schaeffer calls this mode of listening 'reduced' indicates the strength of the 'normal' mode in which sounds are heard in terms of the objects and events which produce them.

In the case of music, listeners are often fully aware of the instruments which produce the sounds, even in cases of recorded or broadcast sound, but unreal sounding bodies are sensed also. The accounts quoted above have referred to waves, gobs, snowflakes and bubbles, all of them, when real, objects with a distinct sonic aspect but not principally conceived as sound-generating objects. More fanciful still is this account from SEM, of listening to the slow movement of 'Beethoven's ninth' (symphony, presumably): 'I remember what it was like one evening, when I suddenly heard – *heard!* – the delightfully beautiful flower wind its way up as if out of an incense holder in front of me' (Gabrielsson 2011: 76). Even when a report explicitly refers to the actual sound source – in this case an orchestra – the sensation can be of a different kind of body entirely: 'The orchestra begins to be like one of those old toasters that we had when I was a child, it glows in the red-hot wires inside, the electricity increases in tension and tiny sounds caused by the heat can begin to be heard' (Gabrielsson 2011: 226).

Often what we sense in sound is not so much the individual objects and events around us as the general environment. To be in a small enclosed space sounds entirely different from being in a large hall or in the open air. Many listening accounts refer to the actual environment – the concert hall, the church, etcetera – and many refer to music engendering a virtual enveloping space. We referred above to the importance of music giving a sense of 'being there', and it is clear that listeners often deliberately choose to listen to specific music in order to transport themselves to a different environment. The portability and interconnectivity of modern multimedia devices mean that individuals are able to access their own music anywhere. An individual can create a chosen sonic environment, affording them the space to retreat into another sphere of experience. Leadbeater (2014) found one of the key functions afforded by music to be the ability to transport the individual to a specific place away from their immediate environment. In particular, participants in the interviews in MAM identified that to cope with the uncomfortable and crowded environments of public transport or the drudgery of the daily drive to work, they selected music to be 'there', anywhere but their actual location. For example, Jonathon (20) engaged with his music during his commute for purposes of relaxation: 'Yes, especially when I'm on the bus . . . I sort of go into a half dream-like state. It's almost like you're dreaming, you're asleep.' The workplace is also a common venue for using music to take the listener out of their immediate environment. Heye and Lamont (2010) carried out a mixed methodological study to explore the function of music through MP3 players at a university in the North West of England. They noted that individuals enjoyed listening to music to create a 'bubble' (cf. Bull 2007), but the bubble was permeable. While participants enjoyed creating their own internal worlds through the music, the outside world, that is, interruptions and conversations with colleagues took precedence. These are cases reminiscent of some of the accounts given above under the heading of 'memory', but the music takes the listener 'there' not to a real, remembered place but to a virtual place more desirable than the one they are actually in.

Conclusions

On the basis of extensive study of listeners' accounts of strong experiences with music, Gabrielsson gave his book the subtitle *Music Is Much More Than Just Music* (2011). The evidence and argument above suggests not only that music is much more than just sound, but that it is *sensed* as more than just sound. In this conclusion we explore two corollaries, about the use of music and alternative realities, and one speculation about technological developments.

It is well established that listeners are not casual in their selection of music to listen to. DeNora (2000), in a qualitative ethnographic study of women's everyday listening habits, identified that women used music as a 'technology of the self'. According to DeNora, the music was utilized as a resource of the self to relive events and past relationships in order to give meaning to their daily lives and enhance the experience of listening to music. In effect, the music appeared to satiate 'an inner need' (Dibben 2002). As explored above, in music a listener senses not just the sounds but they also re-sense – feel – features of remembered experiences associated with the music. Leadbeater (2014) affirmed the position of DeNora and Dibben, but analysis of the MAM interviews suggested that the function of music was not confined to nostalgia alone. So too the analysis above indicates that, through metaphor, motion cognition and the sensing of real or fictive sounding bodies, music can give a sensation of being in a different place. Listeners use music to take them 'there' because of the non-sonic aspects of its sensation just as much as because of its ability to conjure a memory of a different place.

The point is not that the conjuring is a trick which prods the listener into performing mental work to draw these sensations from memory or imagination (although people do both remember and imagine while listening to music), but that these sensations arise *in the hearing of the music*. The music presents for the listener a world accessible to all the senses and not just through hearing. The world is a different one from that of everyday experience, in which an eye is required to see and a nose to smell, so in this musically engendered world, light, smell, space and movement arise without the agency of those sense organs. Music generates an alternative reality, and sometimes a hyper-reality. Just as those non-sonic sensations arise without an evident proximal cause, it would seem that music can be particularly powerful when the source of its sound is not evident; the entire musical world, sound and not-sound, comes from somewhere unknown. It is striking how often in our sources strong experiences of music are associated with music from an unseen source. Two examples from LED can serve as illustrations.

> I went out on the terrace and could hear the sound of violins, guitars, and flutes, in the distance. I came in again quickly and sat down near the window so as to hear it better. It was a charming trio. I have not listened to music with so much pleasure for a long time. (Bashkirtseff [1890] 1985: 15)
>
> We had scarcely trod the stone floor of the chapel, and taken off our hats, when we were startled by a sudden peal from an organ, placed somewhere out of sight, playing a voluntary; this, however, very soon was changed into an anthem, accompanied by the sweetest notes of female voices. We stood in mute wonder, for though we heard much, we could see nothing. (Diary of an Assistant Surgeon 1841: 6–7)

Both of these accounts come from the nineteenth century, and the unseen nature of the source would have contributed to the impression of another reality, sensed only through the music. For modern listeners too, however, it is not uncommon for music to act as a means of access to another reality. In MAM the second author encountered individuals who held exo-identities (i.e. beyond their immediate socio-cultural temporal location and identity) for whom music acted as a conduit to assist in the manipulation and distortion of their own physical, social, temporal and geographical spaces. For example, Elizabeth (British, 19) is an aficionado of Korean and Japanese pop music commonly known as K-Pop and J-Pop, respectively. She is also a member of a Korean dance troupe. Yet despite her blond hair and blue eyes, during practice sessions and performances with the troupe she sees herself as holding a Korean identity. In the mirror she admitted that she sees herself as having oriental features, black hair and dark eyes. Lucy (Lithuania, 18) holds a strong affinity with culture and music of the late 1950s early 1960s and in particular she is drawn towards jazz, swing, blues and the crooners of the period. Yet her exo-identity can only exist as a fantasy. Whereas Elizabeth acts out her fantasy identity within a specific social group, for Lucy her identity is entirely internal. Outwardly she appears to have an entirely normal appearance of a modern young woman, but in her fantasy or exo-identity she sees herself and her immediate environment firmly located in the fashion of that period. In short, her external appearance and modern-day objects, such as cars and computers, are selectively removed from her sphere of conscientiousness. Lucy identifies the songs of Doris Day, Sinatra and Dave Brubeck as conduits to her fantasy identity. She described a particular common scenario which the music creates for her:

> It creates a beautiful image of for example like a pub or something, like that you know and you have all these beautiful girls, dressed nicely and usually a singer, just performing 'that' [the song] . . . I'm like completely

> out, like I can walk the street but I'm completely in the other world for example imagining myself like on a stage performing the song.

It is interesting to note here that the music engenders a sphere of consciousness that is totally removed in all aspects from her immediate environment. So although she may be walking down the street in twenty-first century Britain, she admits that she isn't aware of the cars and the immediate environment at all, but she has been relocated by the music to a stage singing.

Unlike the nineteenth-century listeners whose reports in LED were quoted above, modern listeners are used to hearing music with no instruments or players near, because most music is now heard reproduced through loudspeakers. An unseen source is the norm in musical experience. Furthermore, the manipulations of sound involved in the processes of recording, editing and production often create a final sound which can correspond to no possible actual reality. Sounds are synthesized which no real instrument can produce. Even if they sound instrument-like, they can have a precision of tuning and steadiness of tone which is a physical impossibility in a real instrument. A mix of levels and reverberations on different tracks can produce an impossible composite: a singer appears to whisper into your ear in your living room, sounding just as loud as a string orchestra which appears simultaneously to be playing in a voluminous church and a drum kit which sounds to be down a corridor somewhere. Then a moment later the singer is, as if magically, no longer whispering in your ear but belting from a stage in front of you, but no louder than she was before.

The four mechanisms of non-sonic sensation identified here – memory, metaphor, motion cognition and sounding bodies and environments – depend for their effect on a listener's implicit knowledge of where and when sounds come from. A listener knows, from experience, what kind of body is likely to be the source of a sound, in what sort of environment and with what sort of movement. This knowledge allows the listener to understand and formulate metaphors about sound by reference to other things with similar shape, pattern or movement. When listening to a performance of Stockhausen's *Kontakte*, for example, a piece for piano, percussion and tape, one can see the hitting and scraping which produce some of the sounds. But the electronically produced sounds in the tape part are equally heard as scraping and hitting sounds, regardless of the fact that one does not see anything scraped or hit and that this is not how the sounds were actually produced. However, in the twenty-first century, when music is solidly associated with sound from an unseen source manipulated in ways to make it free from the constraints of reality, music becomes dissociated from real-world sound, and the mechanisms of metaphor, motion cognition and sounding bodies and environments might cease to apply. Perhaps in the future the only non-sonic sensations of music will be of the first kind: evocation of things sensed when the music was heard before. To gain success through the kind of powerful non-sonic sensations examined here, a piece of music will then have to be accompanied by strong sensations at its first hearing, so that these can have their effect when brought to mind as the music is heard subsequently through headphones on a commuter train. Is this one of the drivers of the modern emphasis on beautiful performers, stylish videos, spectacular performances and bucolic venues?

Notes

1 The Listening Experience Database, http://www.open.ac.uk/Arts/LED/ (accessed 11 August 2016).
2 The BRECVEM model lists seven elements: brain stem reflex; rhythmic entrainment; evaluative conditioning; emotional contagion; visual imagery; episodic memory; musical expectancy.

References

Bashkirtseff, M. ([1890] 1985), *The Journal of Marie Bashkirtseff*, translated by M. Blind. London: Virago.

Bull, M. (2005), 'No Dead Air! The iPod and the Culture of Mobile Listening'. *Leisure Studies* 24(4): 343–355.

Clarke, E. (2005), *Ways of Listening: An Ecological Approach to the Perception of Musical Meaning*. Oxford: Oxford University Press.

Clayton, M. (2012), 'What Is Entrainment? Definition and Applications in Musical Research'. *Empirical Musicology Review* 7(1–2): 49–56.

Copland, A. ([1943] 2013), Letter from Aaron Copland to Leonard Bernstein, 11 April 1943. In N. Simeone (ed.), *The Leonard Bernstein Letters*. New Haven, CT: Yale University Press, p. 122. Extract in *The Listening Experience Database*. Available at http://data.open.ac.uk/led/lexp/1388235301166 (accessed 11 June, 2015).

Davies, J. B. (1978), *The Psychology of Music*. London: Hutchinson.

DeNora, T. (2000), *Music in Everyday Life*. Cambridge: Cambridge University Press.

Diary of an Assistant Surgeon, No. I (1841), *The Asiatic Journal and Monthly Register for British and Foreign India, China, and Australasia* 35: 4–14. Extract in *The Listening Experience Database*. Available at http://data.open.ac.uk/page/led/lexp/1374143475 (accessed 30 June 2015).

Dibben, N. (2002), 'Gender Identity and Music'. In Raymond Macdonald, David Hargreaves and Dorothy Miell (eds), *Musical Identities*. Oxford: Oxford University Press, pp. 117–134.

Gabrielsson, A. (2011), *Strong Experiences with Music: Music Is Much More than Just Music*, translated by Rod Bradbury. Oxford: Oxford University Press.

Godøy, R. I. and M. Leman (eds) (2010), *Musical Gestures: Sound, Movement and Meaning*. Milton Park: Routledge.

Greasley, A., A. Lamont and J. Sloboda (2013), 'Exploring Musical Preferences: An In-Depth Qualitative Study of Adults' Liking for Music in their Personal Collections'. *Qualitative Research in Psychology* 10(4): 402–427.

Heye, A. and A. Lamont (2010), 'Mobile Listening Situations in Everyday Life: The Use MP3 Players While Travellling'. *Musicae Scientiae* 14: 95–120.
Juslin, P. and D. Västfjäll (2008), 'Emotional Responses to Music: The Need to Consider Underlying Mechanisms'. *Behavioural and Brain Sciences* 31(5): 559–575.
Krause, A. and D. Hargeaves (2012), 'myTunes Digital Music Library Users and their Self-Images'. *Psychology of Music* 45(5): 531–544.
Lakoff, G. and M. Johnson (1980), *Metaphors We Live By*. Chicago: University of Chicago Press.
Larkin, P. (1992), *Selected Letters of Philip Larkin 1940–1985*, edited by A. Thwaite. London: Faber & Faber. Extract in *The Listening Experience Database*. Available at http://data.open.ac.uk/led/lexp/1387188546771 (accessed 24 June 2015).
Larson, S. (2012), *Musical Forces: Motion, Metaphor and Meaning in Music*. Bloomington, IN: Indiana University Press.
Leadbeater, R. (2014), 'Magpies and Mirrors: Identity as a Mediator of Music Preferences across the Lifespan'. PhD, Lancaster University, Lancaster.
Marks, L. E. (1975), 'On Coloured-Hearing Synesthesia: Cross-Modal Translations of Sensory Dimensions'. *Psychological Bulletin* 82(3): 303–331.
Marsden, A. (2014), 'Echoes in Plato's Cave: Ontology of Sound Objects in Computer Music and Analysis'. *Proceedings of International Computer Music Conference & Sound and Music Computing Conference*, Athens, pp. 41–46.
Neville, J. E. H. (1930), *The War Letters of a Light Infantryman*. London: Sifton, Praed & Co. Extract in *The Listening Experience Database*. Available at http://data.open.ac.uk/led/lexp/1389645864656 (accessed 11 June 2015).
Schaeffer, P. (1966), *Traité des objets musicaux*. Paris: Éditions du Seuil.
Todd, N. P. M., D. J. O'Boyle and C. S. Lee (1999), 'A Sensory-Motor Theory of Rhythm, Time Perception and Beat Induction'. *Journal of New Music Research* 28(1): 5–28.
Tomes, S. (2004), *Beyond the Notes: Journeys with Chamber Music*. Woodbridge, Suffolk: Boydell Press. Extract in *The Listening Experience Database*. Available at http://data.open.ac.uk/page/led/lexp/1402317533198 (accessed 29 June 2015).

Part 3

Vision, Touch and Technologies of Sense

9

Art Spectatorship and Haptic Visuality: An Eye-Movement Analysis Exploring Painting and Embodied Cognition

Beth Harland and Nick Donnelly

Introduction

A painting is a highly coded 'world', which we interpret through engaging with its syntax, composition and style. It has agency in that it *makes* something in the world rather than simply representing the world. Of course, art works do have a representational function, they can be *read*, but the form of their agency is complex in that it also operates at the level of *affect*. Here affect refers to intensities in bodily state, variously elaborated in philosophy, social science and art theory, and places emphasis on the activation of sensation and bodily experience: '[F]ollowing Spinoza, we might define affect as the effect another body, for example an art object, has upon my own body and my body's *duration*'(O'Sullivan 2001: 126). In acknowledging that a painting creates affects, or as Deleuze and Guattari (1994) would say, a *bloc of sensations* that is reactivated by the spectator, our attention needs to turn to our encounter and physical interaction with the work.

For cognitive science, as well as art theory, affect is important in developing an understanding of embodied cognition in which senses co-mingle. In what follows we utilize methods from both of these disciplines to explore the experience of the art spectator in relation not simply to vision but also touch and the notion of a 'haptic visuality' (Marks 2000). The ways in which tactility can be experienced through looking is discussed with reference to two artists whose paintings present us with a particularly rich experience in this respect, and who are linked, through aspects of their practices, across the divide of two centuries: Velazquez and Manet.

We introduce a case study of experimental work using eye-tracking and verbalization, with Manet's *A Bar at the Folies-Bergère* as a stimulus. After first outlining the context for exploring this work from the perspective of multisensory response, we present the data from this study and offer interpretations. The resulting discussion begins to address the impact on spectator experience of a haptic stylistic approach to painting, and the impact of viewing the original *Bar* painting as against a reproduction of it. Differences in patterns of inspection are explored through two comparisons: first, we analyse data from experts and novices in pictorial spectatorship while viewing the original painting in situ, under free-viewing conditions[1] as against the same group viewing the painting following a specific task instruction. Second, we explore data from novices while viewing the original painting in situ, as against novices viewing a photographic reproduction of the painting. We are interested in whether the painting can evoke a particular type of seeing, one which moves beyond the singularly visual and into the tactile, and to what extent this relies upon a direct experience of the actual painting. Our aim is to examine viewers' experience of a sensation of tactility, and the idea that possibly other senses than vision can also be activated in encounters with actual paintings in a way that is less pronounced, or virtually neutralized, when looking at reproductions of those works. We see this as a method for further exploration of the multisensory dimensions of spectatorship and the qualitative difference of viewing an actual painting as opposed to a reproduction.

Context

There has been a recognition by cultural theorists in recent times that several centuries of European ocularcentrism, in which vision is both dominant and separate as a sense, needs to be challenged (see Jay 1993). Some have referred to the categories 'haptic' and 'optic' devised by Alois Riegl at the beginning of the twentieth century as a means of developing a relation with touch in the act of seeing. Haptic space is defined by close vision, while optical space indicates a more distant, detached view, and thus in terms of Western art, relates to the dominant convention of linear perspective. Jay explores the impact of perspectival vision on the construction of the spectator's position, through which the multiple vantage points of the medieval view were replaced 'by one sovereign eye . . . a monocular unblinking fixed eye (or more precisely, abstract point), rather than the two active, stereoscopic eyes of embodied actual vision, which give us the experience of depth perception' (Jay 2000: 54–55).

The term 'haptic visuality' was introduced by Laura Marks to describe certain filmic images that propose an experience of looking involving multiple sensory impressions: '[I]f vision can be understood to be embodied, touch and other senses necessarily play a part in vision'(Marks 2000: 22).

We propose that the notion of a haptic visuality is an interesting one to apply to spectator experience of certain paintings, focusing on Manet but beginning with Velazquez, who was working in the period immediately after the Renaissance, when the scopic regime of perspective became established.[2]

The Renaissance period is a complex one in terms of the senses and the development of painterly representation. As well as setting perspective and mathematics to work in various forms, there were ways in which the full range of our senses were both depicted and evoked. This was a period in which notions of the senses began to alter with increasing urban growth, new religious cultures and technological innovations (in painting, specifically, the introduction of oil painting as well as linear perspective). Though the notion of *aesthesis*, meaning our complete sensorial experience and the way in which we know through our bodies, goes back to Aristotle, the conception of the senses as interconnected was strong in this period. There are instances of painters reflecting upon inter-sensory relations, particularly sight and touch, an example of which can be seen in the description of a contest between a number of seventeenth-century Dutch painters. In this contest, Hoogstraten, a pupil of Rembrandt, selects the artist van Goyen for praise because he did not devise his paintings in advance, as was the prevailing method, but allowed them to emerge in the process of painting. The approach of van Goyen, including his liking of impasto, thick paint directly applied with fingers as well as brushes, is elsewhere characterized less positively as one in which the mind and the eye are placed within the hand. This has been seen as 'a fine instance of an early modern painter's haptic visuality and through such interconnectedness, of directly enhancing the viewer's sensory and emotional engagement' (Roddenberg 2014: 7).

Roddenberg makes a case for further attention to be given to contextualization in studies of history and cognition, as we see, for example, in work on 'situated cognition' (see Robbins and Ayede 2009): 'The socially and environmentally contextualized body thinks along with the brain' (Scheer in Roddenberg 2014: 17). Yet, as David Howes (2014: 1) notes, a strong hierarchy of the senses had developed, the emphasis on sight in Western society giving rise to the notion that this was the noblest of the senses, linked to intellectual enlightenment. In these terms however, the Renaissance can be seen as 'setting the importance of sight in relation to its ability to provide the ground for multisensory anticipations of the world' (Quiviger 2014: 174). Earlier established signs in painting had begun to prompt viewers towards considering their own sensory experiences and there was an increasing move towards realism, one that represents a 'shifting from the vocabulary of signs to representations evoking textures and tactile sensation' (Quiviger 2014: 176). Quiviger's account argues that, following the focus of Renaissance artists on figuration, painters became more interested in the expression of sensation, although the sensory world in painters' work has been little studied in the post-Renaissance period. As a backdrop to the work of Velazquez in the Baroque period that followed, this provides a useful context. She also makes the point that the early moderns 'believed in the ability of the imagination to make present what was not', and that this belief in images to represent and stimulate, to evoke multisensory response, might be seen in relation to neuroscientific theories of mirror neurons today (Quiviger 2014: 200). While the study of separate individual senses has been dominant in psychology, Howes (2014: 154) makes the point that 'in recent years a more interactive, relational approach to the understanding of how senses function has begun to take shape'. Our study takes this approach, utilizing experimental psychology to explore multisensory aspects of pictorial spectatorship.

The haptic qualities that we see in paintings by Velazquez, and later in Manet, are evoked through showing the viewer something particular about the surface of an object: the way the light catches it; the density of the material; the distinct difference between one surface and another. This sense of being 'shown things' seems to evoke sensations that we may take for granted in most usual situations, perceptions with cognitive significance but also coloured by affect that we may not necessarily remark on ordinarily because of the complexity, and yet familiarity, of lived moments which follow swiftly one from the other. A painting halts or slows this flow and gives us, in the case of the examples we are focusing on, a view of fleeting phenomena that is orchestrated specifically to remark them. This is where the painting differs from a photograph; it is in the editing involved in painting a scene as opposed to photographing it that time is controlled differently. The record of time and the details of the visual field operate indexically in a photograph,[3] whereas in a painting, the choice of inflection is entirely different and operates in a more transformative manner. In the paintings of Velazquez, the senses are collectively evoked, vision is not separated from touch: when looking at Velazquez's *Las Meninas* we see the boy place his foot playfully on the dog's back, but we also experience something of the pressure, weight and sense of touch, somehow jointly applying to both the boy's foot and the dog's back. It is the precise 'marking' of this tactile moment, an event in a world, that is remarkable. The surfaces depicted have a 'summary' quality in his paintings, the detail is 'just-enough' to convey this particular quality. What we will call this 'just-enoughness' indicates a quality of depiction that is highly evocative of the particular surface depicted. This is achieved without giving us the level of detail that the eye at the point of fixation (when the area of the retina with sufficient cells to provide highly detailed information is operative), or indeed the photograph at the point of sharp focus, would record. Brown (2008: 163) describes Velazquez as 'an artist who is creating a new way to paint, based on inference not description, in which the spectator is compelled to become a participant in the process of creation and not merely an observer'. A similar point is made in an experimental psychology study by DiPaola et al. (2010: 146) with reference to Rembrandt's paintings: '[T]extural agency techniques help to guide the viewer's gaze through the "act of finishing the painting" as a personal and subjective mental act, rather than experiencing the artwork in the more mechanical way one might view a uniformly detailed photograph.' Also highlighted in DiPaola's study is the point that what the authors call 'textural agency' in Rembrandt began with the late paintings of Titian: 'Noted art historian David Rosand described the appeal of these late paintings as "tactile as well as visual, inviting us to touch as well as to look"' (DiPaola 2010: 147). Titian was a painter who also influenced Velazquez[4] and at a similar point historically, as Velazquez and Rembrandt were working roughly parallel in time.

Brown (2008: 152) describes a passage in Velazquez's London portrait of Phillip IV as 'notational' and providing 'the minimal amount of definition required to reproduce the sparkling highlights of the silvery embroidered costume'. It would seem reasonable to suggest that the transformative nature of this 'just-enoughness' in paintings such as Velazquez's and later, Manet's, relies to some extent upon the direct experience of the painted surface, its textures and presence, and that the reproduction rather takes us back towards the type of experience that photography of the original scene would offer.

Velazquez's paintings seem to many to evoke the almost startlingly real presence of the figures and objects he portrayed, and yet in such a way that the artistry involved is difficult to pin down. Accurately described by Alpers (2005: 154) as a 'dissembling' of the painting's art, which she also picks up in Kenneth Clark's remarks on spectating Velazquez's work as, while moving back and forth between the casual brushwork of the close-up view and the 'real appearance of the painted world distantly viewed', there is a difficulty of locating the sensory effect achieved. The way in which the execution of the painting closely (if mysteriously) registers life itself, is again confirmed in the absence of composition – the fact that the pictures seem hardly to have been composed (Alpers 2005: 154).

There is much documented evidence that Manet considered Velazquez to be 'the greatest artist there has ever been' (Letter to Baudelaire, Wilson-Bareau 1991: 36), having studied his work on a trip to Madrid in 1865. The similarities between their ideals and techniques include the central importance of the portrait and the use of gesture, but also 'the painting of cloth' (Alpers 2005: 226), which clearly indicates that Manet noted the way in which visual information is distilled in Velazquez's painting of surfaces and textures. This interest is described by Manet's friend and commentator Antonin Proust as residing in the economy and frankness with which the paint is handled. We should note a trajectory in painted depiction towards more abbreviated means, from the sixteenth century onwards, leads to interesting examples in works by contemporary figurative painters such as Wilhelm Sasnal, Luc Tuymans and Marlene Dumas, though a full discussion of this development is beyond the scope of this chapter.

Case study

In our original experimental study of Manet's *A Bar at the Folies-Bergère* (Figure 9.1), conducted in 2012 in situ at the Courtauld Gallery, London (Harland et al. 2014), the intention was to ascertain whether the complex 'double relation' (Fried 1996) in the picture's forceful address to the viewer, which is described in art theory as bringing into focus the role of the spectator themselves as well as the subject of the painted scene, is in reality experienced by the viewer. The study found that the extent to which this was the case varied across novices and experts in art spectatorship, with only the experts recognizing that the visual puzzle set up by the reflections in the mirror behind the bar positioned them as viewers in this particular way. However, something of the 'double relation' effect is picked up by novice viewers, through the ambiguity of the barmaid's gaze. This gaze, characteristic in Manet's work, has been explored in a further study we have conducted of his portraits. We note that the 'double relation' in many of his works is primarily the result of the sitter's gaze appearing distracted, misaligned and highly ambiguous to the viewer, and this is something that is not only registered by those with expertise in art spectatorship, but is also familiar to all in acts of social cognition.

A number of questions arose from this study of *A Bar at the Folies-Bergère* around the difference in spectator experience of the actual painting

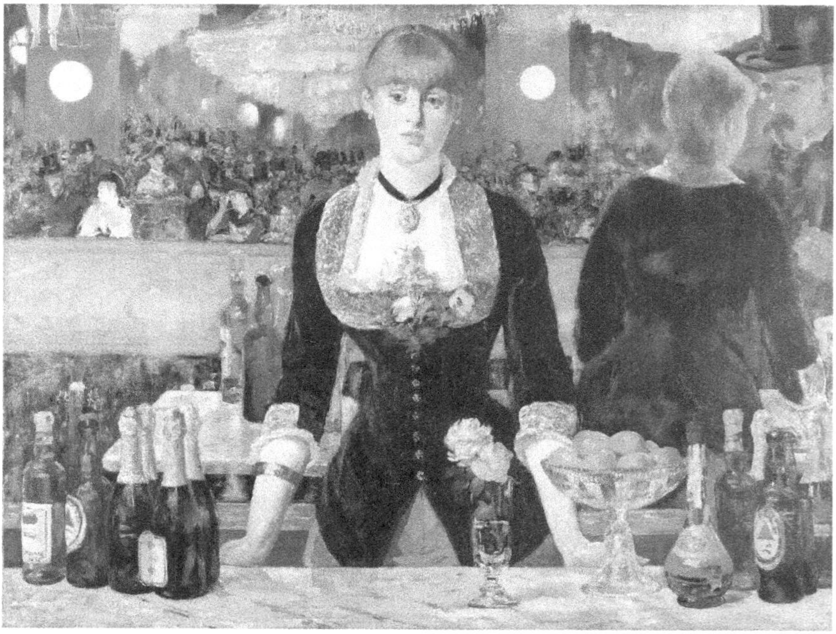

FIGURE 9.1 Edouard Manet, *A Bar at the Folies-Bergère*, 1882. Courtesy the Courtauld Gallery, London.

and of a to-scale reproduction of it. The question of whether the patterns of inspection of participants differ in response to the painting itself in situ and its photographic reproduction has a number of implications, but here we focus on what it tells us about the extent to which the act of spectatorship is multidimensional in sensory terms. We asked: does textural agency (DiPaola 2010) influence spectatorship in this painting and does the presence of the texture in the actual painting have an impact on what viewers look at, as compared with the reproduction?

Method

Four expert and four novice spectators viewed the original painting in situ at the Courtauld Gallery, and sixteen novices viewed a to-scale reproduction of the picture in the lab. All spectators had their eye movements and speech recorded as they described the image and their response to it. Eye movement data was recorded using a uniquely designed perambulatory, head-mounted eye tracker consisting of a camera pointing towards the scene and one directed towards one eye, mounted onto a pair of goggles.[5]

Eye movement and voice recordings were taken as participants free-viewed the painting and then in response to the question: 'To what extent do you feel included in or excluded from the scene?'

Results

To explore eye movements during the task, the painting was coded into regions of interest (ROIs). ROIs were defined on the basis of figures, objects, object clusters and regions (see Figure 9.2). We report the total viewing time to each region.[6] The eye movement data are summarized in Figure 9.3. The small numbers of participants able to view the painting in situ make formal statistical analysis of these data difficult. In the present study we considered means (averages) as being different if the standard errors (a measure of variation around means) for the means being compared did not overlap.

Observation 1: Comparing expert and novices spectatorship of the actual painting

In order to consider the questions outlined, we can explore *A Bar at the Folies-Bergere* as an image with different 'affordant' properties, according to J. J.Gibson's definition of affordance as what is offered to us in an interrelation with our environment, the term '*implies the complementarity of the animal and the environment*' (Gibson 1979: 127). We here label these levels of affordancy as:

1. Graspability
2. Social significance
3. Visual puzzles (the mirror reflections, the trapeze)

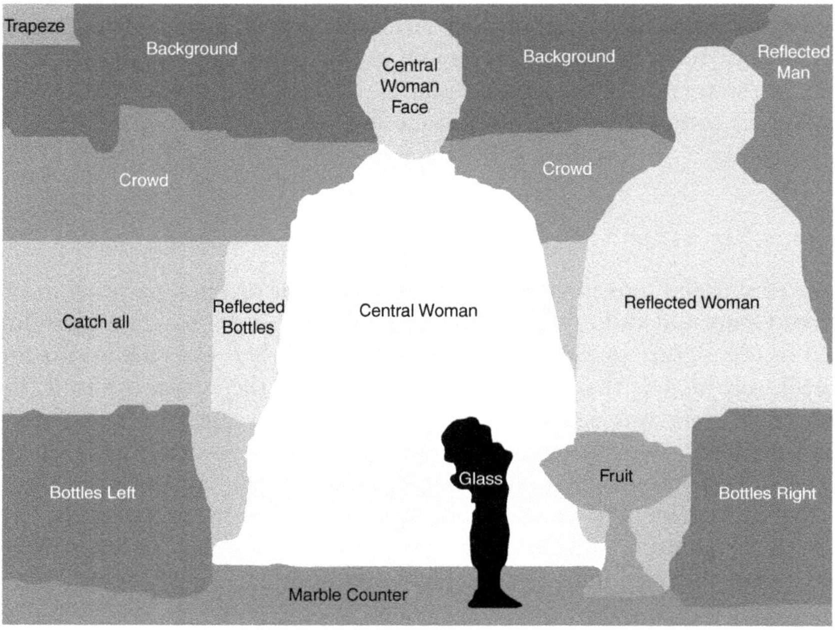

FIGURE 9.2 *The painting segmented into regions of interest.*

In freeviewing, we can be confident that experts looked more at the reflected bottles, the trapeze and the reflected man than novices. All these attributes of the painting fall within affordancy 3.

In response to being asked a question about their sense of inclusion and exclusion, experts looked more than novices at the triad of the woman's face and the reflected man and woman. The experts also attended more than novices to the fruit and glass (containing flowers). We conclude that here experts attend to the affordances of graspability (affordancy 1) and social significance (affordance 2). The shift in the strategy of experts across conditions was evident in their verbal reports.

Observation 2: Comparing novices' spectatorship of the actual painting as against the reproduction of the painting

In the freeviewing task, novices engaged more with five aspects of the painting when viewing the original compared with the reproduction. Areas

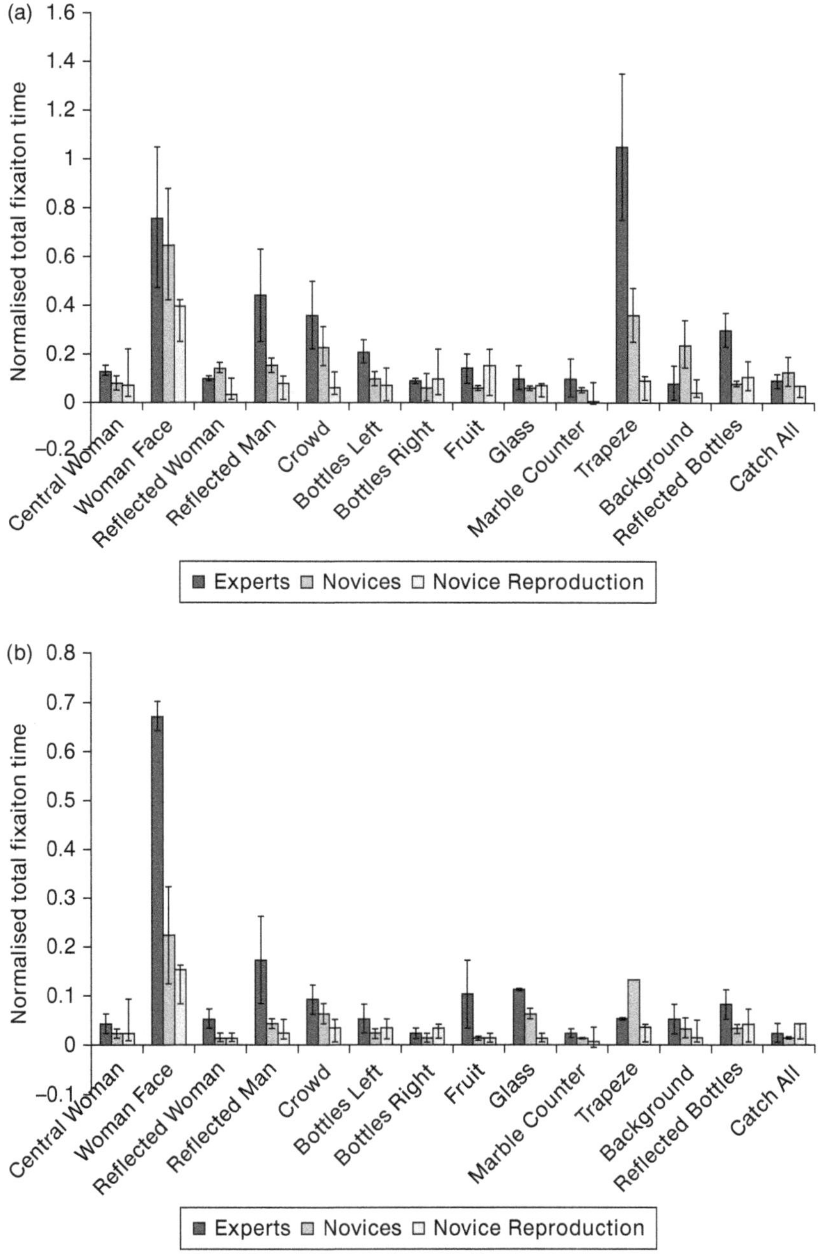

FIGURE 9.3 *Eye movement data from freeviewing (Panel A) and inclusion/exclusion (Panel B) conditions.*

in the upper part of the painting (background crowd, trapeze, reflected woman) and lower part of the painting (marble counter, glass) drew more attention in the original than the reproduction. While the lower region draws attention through its fine detail, the upper region does so because the painting is more textural than its reproduction. In fact, the whole of the reflected area behind the bar is rendered in a looser way, the non-reflected elements are painted in more detail, with finer, less-textured brushwork. The scattered brushwork of the textured crowd draws spectators' attention only in the presence of the painting.

In the inclusion/exclusion task novices look more at the glass and the trapeze in the original painting than in the reproduction. As with experts, consideration of inclusion and exclusion diminished inspection of the background. It may be that the painting of the glass better afforded direct interaction than did its reproduction (affordance 2). Alternatively, given that this effect was limited to the glass, it may simply be that the reproduction failed to capture the reflective quality of the glassy lustre, reducing its salience.

Interestingly, novices attend more to the trapeze in the real painting than the reproduction, and they do so in both the freeviewing and inclusion/exclusion tasks. This is likely to result from the impact of this unusual object in a bar scene being more readily noticeable in the actual painting and somewhat less defined through texture and colour in the reproduction, as is the rest of the background.

Discussion

With respect to the present question of art spectatorship and eye movements, our case study has revealed two important points. First, viewing the painting rather than the reproduction does have an impact on the spectatorship of novices and this can be described largely in terms of the enhanced sense of space that is experienced in the original. The depth of field, communicated both through the presence of fine detail in the foreground and textural agency in the background of the painting, is more readily conveyed by the actual painting. Regions of the painting present fundamental differences to the viewer in relation to the low frequency visual processing of roughly painted areas and high frequency of fine brushwork: 'low-spatial-frequency information, which is transmitted very rapidly to many regions of the visual system . . . [helps] orient the eyes to points of possible interest' (DiPaola 2010: 145). The salience of the crowd in the original painting is largely lost in the reproduction and we suggest that this is as a result of loss of texture which thus impedes the capacity of the painting to operate as haptic visuality. A novice's sensitivity to the bottom-up (or stimulus-driven) cues to depth works against the role of a reflecting mirror as, for them, the cues to a mirror are weak and they do not have confidence in interpreting the scene as showing a reflection. It seems that understanding the presence of the mirror in the painting requires applying prior knowledge to its perception (so-called top-down perception). Evidence for this is in the importance of the triadic figure relationship for experts but not novices. Only experts see and consider the three figures as a triad. They alone understand the painting as showing a reflection and the implication that the trio of figures has for them as spectator, that is, that they themselves take the place of the man and become aware of the 'double relation' (Fried 1996) of the painting's address to them.

Second, we find that when tasked with considering how the painting includes and excludes them, experts do change their viewing strategy. Here we see evidence of experts processing all three of the affordances we outlined: for them the painting affords grasping, social significance and the visual puzzles when they are tasked with determining inclusion and exclusion, but not when merely freeviewing the painting. The evidence for profound changes in strategy with novices is much weaker. We noted above how the failure to understand the unseen mirror limits the possibilities for shifting strategy. Evidence of a shifting strategy in novices was restricted to a focus on the glass, suggesting some partial sensitivity to the affordance of grasping.

In conclusion, the data show two things. First, seeing the painting rather than a reproduction influences the spectatorship of novices through the additional bottom-up perceptual information of increased textural definition in the painting. Second, prior knowledge of the painting qualitatively changes how it is perceived by spectators. Spectatorship is a function of bottom-up and top-down influences on perception and these influences can be laid open by exploring eye movements.

In terms of the impact of viewing the actual painting over a reproduction, the increased saliency of the crowd is the most important aspect. It is likely that the main driver of this difference is the effect of textural agency that might be said to involve the viewer in the mental act of 'finishing' the painting. The technique of indicating a summary representation of objects and surfaces, with just enough information to indicate their particular quality, contributes to this sense in which the act of spectatorship becomes proactive. This approach, which we see in the paintings of Velazquez, who was so influential in the development of Manet's style, makes a particular appeal to the viewer, in part through evoking a sense of tactility, in other words to a haptic visuality. We suggest that when viewing a reproduction of the painting, the flattening of the image that occurs when certain textual cues become less clear, does have an impact on the haptic space that is palpable in the original painting. This impact is noted for all types of viewers, though experts appear more attuned to the textural agency of the painting and experience a stronger sense of haptic visuality than do novices.

The radically new mode of address to the viewer introduced by Manet's paintings, which Fried (1996) calls 'facingness', is one by which the spectator is challenged. These paintings require interpretive agency; they evoke a world in which the agent (spectator) acts, which introduces both freedom and pressure upon them. *A Bar at the Folies-Bergère* is a striking example of this, in part through the visual puzzle it sets up in the reflected figures, but also through its haptic qualities. These artworks, being objects as well as in some sense worlds of their own, contain multiple moments of time, developed during both their production and viewing. The patterns of pictorial inspection that unfold in different viewing conditions can tell us much about the factors that influence our viewing experience and, with further study, can reveal more about the nature of multisensory, embodied cognition in art spectatorship.

Notes

1 In freeviewing the participant is simply asked to look at the painting without being given a question to consider.
2 See M. Jay (2012) 'Scopic Regimes of Modernity Revisited', in I. Heywood and B. Sandywell, *The Handbook of Visual Culture*, pp. 102–114.
3 Charles Peirce's term 'indexicality' describes the physical relationship between the object photographed and the photographic image.
4 Velazquez knew Titian's paintings from Philip IV's collection in Madrid, and in 1629 he went to Italy to study the works of the Italian masters. As Lopez-Rey (1999: 77) notes, he was influence particularly by Venetian painters, Titian most of all: he 'seized upon the peculiarities of Titian's brushstroke'.
5 Videos were recorded at 30Hz (sampling every 33.3 ms). The resulting video feeds were recorded onto a Lenovo X201 tablet laptop, using the University of Southampton's EyeCalibrator software. To optimize gaze-point estimation, a five-point calibration was achieved by aligning participant gaze with the four corners of the painting and the locket around the neck of the central woman.
6 The data were normalized by ROI surface area of the appropriate ROI. This was done in order to ensure they reflect the importance of ROIs rather than their size.

References

Alpers, S. (2005), *The Vexations of Art: Velazquez and Others*. New Haven and London: Yale University Press.

Bacci, F. and D. Melcher (eds) (2011), *Art and the Senses*. Oxford: Oxford University Press.

Brown, J. (2008), *Collected Writings on Velazquez*. New Haven and London: Yale University Press.

Cerf, M., E. P. Frady and C. Koch (2009), 'Faces and Text Attract Gaze Independent of the Task: Experimental Data and Computer Model'. *Journal of Vision* 9(12): 10, 1–15.

Deleuze, G. and F. Guattari (1994), *What Is Philosophy?* London: Verso.

DiPaola, S., C. Riebe and J. T. Enns (2010), 'Rembrandt's Textural Agency: A Shared Perspective in Visual Art and Science'. *Leonardo* 3(42): 145–151.

Fried, M. (1996), *Manet's Modernism; or, the Face of Painting in the 1860s*. Chicago and London: The University of Chicago Press.
Harland, B., J. Gillett, C. M. Mann, J. Kass, H. J. Godwin, S. P. Liversedge and N. Donnelly (2014), 'Modes of Address in Pictorial Art: An Eye Movement Study of Manet's Bar at the Folies-Bergère'. *Leonardo* 47(3): 241–247.
Howes, D. and C. Classen (2014), *Ways of Sensing: Understanding the Senses in Society*. London: Routledge.
Jay, M. (1993), *Downcast Eyes*. Berkeley: University of California Press.
Jay, M. (2012), 'Scopic Regimes of Modernity Revisited'. In I. Heywood and B. Sandywell (eds), *The Handbook of Visual Culture*. London and New York: Berg, pp. 102–114.
Lopez-Rey, J. (1999), *Velázquez, Catalogue Raisonné*. Vol 1. Cologne: Taschen.
Marks, L. U. (2000), *The Skin of the Film*. Durham and London: Duke University Press.
O'Sullivan, S. (2001), 'The Aesthetics of Affect: Thinking beyond Representation'. *Angelaki, Journal of the Theoretical Humanities* 6(3): 125–135.
Quiviger, F. (2014), 'Art and the Senses: Representation and Reception of Renaissance Sensation'. In *A Cultural History of the Senses*. Vol 3. London: Bloomsbury.
Robbins, P. and M. Ayede (eds) (2009), *Cambridge Handbook of Situated Cognition*. Cambridge: Cambridge University Press.
Roodenburg, H. (ed.) (2014), *A Cultural History of the Senses*. Vol. 3. London: Bloomsbury.
Wilson-Bareau, J. (1991), *Manet by Himself*. New York: Little, Brown and Company.

10

Sensing Atoms and Bits

Paul Coulton

Introduction

It was Milgram, Takemura, Utsumi and Kishino who introduced the Virtuality Continuum in 1995 (Milgram et al. 1995) and highlighted that the distinction between real and virtual[1] was increasingly not a hard boundary, but one in which both the real and the virtual coexisted. However, in the intervening years our experience of this continuum has increasingly taken place through flat glass screens that primarily address our senses of sight and touch. With the emergence of the so called Internet of Things (IoT) as a global infrastructure of networked physical objects, or 'things', that are readable, recognizable, locatable, addressable and/or controllable via the Internet (Coulton, Burnett, Gradinar, Gullick and Murphy 2014), designers will be able to consider interactions that can encompass all of our senses relating to the real and the virtual aspects of these objects as they are constructed from both 'Atoms and Bits'.

While the physicality of these things will undoubtedly allow a richer range of sensory experiences to be created, the design challenge of ensuring the interactions are perceived by and understandable to users is a complex task. This is because, as users, our understanding of interactions is based not simply on the sensory information we receive in relation a particular action. Rather, this understanding is established from our perception of what 'should' happen in relation to the action, which in turn is based upon our existing understanding of the these objects operating in a particular context. As Richard Langton Gregory states:

> Perception is not determined simply by the stimulus patterns; rather it is a dynamic searching for the best interpretation of the available data . . . The senses do not give us a picture of the world directly; rather they provide evidence for checking hypotheses about what lies before us. Indeed, we may say that a perceived object is a hypothesis, suggested and tested by sensory data. (Gregory 1997)

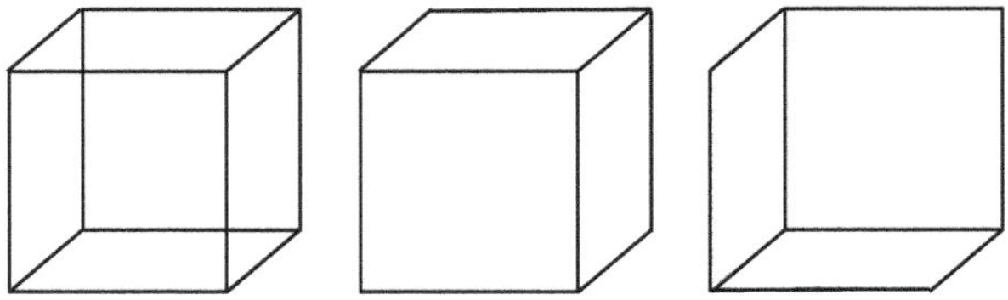

FIGURE 10.1 *Necker cube.* © Paul Coulton, Lancaster University.

An important aspect of this is the distinction between what information we passively sense and what meaning we may actively perceive from this information. As an example of this, Gregory highlights the Necker Cube, shown on the left of Figure 10.1, which presents the observer with two different hypothesis, shown in the centre and on the right, with no indication of which interpretation is correct.

While product design and user interface design have developed an understanding of user perception when designing real and virtual objects, respectively, they have rarely been combined, and designers addressing the design of things that encompass both must therefore develop new practices that draw from both of these disciplines. In this chapter, I will present a discussion of the new design sensibilities required for things comprised of, and residing within, a world of Atoms and Bits.

A World of Atom and Bits

The creation of the Virtuality Continuum (Milgram et al. 1995), shown in section (a) of Figure 10.2, highlighted that there was/is considerable opportunity to blur the boundaries within the hybrid/mixed reality that is situated between the real and the virtual. While a continuum suggests a range of possibilities, in intervening years research and development has primarily considered either virtual reality, or the two intermediate states of Augmented Reality (AR) and Augmented Virtuality (AV). AR represents a specific point on the continuum that describes virtual objects that are: dynamically integrated into a view of the real world; in real-time; and correctly situated in three dimensional space (Drascic and Milgram 1996). AV, on the other hand, describes physical objects that are dynamically integrated into, and can interact with, a virtual world in real-time (Drascic and Milgram 1996).

More recently research attention has predominantly focussed on AR implemented on mobile phones (Čopič Pucihar and Coulton 2014) although VR has recently undergone a resurgence of interest with the appearance of low cost VR Head Mounted Displays (HMD), such as the Occulus Rift.[2] In terms of the characterization of human activity within the continuum, it is predominantly expressed as either liminal or liminoid as shown in section (b) of Figure 10.2. Liminal refers to a threshold and is used to indicate that a being is between two states, neither here nor there, whereas liminoid

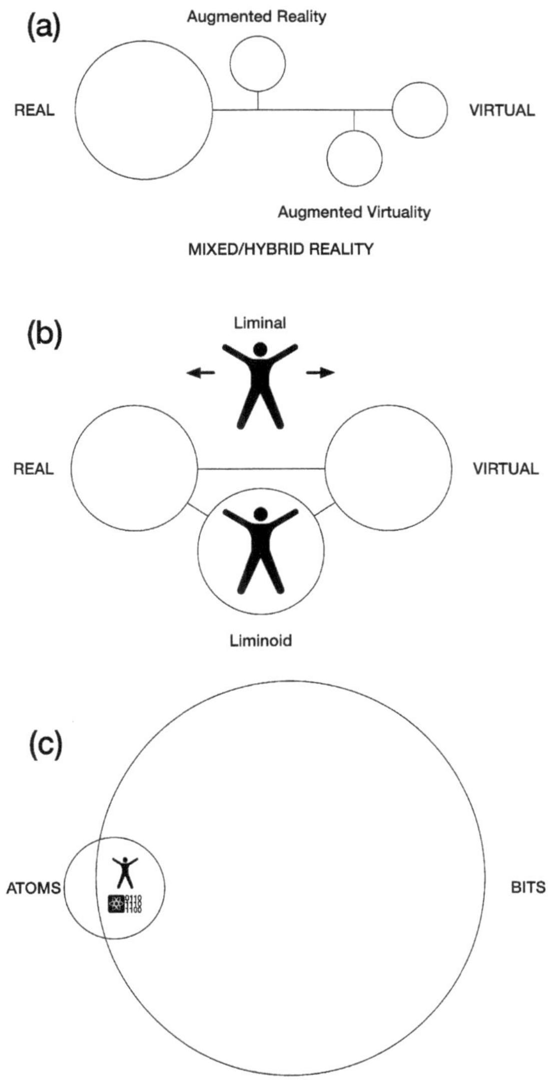

FIGURE 10.2 *Representations of hybrid worlds.* © Paul Coulton, Lancaster University.

represents activities outside normal life, such as theatre. This shared characterization of separation is likely due to a number of factors but has arguably been enhanced by the early representations of virtual reality as an alternative, and largely separate, world, and that our experiences of mixed reality have been predominantly mediated through computer screens. Given the proliferation of wireless infrastructures and networks, we are now living in what Anthony Dunne described as the 'electrosphere' (Dunne 2005), and since these networks are controlled by computer algorithms, we have effectively added a layer of code to much of our physical world. This layer of code also facilitates our access to the Internet which, with the advent of the IoT, is no longer going to be principally available through screens, but increasingly more mundane everyday objects. Thus the characterizations of liminal and limnoid no longer seem applicable as the Internet 'will no longer be a space we visit but the place we live in' (Coulton 2015) as represented in section (c) of Figure 10.2.

If designers are to design for such a world, they must develop new ways of framing the objects, interactions and spaces that make such worlds. In the following sections I will consider such characterizations.

Things Made from Atoms and Bits

Due to the extensive range of design possibilities, there is currently no accepted way of classifying IoT objects in order to contextualize them alongside objects more generally. It is therefore useful to draw upon the work of science-fiction writer Bruce Sterling, who characterizes objects into their varying human–object relationships in his non-fiction book *Shaping Things* (Sterling, Wild and Lunenfeld 2005). These characterizations are shown in Figure 10.3 and are defined as:

- *Artefact:* artificial objects, made by hand, used by hand, and powered by muscle.
- *Machine:* complex artefacts with integral moving parts with a non-human/non-animal power source.
- *Product:* non-artisanal uniformly mass produced artefacts supported by large transport, finance and information infrastructures.
- *Gizmo:* user alterable and programmable multi-functional objects commonly linked to network service providers.
- *Spime:* networked objects with extensive and rich informational support that are designed on screens, fabricated on screens and tracked in space and time throughout their lifespan.
- *Biot:* an entity that is both object and person that provides data to the network.

Of these characterizations it is the Spime that many IoT researchers have been drawn to (Coulton et al. 2014) and Sterling identifies the dawn of the

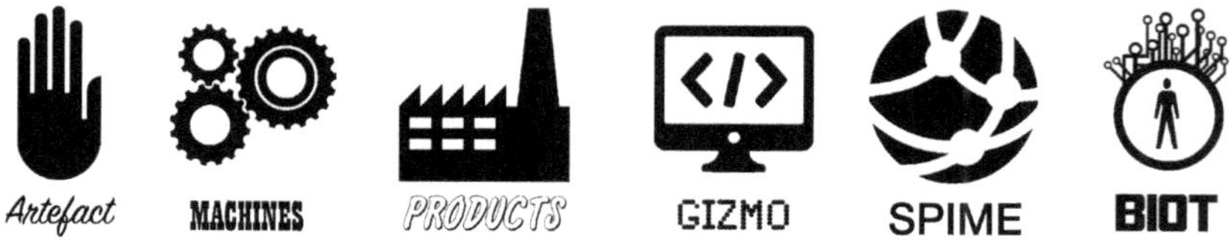

FIGURE 10.3 *Human–object relationships.* © Paul Coulton, Lancaster University.

Spime in relation to the US Department of Defence decision to require all of its suppliers to fit Radio Frequency Identification (RFID) tags to all military supplies (Sterling et al. 2005). This decision, which has subsequently spread to commercial inventory systems, means that objects can be tracked through space and time, and with the majority of such objects being designed and fabricated digitally, our potential knowledge of such objects can go from 'cradle to grave'. This view is particularly attractive for those striving to produce more sustainable products, as Sterling also describes Spimes as 'enhanceable, uniquely identifiable, and made from substances that can and will be folded back into the production of future Spimes' (Sterling et al. 2005).

While this characterization of things is useful, advances in 3D printing, open-source operating systems, open hardware and improved connectivity means that designers and researchers are in a position to experiment with the creation of objects that can be hybrids of these classifications. To illustrate this point, the following section presents a case study of a novel hybrid thing/service termed the 'Physical Playlist' (Burnett et al. 2015).

Physical Playlist

When people share a mixtape,[3] it created an emotional and physical connection between people that shared digital content does not. This connection derives from the fact that objects and artefacts often symbolize something more than their intrinsic value and this symbolism can be preserved over the years. Our personal associations with objects gain subjective meaning based on the memories that we have about them, although such memories are generally hidden and intangible (Csikszentmihalyi and Halton 1981). As mp3 emerged soon after the writeable compact discs (CD), the CD never established itself as a shareable treasured object akin to the mixtape and in the subsequent years nothing has emerged that is viewed in the same way. It was this realization that produced the initial inspiration for creating a new form of digital media compilation that offers the lost tangibility of original mixtape (Burnett et al. 2015). The physical playlist project created a system to explore users' experience of a physical shareable personalized object that has digital content embedded within it. Thus it differs from those projects that have used objects as a means of storing memories, such as Memory Boxes (Frohlich and Murphy 2000), as the object itself is also an embodiment of the time and effort the creator took to personalize the gift thus making it more meaningful than a purely digital playlist.

The project has resulted in two components; the physical shareable objects themselves, and a bespoke media content player designed to ensure that the content of the physical playlist is presented to the user in the sequence in which the creator intended. The current physical playlist takes the form of a 'charm' bracelet and contains customizable 'widgets' that house a small Near Field Communication (NFC) tag (approx. 10mm in diameter and 2mm thick) to store the digital information. The playlist

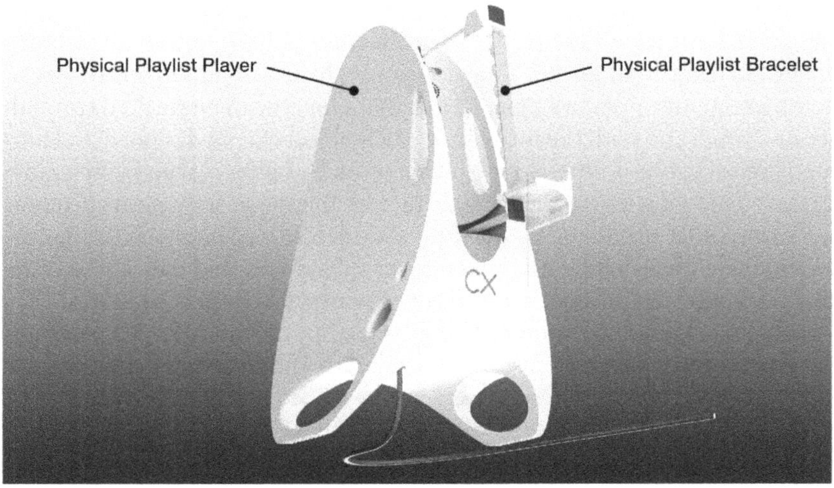

FIGURE 10.4 *Physical playlist.* © Michael Stead, Lancaster University.

creator embeds a link to their chosen digital content within a 'widget' using a bespoke Android application, which currently supports media from BBC iPlayer, Spotify and YouTube. The player (shown in Figure 10.4) also contains an NFC reader that moves up and down a rotating rod to read the physical playlist which is held by two brackets on the player as shown. The player streams the associated media through an attached monitor.

While the mixtape offered elements of personalization, the flexibility of the potential objects that can be combined to form a physical playlist is considerably greater as they can take almost any form. Further, as the playlist is digital enabled they can also be made to utilize other information from the Internet. For instance, they could be made such that they could only be played on a specific day, such as a birthday, or at a specific time, or when the weather is warm and sunny, thus allowing the creator to produce a very unique personalized experience.

In terms of our previous discussion on the characterization of 'things', the physical playlist would not fit in. This is because it is made by hand and contains no moving parts, which would characterize it as artefact, yet the NFC tag and subsequent reading by the player means it can be tracked through space and time which are characteristics of Spime.

This example highlights that considering interaction with a 'thing' alone may be insufficient for designers and they must consider the overall context within which the interaction takes place.

Interacting with Atoms and Bits

In terms of enabling how users may interact with the world, there are a vast array of processes, models and frameworks through which a designer might consider approaching a given design. However, in this chapter I have chosen to illustrate the issues through the sketch by Bill Verplank (2009), recreated in Figure 10.5, which describes the interaction designers' role as having to answer three basic questions in relation to the user: How do they do? How do they feel? How do they know?

Verplank distils 'How do they do?' into a consideration of whether the interaction is either continuous, as in pulling or pushing a handle or joystick, or discrete as in pressing a button or buttons. Not only are both of these modes of interaction applicable and available to designers, they must also extend their thinking to consider that these interactions can also be implemented as a combination of real or virtual interactions. Designers must, therefore, consider carefully how such interactions are used and combined so that they are successfully perceived by the user.

Verplank is considering 'How do they feel?' in relation to how it is presented to the user's senses through a particular medium. This is a utilization of Marshal McLuhan's definition of media as 'any technology that . . . creates extensions of the human body and senses' (McLuhan and Zingrone 1996). McLuhan categorized media in terms of a temperature range, whereby a hot media, such as print, is one that dominates one particular sense absorbing our attention and leaving little room for participation, while a cool media engages across a number of our senses and allows greater exploration by the user (McLuhan, Fiore and Agel 1967). We will return to this consideration of how we engage with our senses in the forthcoming section 'Bandwidth of the senses'.

Verplank illustrates his final question of 'How do they know?' in terms of 'paths' and 'maps' and subsequently argues that often the most

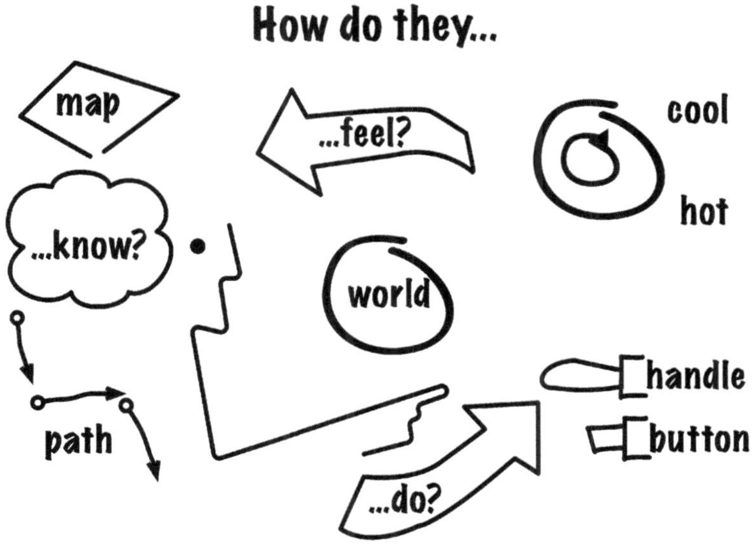

FIGURE 10.5 *Interaction design.* © Paul Coulton, Lancaster University.

successful interactions combine both (Verplank 2009). Note this categorization is derived from Kevin Lynch's work on the legibility of cities in which he considered how people developed an understanding of the layout of a city (Lynch 1960). 'Paths' are step-by-step instructions that guide the user through an interaction and are generally regarded as the easiest form of interaction to design as the user only needs to know one step at a time. They are typically used in situations that require immediate action, such as emergency exit procedures, by users who are likely to be experiencing the required interaction for the first time. 'Maps', on the other hand, represent knowledge obtained directly through the interaction, during which users construct coherent mental models from which tasks and uses can be inferred. The knowledge maps are built from the interactions performed by the users in multiple scenarios using objects and systems that provide similar interactions. Thus the interaction design requires consideration of how users may construct their mental model when interacting with hybrid digital/physical spaces. It is therefore important to consider this in more detail, and I present such a discussion in the following section.

Affordances, Cultural Conventions and Signifiers

The term 'affordance' is used to define the actionable properties between the world and an organism. The original concept is generally attributed to James Gibson (May 2010), who gave the example that, while a flat surface affords 'sitting', a 'pointy' one would not (Gibson 1977). The important aspect of Gibson's definition was that the affordance of the object exists whether it is acted upon or not.

The concept of affordances was most notably developed for design by Donald Norman who extended from what he regarded as Gibson's 'real' affordances (ones that exist) to include 'perceived' affordances (ones that are expected) (Norman 2002). Norman argued that affordances 'play very different roles in physical products than they do in the world of screen-based products' (Norman 1999) and unlike Gibson he considered affordances were often dependent on the cultural experience of users.

Norman also distinguished between the properties of an object that are controllable by the designer and those that are fixed. Norman argued that in the case of real objects, both the real and perceived affordances are controllable by the designer, whereas for screen-based interaction generally only the perceived affordances are under the direct control of the designer, 'as the computer system comes with built-in physical affordances' [Norman 1999]. Bill Gaver extended upon Norman's discussion, stating that 'affordances exist whether or not they are perceived, but it is because they are inherently about important properties that they "need" to be perceived' (Gaver 1991) and introduced the notion that affordances may be: 'hidden' – from the user if they are not perceived; or 'false' if perceived but not actionable. Dan Saffer suggests hidden affordances may actually be created deliberately as part of the design process and could therefore be regarded as 'discoverable' (Saffer 2013) in recognition that designers may deliberately allow them to be revealed through accidental use or deliberate exploration. Coulton et al. suggest that this is similar to the practice of game designers leaving hidden elements, or 'Easter eggs', within their games to be discovered by accident, and that this practice hints at a possible interesting opportunity yet to be applied in the creation of physical/digital objects (Coulton et al. 2014).

Although affordance has proved a popular concept, it is not without its critics who, while acknowledging their usefulness within the practical design process, reject their simplicity and argue that in reality 'objects have a potentially an unlimited set of properties and affordances' (Hornecker 2012). While I agree with this analysis, I believe it is still a very useful way for designers to address Verplank's question of 'how does the user know?'

When Norman discussed affordances he also introduced 'cultural conventions' (Norman 2002) which serve to constrain user interaction and derive from users' conventional interpretations of how they should interact with a particular artefact. Norman subdivides these cultural conventions into physical, logical and cultural constraints. Physical constraints are related to the artefact. For example, computer software limits the movement of the cursor to the edges of the screen. Logical constraints are when users make judgements to deduce the nature of the interaction. For instance, in a video game with a human avatar the player might assume it can perform the physical actions that a typical human might perform. Cultural constraints are conventions shared by a cultural group. An example of a cultural convention would be that whereby Japanese Manga comics are read back to front and left to right. The challenge for designers is in understanding which conventions they might inherit when designing an artefact of a particular form.

It is notable that in 2008 Norman evolved his consideration of affordances and cultural conventions to include 'signifiers', in response to what he perceived as misunderstandings by designers of perceived affordances (Norman 2008), particularly in the case of the situations or context in which an interaction takes place. Norman stated that 'as we move from the world of standalone objects to social structures, complex, intelligent products, and a heavy dominance of services, then new principles are needed', which is highly relevant to the hybrid digital/physical situations considered in this chapter which often have physical objects connected through a wider computer network.

Norman considers signifiers are the clues in the physical or social world that can be interpreted meaningfully even when the signifier is an accidental by-product of actions within a particular context. For example, if you are rushing to catch a train and you arrive at an empty platform you may perceive that you have missed the train. However, this signifier may not be reliable, as stations in rural locations may not get many passengers. Sometimes the signifier is a trail or trace of previous behaviour, such as the 'desire lines' made by people's footsteps across grass, which represent a more convenient route than the pavement.

It is important to consider that the discussion of perception up to this point has primarily considered it from an environmental perspective, in which our behaviours are learnt, whereas other perceptions may be considered as the result of human evolution. This is the view promoted by evolutionary psychology – that humans have evolved a set of cognitive adaptations in response to recurring problems in the ancestral environment. Such a consideration has been promoted within design in the form of a set of design principles, such as anthropomorphic form, baby-face bias, contour bias, attractiveness bias and savannah preference (Lidwell, Holden and Butler 2010]. For example, savannah preference suggests that the majority of people tend to prefer environments that are open with scattered trees, water and uniform grassiness than other natural environments that are simple, such as a desert; dense, such as a jungle; or complex, such as mountains. It is claimed that this preference is based on the belief that early humans who lived on savannahs enjoyed a survival advantage. While these evolutionary notions could have an influence over aesthetic design considerations, it is likely that environmental characterizations are the more useful framings for design in the context of atoms and bits.

Overall it is important to note that if users are to function within a complex social and technological world of Atoms and Bits, they will need to be able to develop the mental models of what things mean or how they operate. Therefore it is the role of designers to provide these clues by developing new understandings and techniques.

Bandwidth of the Senses

The previous discussion on affordances, cultural conventions and signifiers drew extensively on notions of perception, and in this section we will be primarily concerned with the associated term of sensation. While sensation and perception are complementary processes and often used interchangeably in everyday language, they are actually very distinct. Sensation is often considered as passive, as we don't consciously engage with the process in which information from the outside world is brought into the brain. Perception, on the other hand, is an active process of translating the information brought to the brain by the senses into something meaningful. Therefore, while we have arguably already addressed perception in the previous section, we have yet to engage directly with sensation.

Although there are many ways in which we could consider sensation and the senses, here I will draw primarily from the work of physicist Tor Nørretranders who characterized human senses in terms of an information bandwidth (Nørretranders 1991). Nørretranders presents the information rates or the different senses expressed in terms of bits per second (bps) as would typically be used in relation to sensors connected to digital

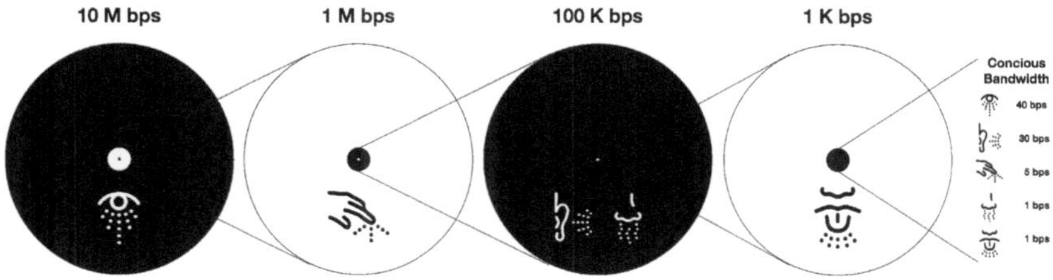

FIGURE 10.6 *Bandwidth of the senses.* © Paul Coulton, Lancaster University.

system. The values are calculated based on the number of receptors in each sensory organ, how many nerve connections send these signals to the brain, and how many signals each connections sends per second. Although other researchers present different versions of these values, they are similar is size and the relative differences between senses is very consistent and Nørretranders' values are used in Figure 10.6. In addition, this figure also includes bandwidth values for the information from the senses that we consciously perceive which is considerably lower.

For example, while the eyes relay visual information at a rate of approximately 10 million bps the brain is only able to consciously perceive 40 bps. While this might suggest a great deal of information is discarded this is not the case as the extra information (exformation) (Nørretranders 1991) may be being perceived and it is just that we are not consciously aware of it. This is perhaps most easily illustrated through the concept of 'muscle memory' whereby when a physical movement is repeated over time, a long-term memory is created allowing it to be performed without conscious effort. There are other examples found in many everyday activities that often become automatic, such as riding a bicycle, typing on a keyboard, typing in a password, playing a musical instrument, etcetera. This perhaps adds the criticism of affordances in that they are not directly perceived but rather they acquire meaning through use (May 2010). Overall it is therefore useful for designers to consider how a thing is sensed separately from how it is perceived. For example, colour blind users sense visual information differently but they may derive the same meaning.

Where the Interaction Is

As was previously highlighted, it is important that designers consider not only the interaction itself, but how the space within which the interaction occurs changes the nature of the resulting experience. Although we are not specifically concerned with games, a useful framing for spaces of interaction is provided by Jesper Juul in his book *The Casual Revolution* (Juul 2009) in which he describes the overall space in which a game is played as player space, screen space and three-dimensional (3D) space. He used this division to highlight that in games using gestural controllers, such as Wii

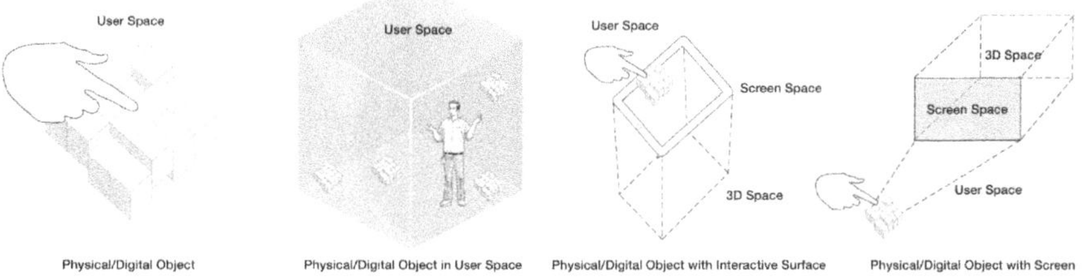

FIGURE 10.7 *Four possible interaction scenarios.* © Paul Coulton, Lancaster University.

Sports, the player space plays a much more significant role than many more traditional console games (Juul 2009). Dividing space in terms of where a user's focus may be directed at a particular instance allows designers to consider where and how the interaction takes place, and where and how feedback on that interaction should be presented to the user. For example, in Figure 10.7, I illustrate four possible interaction scenarios:

- Object Space: In this scenario, the IoT is the focus of the user's interaction and all affordances would be associated with the object.
- Objects in User Space: In this scenario we expect multiple objects to be used to enhance the physical space. While a screen might form part of this scenario, the objects would not operate with it directly.
- Object with Tablet: In this scenario, the screen of the tablet provides a surface through which the physical objects interact with a virtual world that could be represented as either 2D or 3D space (Coulton et al. 2014).
- Object with Screen: In this scenario, movements of the physical object are transferred to the screen via a wired/wireless link and as with the previous case the virtual world can be represented as either 2D or 3D space (Coulton et al. 2014).

It is important to note that although these scenarios are representative of just some of the current implementations involving objects, they are not the only possibilities, and designers are also free to configure such interaction spaces as they desire which will also have implications on the type of sensory information used.

Conclusions

In this chapter I have considered the challenges for designers in creating meaningful interactions in a world that is increasingly constructed of both Atoms and Bits as we continue to add layers of code atop our physical world. This consideration moves beyond previous characterizations that have often presented hybrid digital and physical worlds through notions of traversing between states, or as separate spaces, to one which represents our everyday lived experience whereby the Internet is no longer the space we visit but the place we live in. In particular, it has focussed on developing potential design frames that address how users both sense and perceive such worlds.

To explore interactions within these worlds we have focussed on interacting with digital/physical objects using Sterling's characterization of human–object relationships. Although it is Spimes and Biots that may be considered most relevant due to their association with the IoT, I have highlighted that Sterling's characterizations should be viewed as specific instances rather than as a taxonomy, as many objects, such as the Physical Playlist discussed, can combine elements from across Sterling's descriptors.

Starting from Verplank's model of interaction design in which he considers designers are aiming to provide answers to three questions of 'How does the user do?' 'How does the user feel?' and 'How does the user know?' we have examined each of these questions in relation to hybrid physical digital spaces. The first question is the easiest to consider in that while interactions in this context can be implemented either physically or virtually, they can still be considered as either continuous or discrete, and both physical and perceived affordances associated with these interactions will be under the control of the designer.

In terms of 'How does the user feel?' we have considered this using Nørretranders' discussion of the bandwidth of the senses. This allows us to separate the notion of what a user may sense from what they might actually perceive. Therefore I have argued that 'How does the user sense?' might be a better framing of Verplank's second question for designers in this context rather than 'How does the user feel?' This separation allows us to frame the final question as 'How does the user perceive?' rather the 'How does the user know?' and while paths and maps are still useful metaphors for the revised question, designers should not only consider real and perceived affordances but also cultural conventions and signifiers. Thus my suggested framing of designing for interaction in the context of hybrid digital spaces is shown in Figure 10.8.

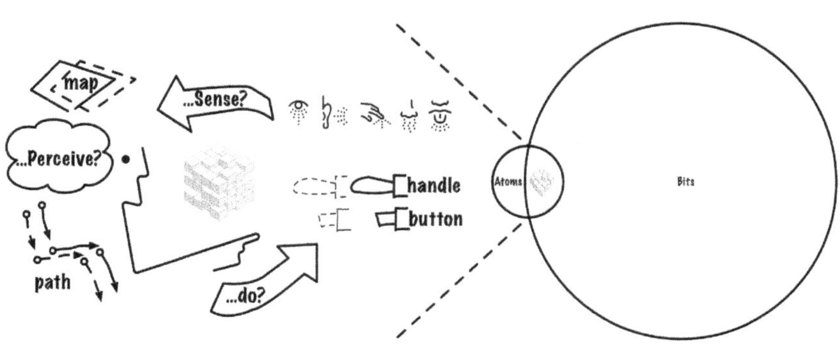

FIGURE 10.8 *Interaction in a world of atoms and bits.* © Paul Coulton, Lancaster University.

However, it is important to note this framing is not intended as a fixed set for rules or a recipe to follow, but is intended to open up a discursive space through which designers can build and criticize, while developing the design techniques and evaluation methods that will be required when developing interactions for a world of Atoms and Bits.

Notes

1 Virtual is used to denote something that does not physically exist but made by software to appear to do so.
2 The Rift is a virtual-reality head-mounted display developed by Oculus VR.
3 A mixtape is the generic name for a compilation of songs recorded on any audio format, although is primarily associated with compact audio cassettes from the 1980s. Their production is often associated with them being created as a romantic gift for someone you were attracted to.

References

Burnett, D., A. Gradinar, J. Porter, M. Stead, P. Coulton and I. Forrester (2015), 'Physical Playlist: Bringing Back the Mix-Tape'. Proceedings of International Conference on Human–Computer Interaction – INTERACT 2015.

Čopič Pucihar, K. and P. Coulton (2014), 'Exploring the Evolution of Mobile Augmented Reality for Future Entertainment Systems'. *Computers in Entertainment (CIE)* 11(2): 1, 12.

Coulton, P. (2015), 'Playful and Gameful Design for the Internet of Things'. In A. Nijholt (ed.), *More Playful User Interfaces: Interfaces that Invite Social and Physical Interaction*. Singapore: Springer, pp. 151–173 (Gaming Media and Social Effects).

Coulton, P., D. Burnett, A. Gradinar, D. Gullick and E. Murphy (2014), 'Game Design in an Internet of Things'. *Transactions of the Digital Games Research Association* 1(3).

Csikszentmihalyi, M. and E. Halton (1981), *The Meaning of Things: Domestic Symbols and the Self*. Cambridge: Cambridge University Press.

Drascic, D. and P. Milgram (1996), 'Perceptual Issues in Augmented Reality'. In *Electronic Imaging: Science & Technology*. International Society for Optics and Photonics, pp. 123–134.

Dunne, A. (2005), *Hertzian Tales: Electronic Products, Aesthetic Experience, and Critical Sesign*. Cambridge: MIT Press.

Frohlich, D. and R. Murphy (2000), 'The Memory Box'. *Personal Technologies* 4(4): 238–240.

Gaver, W. W. (1991), 'Technology Affordances'. In *Proceedings of the SIGCHI Conference on Human Factors in Computing Systems*, ACM, pp. 79–84.

Gibson, J. J. (1977), 'The Theory of Affordances'. In R. E. Shaw and J. Bransford (eds), *Perceiving, Acting, and Knowing*. Hillsdale, NJ: Lawrence Erlbaum Associates.

Gregory, R. L. (1997), *Eye and Brain: The Psychology of Seeing*. Originally published in 1966 and updated by Princeton University Press.

Hornecker, E. (2012), 'Beyond Affordance: Tangibles' Hybrid Nature'. In *Proceedings of the Sixth International Conference on Tangible, Embedded and Embodied Interaction*, ACM, pp. 175–182.
Juul, J. (2010), *A Casual Revolution: Reinventing Video Games and Their Players*. Cambridge, MA: MIT Press.
Lidwell, W., K. Holden and J. Butler (2010), *Universal Principles of Design, Revised and Updated: 125 Ways to Enhance Usability, Influence Perception, Increase Appeal, Make Better Design Decisions, and Teach through Design*. Beverly, MA: Rockport Publishers.
Lynch, K. (1960), *The Image of the City*. Vol. 11. Cambridge, MA: MIT Press.
May, M. (2010), 'Beyond Affordances – Why Direct Perception Is Not Enough in Design Engineering'. In Proceedings of CEPHAD 2010 Conference, Copenhagen (www.dkds.dk/Forskning/Projekter/CEPHAD) (accessed 17 October 2016).
McLuhan, E. and F. Zingrone (eds) (1996), *Essential McLuhan*. New York: Basic Books; 1st ed.
McLuhan, M., Q. Fiore and J. Agel (1967), *The Medium is the Massage*. New York: Bantam Books.
Milgram, P., H. Takemura, A. Utsumi and F. Kishino (1995), 'Augmented Reality: A Class of Displays on the Reality–Virtuality Continuum'. In *Photonics for Industrial Applications*. International Society for Optics and Photonics, pp. 282–292.
Norman, D. A. (1999), 'Affordance, Conventions, and Design'. *interactions* 6(3): 38–43.
Norman, D. A. (2002), *The Design of Everyday Things*. New York: Basic Books, 2002.
Norman, D. A. (2008), 'The Way I See It: Signifiers, not Affordances'. *interactions* 15(6): 18–19.
Nørretranders, T. (1991), *The User Illusion: Cutting Consciousness Down to Size*. New York: Viking.
Saffer, D. (2013), *Microinteractions: Designing with Details*. Sebastopol, CA: O'Reilly Media.
Sterling, B., L. Wild and P. Lunenfeld (2005), *Shaping Things*. Cambridge, MA: MIT Press.
Verplank, W. (2003), Interaction Design Sketchbook: Frameworks for Designing Interactive Products and Systems. Available at https://ccrma.stanford.edu/courses/250a/lectures/IDSketchbok.pdf (accessed 7 June 2015).

11

Drawn Away from Vision: Encounters with the Unseen

Sarah Casey and Gerry Davies

Introduction

Since the Renaissance, drawing has been allied with the production of knowledge not only to record and communicate observations, but as an integral part of making observations themselves, that is, as a method to direct and focus attention on the visible world and as a tool to craft an image. Yet, throughout its history, drawing has been used to visualize information at the limits of human vision.

Drawing has assisted scientists in seeing subjects whether it be the distant, for instance, in astronomy and Galileo's moon drawings, or the minute, as in Robert Hooke's wonderful *Micrographia*; it has made the very complex comprehensible, as in Wenceslaus Hollar's topographical studies and maps of London, or made information that is hidden from sight behind a barrier visible, for instance, the inner workings of the human and animal body as in the works of George Stubbs and Versalius.

Surveying both historical and contemporary drawing, we can see a range of ways that drawing approaches the barely visible, and along the way identify strategies that enabled artists and others to direct their drawing to extend their visual capacity.

As artists working with drawing in contexts where vision is challenged, our particular interest is to examine strategies to capture information at the limits of vision. The question we consider here is how might graphic strategies be deployed to address not just the barely visible, but to approach phenomena, effects and information available to other senses, that is, beyond the scope of vision. What can drawing do in situations where sight is not the primary means of sensing? What evidence is there that drawing can make us more attuned to other forms of sensory awareness, including sensory absence? We will examine contemporary and historical examples where artists have challenged their awareness and graphic competencies to develop strategies to perceive the non-visual.

The idea that drawing can enable the draughtsperson, be they artist or investigator, to grasp and reflect on, and therefore understand a subject is described by Leonardo Da Vinci in his notebooks. He argues that looking at one of his anatomical drawings conveys more information than watching the anatomist at work. The reason for this, he argues, is that the drawings are the product of multiple dissections – he dissected over ten human bodies to get a 'true and perfect knowledge' of a particular structure (Taylor 1960: 27). By synthesizing information gained over time and compiled from different sources, the drawing can convey more information than a single perspective view of the object itself. What Leonardo points to here is the difference between 'just looking' and the way in which the artist/anatomist has cognitively processed sensory information. The artist draws not only what he or she sees but also his or her knowledge of the visible and its limits.

A variant of this is found in nineteenth-century astronomy. The development of new telescopes had enabled astronomers to 'see' farther, revealing mysterious smudgy forms among the stars, what we now know to be galactic clusters of stars but not then distinguished as such.

On the Rosse project, operational from 1839 to 1880, a team of artists drew their nightly observations. One strategy involved multiple studies of the same phenomena made by the same artist, another saw many studies made by multiple observers of the same object, with the aim that several repeated representations of a feature could be relied upon to show definitive characteristics of the object of study (Nasim 2013). What these examples demonstrate is something quite distinct from a singular objective observational study. Both present drawing as a methodology for amassing and organizing information, designed to 'stabilise' a phenomena, minimizing individual perceptual variation. Here drawing is a critical, multi-layered, intellectual activity, enabling us to 'see' further and to understand – or acknowledge – what we are seeing.

The idea that the activity of drawing itself enables the drawer to 'see' the object of study more clearly was central to the teachings of John Ruskin. In his *Elements of Drawing* (1857) Ruskin offers a simple example of a fundamental principle – of drawing as prolonged study, a form of address which makes us look longer, and more carefully at the world:

> I believe that the sight is a more important thing than the drawing; and I would rather teach drawing that my pupils learn to love Nature, than teach the looking at nature that they may learn to draw.

In other words, drawing was key to developing a keener sense of sight and accordingly empathy with the world (Ruskin 1857). In order to draw a

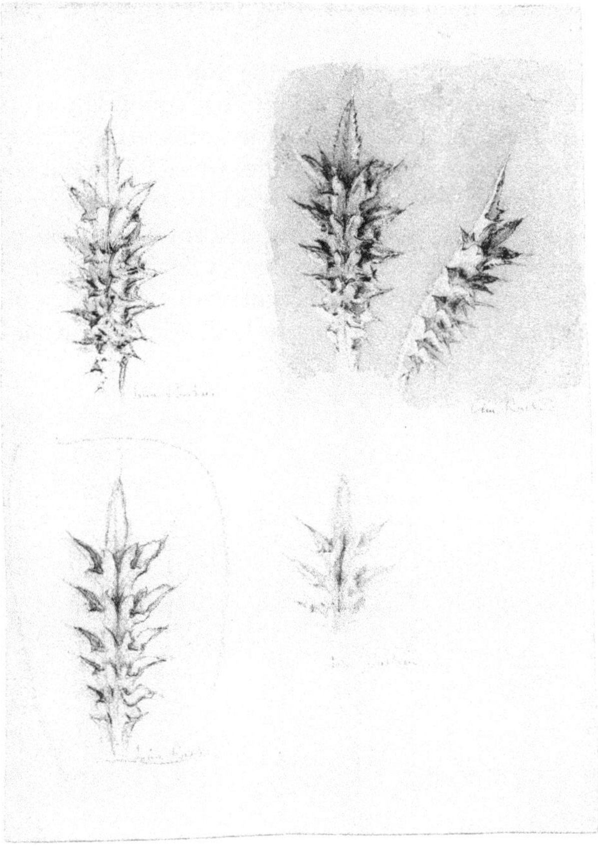

FIGURE 11.1 John Ruskin, *Study of Thistles*. Ink, watercolour and pencil on paper. © Ruskin Foundation (Ruskin Library, Lancaster University).

subject one must look at and scrutinize it to determine the length, weight and quality of line with which to render its image on a sheet of paper – you have to do more than merely look (Figure 11.1). The critical observer purposefully applies a piercing scrutiny and then makes critical decisions on where to place lines and marks. In doing so, fine assessments of the visual qualities of a subject are made: the subject is seen more clearly.

This principle of prolonged looking married to technological advancements, for instance, in telescopes and microscopy, further extends the reach of sight. However, there is more to extending sight than magnification. An example of an alternative strategy is found in the work of Ramón y Cajal, the Spanish neurologist working at the turn of the twentieth century.

Studying the microscopic endings of neural networks, his practice used a range of methods to make visible the unseen, ranging across photographic, histology and chemical staining. Added to these conventional scientific methods, and what makes Cajal fascinating to us is he also had a graphic practices, and made thousands of drawings examining neural cells and fibres.

In his notebook, he wrote that drawing 'forces us to examine the entire phenomenon, thus preventing the details that commonly go unnoticed in ordinary observation from escaping our attention' (De Rijke 2010). In his writing he makes clear his preference for drawing because it enabled seeing things that other methods could not reveal. For instance, a camera is only in focus at one specific depth and the histological slide produced only single slices of information, whereas the eye moves back and forth between different focal points and depths. This is evident in his drawing of a section of the cerebral cortex of a mammal (Figure 11.2) where the right hand side of

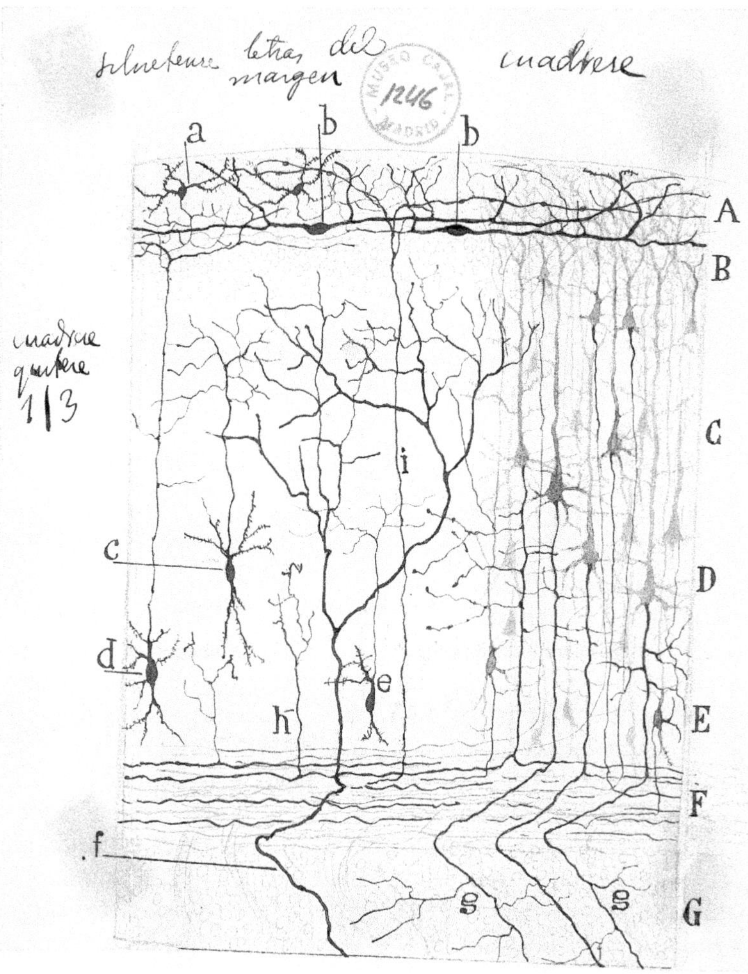

FIGURE 11.2 Santiago Ramón y Cajal, *Diagram of a section of the cerebral cortex of a mammal*. Pencil and ink on paper. © Cajal Legacy, Instituto Cajal (CSIC), Madrid.

the drawing depicts a column of the cortex and a close up detail of individual structures is shown magnified at a different scale on the left hand side of the page. In drawing, Cajal would move his bodily viewing position, tilt and crane his head, switch attention between objects, surfaces and details. The eye, brain and to some extent the body are working together, enabling Cajal to gather and present information garnered from many focal planes and depths onto a single surface. Using drawing, he could both synthesize different views and crucially edit to extract essential information. In other words, Cajal recognized that his drawing was in part mediated though the body, and that the wider responsiveness of the investigator was an essential component in his experimental practice and drawing was a key mechanism in eliciting, ordering and communicating his results.

The Ramón y Cajal example is interesting in that it highlights the contribution and value of embodied knowledge, that is, he expressed a preference for drawing because it encompassed critical decision making and it offered the capacity to synthesize phenomena as it was seen and experienced by him. The limitations of microscope slides reside in providing only a thin slice of information in one plane. Cajal both moved and manipulated them and brought together information from many slides that could not ordinarily have been seen simultaneously. The significance is that subjects are observed and *made to be visible.*

On this evidence, drawing offers the observer a particular visual capacity which was not superseded by developments in photography. This claim is borne out by recent work exploring drawing's value in aiding and extending vision. For instance, the contemporary artist Lucy Lyons uses drawing to reveal previously unseen medical details.

In her project, *Delineating Disease* (Figure 11.3) she worked with pathologists, medical researchers and patients to investigate the rare disease Fibrodysplasia Ossificans Progressiva (FOP) (Lyons 2012). Her subjects are specimens of such repetitive complexity and minuteness which at first sight appear as a uniform pattern. Lyons examines and records the tiny changes of shape and direction of bone growth to see and understand their structural significance. In her drawing she *draws attention* to these changes and, without exaggeration, emphasizes them, whereas the camera treats them as continuous texture. For example, as part of the project she spent many hours patiently drawing details of a skeleton affected by the disease. As a result she noticed that the excessive bone growths which were visually complex and hard to distinguish, could through careful observational drawing be untangled and discerned; Lyons laid bare information so fine as to be lost in photography, which could now be identified, recorded and made visible. The drawings offered insights into the condition which were particularly felt by patients because the drawings rendered details clearly and communicated aspects of their condition more directly than x-rays or scans (Lyons 2012: 5).

So we have seen how drawing has extended and continues to extend the limits of vision. In both contemporary and historical examples of artists and

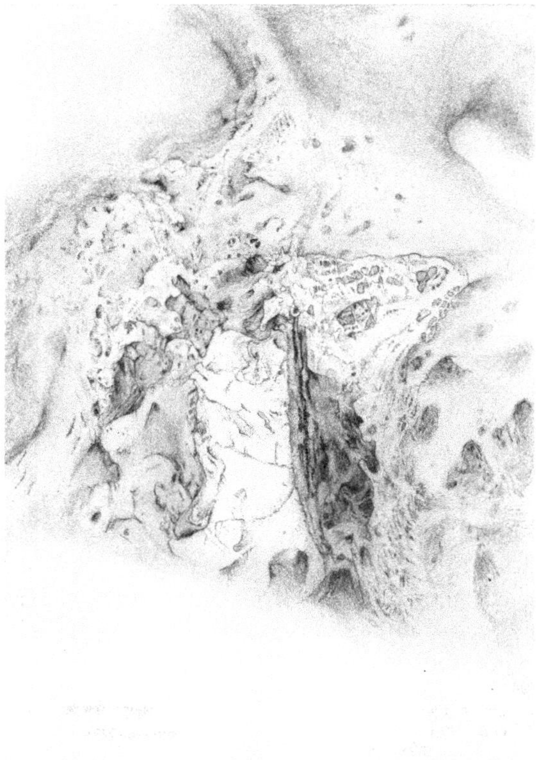

FIGURE 11.3 Lucy Lyons, *Delineation* 50 7646 Excision. Pencil on paper. © Lucy Lyons.

non-artists it is evident that drawing not only helps the drawer to record barely visible information but to actually *see* it. But what can drawing as a visual medium achieve when sight offers us limited means of knowing, for example, in the dark, or when the defining qualities of a subject are non-visual, for instance, if they are auditory or haptic? We turn now to consider how drawing aids non-visual sensory experience and the contribution of the other senses to images which extend our understanding of a subject.

A well know example of the effects of sensory change and adaption in the visual arts is Goya's work after 1792. Affected by his gradual descent into deafness, representations of gesture and hand movement become pronounced. This belies an increased sensitivity to inflections of hand gesture and their role in communications (Tal 2010). Recent research has uncovered the drawings and biography of a lesser-known seventeenth-century artist, the Dutch draftsman Johannes Thopas (c.1626–1690/5) who was born both deaf and mute.

Johannes Thopas was a successful portrait miniaturist who, as a result of this disability, was a ward of his family all his life; he remained unmarried and a comparative outsider to civic and public life (Eckhart

2014). Not only did he live in a silent world but his experience of it was limited. Thopas is interesting, because his work has only recently come to critical acclaim, but also for the way in which his drawings manifest his uncommon sensory experience of the world. Thopas's sheltered and soundless experience is powerfully and palpably sensed by a viewer of his drawings. If deafness heightened Goya's sensitivity to gesture (Tal 2010) then what we find in Thopas is further and more substantive evidence of drawing's capacity to capture sensory experience beyond the visual.

Thopas's deafness and muteness insinuates into the atmosphere of the drawings a sense of silence. His lack of voice and hearing is compensated for with an exaggerated ability to imbue his drawings with the detailed fabric of domestic interiors and evoke the presence and stillness of the sitter.

As a draughtsman with fine appreciation of the exact grain of surfaces, and an extraordinary capacity to see and translate effects of the particular textures of everyday life, he displays heightened concentration on the technical execution of the drawing. Running a magnifying glass across the surface of a Johannes Thopas miniature is an extraordinary experience. Every substance is rendered in microscopic detail, each material is unreservedly itself, and every surface reflects its own qualities of solidity, resistance and manufacture. Made with plumbago – a naturally occurring graphite – on sheets of gessoed velum rarely larger than 20x20 centimetres, the drawings reveal themselves as miracles of relentless observation allied to refined technique. Under magnification, the apparently smooth layered gesso is seen to be a mass of minute scores and scratches, the results of sanding and 'boning' with a burnishing tool to achieve a workable substrate across which Thopas constructs images comprised of millions of tiny graphite marks.

These drawings, made in profound silence, suggest sustained and uniform concentration across the whole composition. The drawing manner is relentlessly calm and measured, sitters are posed fore-square or three-quarter and around them there are few devices or visual convolutions. Poised marionette-like, motionless and with an evenness of gaze, their controlled articulations of arms, meticulous arrangements of hands and fingers play out a visual language of touch and gesture (Figure 11.4).

The effect of this stillness or quietude is not simply a lack, sound missing or suppressed, rather it is the positive creation of silence as an independent quality. The intensity of silence becomes palpable taking on its own weight in the same way that the absent can paradoxically be poignantly present, for example, in the still life that we cannot touch, the fruit we cannot taste.

We also see this silence, or feel its weight in the way that the device of the window is used. In keeping with contemporary convention, a sitter indoors is positioned in front of the window, a portal to the outside world. This framed view of a farmstead or factory is used to indicate property or land owned by the sitter, a birth right, inheritance or acquisition. While convention may dictate Thopas's inclusion of the window, its effect within the image goes beyond the typical didactic role. For instance, the scene of

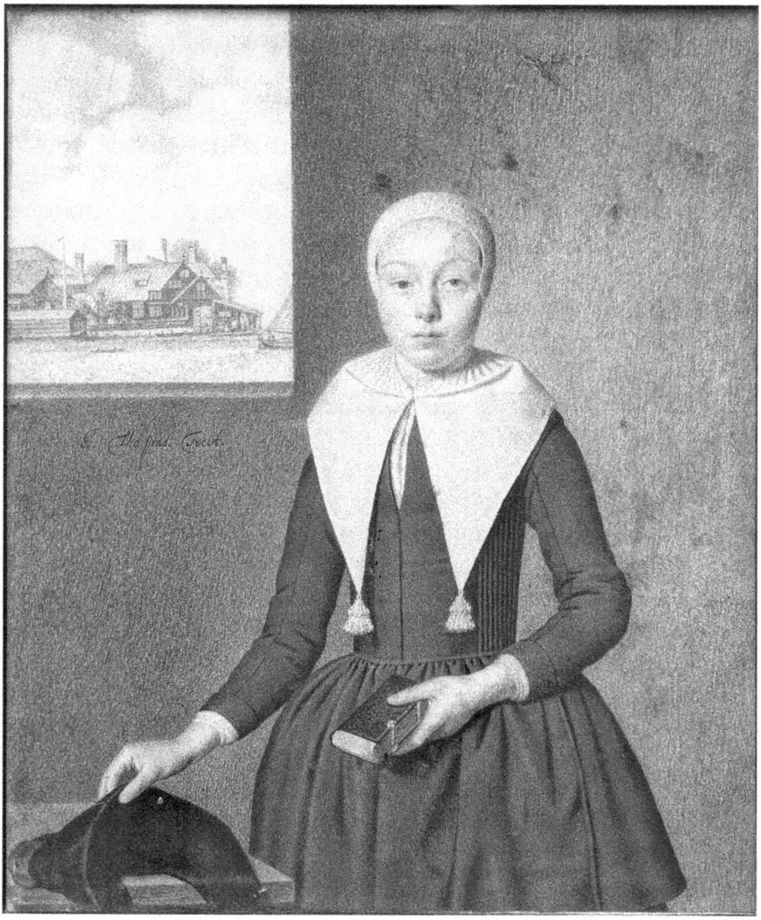

FIGURE 11.4 Johannes Thopas, *Woman Holding a Bible*. Plumbago on vellum. © Zaans Museum, Zaandam.

Portrait of a Woman Holding a Bible appears at quiet remove from the hustle of exterior life. The window contributes to a sense of a hermetically sealed environment: the room is small, dark and sparse, the portal to the outside is compact, and the landscape distant, suggesting a monastic cell. In this way, the window reflects the sensory aesthetics of the image, underscoring the sense of silence within.

Within this silent stage, gesture is also key. Seventeenth-century portrait drawing is alive with mobile hands; fingers point, arms gesture and hands hold objects. Objects and their manipulation are narrative conventions, from gesticulations to subtle indications, and by clutching skulls and wielding pens and paint brushes sitters declare themselves as priests, scholars, artists and much more.

In Thopas, too, we see hands. They are active, but rarely enact dramatic or rhetorical gestures. His sitter's hands are precisely arranged as if they were themselves still lives, self-contained tableaux connected to the person and portrait while suggesting further layers of meaning. In his portraits of single women, hands are particularly pronounced in their muscularity, often slightly over scale and seemingly too large for their bodies, sometimes veined and masculine, yet always assured and capable. Their interaction with objects is by turns firm and delicate, they hold fast to furniture, clutch pens, fans, gloves, fingers part the pages of a book and trace across fabrics. In keeping with convention, the objects held are highly significant. As artefacts they hold cultural and symbolic value designed to project familial and civic ideals of fraternity, temperance and industry. But what interests us here is not so much what each sitter is holding, but the care paid to depicting *how* they are holding it. As with Goya, the record of a subtle inflection of the wrist or finger astutely captures precision of touch, the weight of contact. Thopas displays alertness to the visual cues of touch and tactility, a hand rests on a bible, caresses a cloth cap, as viewers we 'feel' these touches in a manner not seen in the genre of plumbago drawings. Likewise in drawing clothing and costume Thopas displays uncommon sympathy to the weight and fold of fabric as it pleats, falls or creases. He renders the dense, dark wools of bodice and jacket as an enfolding protective shell; as a viewer we feel the warmth of protection or the stiff oppressive weight of the folds.

Viewing these exquisite drawings then, we become aware of Thopas's drawing offering an example of translating tactile and aural into graphic form. In Thopas we see evidence of the situated nature of the knowledge – how the drawing is mediated by his specific sensory limitations. What his drawings manifest is not simply the use of iconography to point to sensory information, rather they capture a particular aspect of the subjective experience of the drawer so often valued in drawing, which records and transmits embodied sensory knowledge. In Thopas, 'embodiment' is an unintentional consequence of his lack of speech and hearing. We turn now to consider examples where the artist is purposefully engaged in developing relationships between the graphic and non-visual.

In contemporary Western art we are familiar with examples of exploration of non-visual and conceptual approaches to art making. Ever since modernism's experimentally inclined avant-garde movements, attempts to use drawing to translate or transcribe non-visual phenomena into graphic form are commonplace. In the twentieth century, conceptual art offered approaches for modelling and visualizing systems, sequences, variations even algorithms – for example, in the work of Sol le Witt and Hanne Darboven. These examples each depict an idea, the process is less sensory more schematic; their value is conceptual and largely abstract. Conversely, Kandinsky's depictions of music or Iannis Xenakis's musical scores represent a form of drawing which moves across sensory experience. These are well-known examples of artists who used artmaking to present equivalents of what they felt or knew through another sense; Kandinsky's synaesthesia is well known. But what is of interest here are strategies using drawing as the means of extending our sensory capacity and refining its sensitivity to capture information at the edges of perception rather than simply as a means of translating one sense into another.

Claude Heath is a prominent example of a contemporary artist exploring relationships between sightlessness, touch and drawing. For some years Heath's practice has involved careful staging of drawing experiments in which he restricts his sight. These have taken a number of forms, for example, in the '*blindfold*' drawings. In one series Heath makes drawn studies of three dimensional objects (pot plants and plaster casts) while blindfolded. He sets up his object of study, for example, a plaster cast of the Willendorf Venus and the drawing surface, each with a piece of Blu-Tack in the same fixed location. These are then his starting and stopping points. By using one hand as a marker and measure, he begins at the Blu-Tack, tracing the three-dimensional terrain with his fingers, returning after each pass to his starting position back at the Blu-Tack. All the while, the drawing hand simultaneously translates his direction of travel and the undulations and textures into drawn marks on the page

That touch can be refined as to enable skilful determination of subtle differentiations is evident in the ability developed by people with visual impairment to read Braille. A more vivid example is perhaps the work of Geerat Vermeji, a blind biologist able to identify new species of molluscs through using touch to perceive subtle differences in the shells (Sachs 2005: 40).

Heath has said of these Blu-Tack drawings, which are as much touched as seen, that depriving himself of sight forces his hands to decipher the details of the subject and translate touch into movement, line and visibility. Heath says

> I wanted to see if this sensation of being directly in touch with my subject could be achieved while using my eyes. So I used them as if they were fingertips exploring the surfaces of plants, moving over contours one by one. (Maslen and Southern 2011: 90)

These experiments, and Heath's rather paradoxical drawings made through touch, test claims about conventional relationships between drawing and vision and object and image. Rendering sculptural and three-dimensional properties into two-dimensional graphic form through 'seeing with his fingers' bring to mind Derrida's description of drawing with an eye on the tip of a finger.

> It is as if a lidless eye had opened at the tip of the fingers as if one eye too many had just grown right next to the nail . . . This eye guides the tracing or outline (tracé); . . . the prosthesis of a seer who is himself invisible. (Derrida 1993: 3)

What Derrida elegantly describes is that sensation familiar to many, but intimate to drawing, the accompanying sensation of fingertip contact which duplicates the transition of the eye across a surface. As the gaze travels along the edge of a form the hand duplicates action on the page, translating the virtual touch of the eye to the actual touch of the fingers and drawing instrument.

Heath's drawings, like Kandinsky's, rephrase the tactile into the visual and translate information from one realm to another; three dimensional and sculptural form become touch and line. However, what Heath's drawings don't tell us is about the quality of that touch, whether something is hot, cold, hard, soft or textured.

Sian Bowen

Thopas and Heath offer very different lenses through which to view the relationship between drawing and non-ocular sensing. We identified in Thopas's drawing a particular form of graphic sensibility flowing from his subjectivity and in Heath a deliberate practice of translation. While the former is incidental and the latter deployed as part of a purposeful experiment, these two distinct approaches come together in the practice of the contemporary British artist Sian Bowen.

Bowen has become known for her drawings which explore a tactile engagement with historical artefacts and objects, many of which have been handled over the centuries. Like Heath, touch plays an important role in her practice, as she seeks to find equivalence for tactile sensations with drawing. While her work bears little visual resemblance to that of Thopas, it shares his heightened sensitivity to mark-making and the sense of silence in graphic form.

One of the distinctive qualities of Bowen's work is the techniques and process through which the drawing is made. The aforementioned tactility is bound up with the materiality of the support – typically paper. In Bowen's practice, paper is not simply a support or vehicle for an image. It is rather an integral part of the meaning of the drawing itself. This is perhaps best exemplified in work from the early 2000s, the *Passage* and *Ream* series.

Both series are made using found papers. The *Ream* series of 2002, which includes large scale works depicting hand-held and personal artefacts, such as scissors and combs, on surfaces compiled from collaged recycled papers. The *Passage* series grew out of a residency at Villa Romana, in Florence when Bowen had the good fortune to stumble upon a group of old handwritten letters.

This careworn surface is drawn upon with the processes of piercing, burning, rubbing, folding, each underscoring the physicality of touch. In the *Pledge* sound piece, for example, the drawing is again composed of multiple layers of old hand-written letters, the upper layer burnt through with successive marks made using a special tool leaving a tiny singed hole, as if an acid-laced finger had lingered too long and eaten the page away (Figure 11.5).

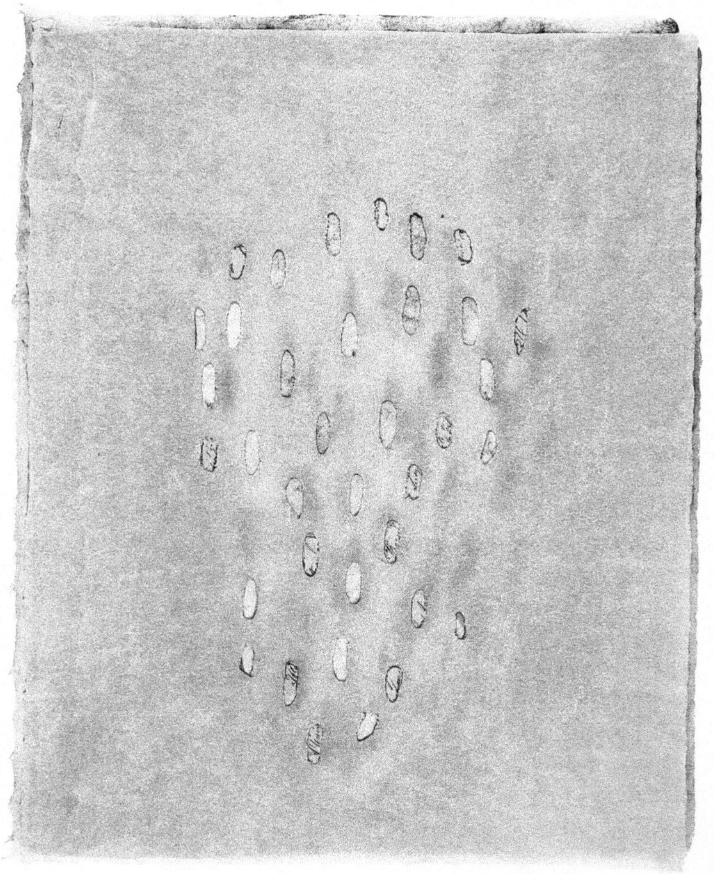

FIGURE 11.5 Sian Bowen, *Pledge Soundpiece*. Ink, pigment, rice starch on paper. © Sian Bowen.

There is a paradoxical juxtaposition of the careful touch, the control and delicacy with which the mark is made, and the association of damage latent in the method of touching – burning or piercing, small actions of damage, a process of drawing which Angela Kingston likens to scarification (Kingston 2000: 34). The surface itself is altered, marked through process, a record of actions upon it as if building up a history of successive touches. The choice of support, and indeed the method of drawing have been critically, thoughtfully, selected to communicate specific qualities of marks left by time and touch.

The writer and art critic Tony Godfrey has described drawing as 'an archaeology of acts of touching' (Godfrey 1990: 9), an idea he revisits in his writing on Bowen, exploring the intimacy between looking and touching in her work. Godfrey makes the claim that 'drawing, like the history of materials, is as much a discourse on touch as sight' (Godfrey 2007: 76).

It is well established that visual mimicry – by observation and representation – is only one way that drawing can depict our view of the world; bodily gestures or systematic process might equally describe ideas or lived experience in graphic form (Downs et.al. 2007: xii). In Bowen's work what we find is a kind of graphic mirroring where the touch of drawing on the page recalls the act of touching in life and touching on the paper, a drawing made through the enactment of movements or manual activities in graphic form that we have elsewhere termed 'performative mimesis' (Casey and Davies 2014: 9).

John Berger identifies this quality of 'imagined touch' in a viewer's experience with reference to a Watteau drawing. He argues that in viewing we imagine the way in which these delicate marks were rendered like stroking a butterfly's wing (Berger 2007: 39). Viewing the drawing is a visual experience but embedded within the marks (and our understanding of them) is a range of sensory knowledge. With Bowen's work, sight and touch are so intimately bound up and interrelated that one does not exist without the other. Bowen's drawing offers not only visual experience but a haptic one. Her drawings do not illustrate or translate another sense, rather they call into play other distant or unrelated senses and we *imagine* touching the object. She presents us with a visual equivalent of how a subject feels to touch.

If, as we have argued, Thopas's drawings evoke qualities of 'solidity, resistance and manufacture', then Bowen's handling of her materials gives a viewer an impression of the tactile qualities of the artefacts she draws, from the pressure of touch to the resistance of texture. While Thopas 'pictures' touch through nuanced depiction of his subjects' hand gesture, in Bowen's work the touch, or the visible trace, is latent in the drawn mark alone, the contact of the instrument on the page indexically recalls the act of touching.

Similarly, the pervading sense of silence identified in Thopas's drawing is also manifest in Bowen's work. Godfrey again has likened Bowen's work to the genre scenes of Chardin or Geogre de la Tour, depicting the absorption of human subjects in manual activities, recalling the ritual of early catholic ceremony and the stillness and quiet of monastic solitude (Godfrey 2000: 9–10). Michael Fried too identifies 'absorption' in the work of both Chardin and Greuze. In each, we see figures engaged in pursuits of the mind and hand, gesturing and gazing meaningfully in measured compositions (Fried 1998: 10). However, Bowen, unlike Chardin and for that matter Thopas, is working in a largely abstract visual language; she achieves a sense of absorption without recourse to figurative or theatrical device.

As with Thopas, this is not 'actual' silence, but recalled or experienced silence depicted. A drawing on paper – in its essence – has no capacity to be audible. What each has done is translated their viewing experience into graphic form – this experience is not uni-sensory, that is, purely visual – but mediated via several senses. Thopas, who was profoundly deaf, experiences his subjects in quiet isolation and as a result his depictions are suffused with silence. Bowen working in sustained silence, almost meditating on her object, identifies that 'the quietude intrinsic to the process of making my work winds its way into the experience of viewing' (Bowen 2012: 143). As a viewer, our experience is quiet, and our attention is drawn to detail and the diligence of the ritual of making. This is evident in Bowen's drawings, which are subtle. Marks and even images are easily overlooked, a visual quality which writers on art have long described as 'quiet'.

The silence of absorption in Bowen is not the result of staged figures in a genre scene acting out silence or absorption. It is not allegory or the personification of a quality or virtue. Neither is it analogy, as when blue is associated with cold or sweeping gestures with passion. Rather, the spacious, orderly divisions and massed accumulation of single marks call the viewer to patiently experience the visual through counting and measurement, and we are invited to weigh, to assay, a quality of silence by their number distribution and balance.

We may well ask how is it that we depict 'silence' in drawing, a medium which is in itself, mute? Michael Fried suggests a form of sensory substitution, where one sense can stand in for the other (Godfrey 2007: 76). He gives the example of the depiction of a blind person to indicate deafness. Certainly there is a slippage. We describe paintings as 'quiet' and 'still' in a metaphorical sense and use the term 'muted' to refer to a subtle pale colour palate. Returning to Thopas and Bowen we can see that stillness, carefully executed mark-making and muted tones do seem to equate to a sense of silence. There is a similitude or visual equivalence. However, what we contend is that the implicated idea of silence goes beyond equivalence or a substitution of one sense for another. With Thopas, and to an extent Bowen, there is more than simply saying that colours are cold or that marks are quiet, but rather that the way the drawing represents its subject conveys, along with visual information, a sensing of deep, enduring silence, perhaps the silence of absorption. What we find in Bowen and Thopas is a sense of 'seeing' as something more than merely visual. Drawing presents us with 'seeing' as a 'bouquet' of all the senses (Connor 2005: 323) where it is unclear where one sense stops and the other begins.

Peter Matthews

If in Bowen and Thopas we see drawing 'capturing' (itself a tactile metaphor) non-visual information in graphic means, British artist Peter Matthews' 'ocean' drawings further synthesize multisensory information. Matthews has developed a graphic script that works as a lingua franca capable of rendering information from an array of senses and sources into a common language and onto a shared surface, so that they can be grasped simultaneously. Unlike Heath's practice, these are not controlled experiments, testing out the capacity of a particular sense against another; his drawing practice is a contingent activity open to the vagrancies of weather and tidal forces in which his entire body is immersed.

Matthews travels widely from the Pacific to the Atlantic to draw in the ocean for hours on end, tracking and transcribing phenomena experienced, such as temperature, tidal patterns and the pull of waves. This information is encoded and laid down in glyphs and ideograms. These are mixed and overlaid with observations of events and occurrences, such as the passing of sea birds, clouds and flotsam, some transcribed as recognizable images some as non-representational gestures, others as text. His drawing observes the natural environment as it moves and changes. He says, 'There's a constant interplay between what one feels physically and what one observes visually' (Matthews 2015). His drawing is a form of perceiving with the whole body, the eyes supplemented by the other senses into multisensory perception. Alongside physical and environmental forces, his drawings include graphic notation of his sensing of time, both internal and as he charts the passage of the sun across the sky (Figure 11.6).

Working at the margins of what is possible, alone in demanding environments, Matthews is acutely aware of a 'synesthetic and kinaesthetic relationship with body in the landscape'. When utterly immersed his drawing is transformed. He says it is 'at that point of visual and visceral arrival that a completely new visual mark making language is created and it's often done in a state of trance so I'm not thinking at all or seeing what the marks on paper look like' (Matthews 2015).

The drawings are combinations of chance and accident, of intentionally directed drawing and drawing intentionally freed to be a graphic stream of bodily-ness and stream of consciousness. The mark-making is at turns ecstatic and sonorous. Tipped instruments trace lines and tracks, points jab and stab to leave dots, flicks and ticks. Busy, nimble lines wander off alone, while others enfold and mass together or assemble into patterns and zig-zags. Alongside these marks we see the ocean has played its part; liquid ink and pigment diluted with sea water swell into softer, larger forms, and tone and colour bleed together. If we were in any doubt, saturated paper, erasures, tears and the rust marks of nails attest to the environment and origin of these drawings.

Alongside gathering information about his surroundings, he is also sensing himself as a recording instrument; immersed as he is for long periods of time, he measures the cold, his waning strength and tiredness. Matthews describes his practice as 'Experiencing the observable and observing the experiential' (Katchadourian 2010: 7). Submerged and engrossed, Mathews draws for extended periods of up to fourteen hours, gradually becoming more attuned to the environment and its forces. He is, in effect, drawing through his physical body. Sight, skin, musculature and the sense of proprioception join to form a conduit for a wider sensibility, permitting him to 'observe' his holistic sensory experience.

Expanding his engagement Matthews sees the drawing board as an active prosthesis for extending touch beyond the body. He says 'the drawing board becomes a highly sensitive extension of my body when in the ocean . . .the board becomes a way to remain buoyant and in tune with a

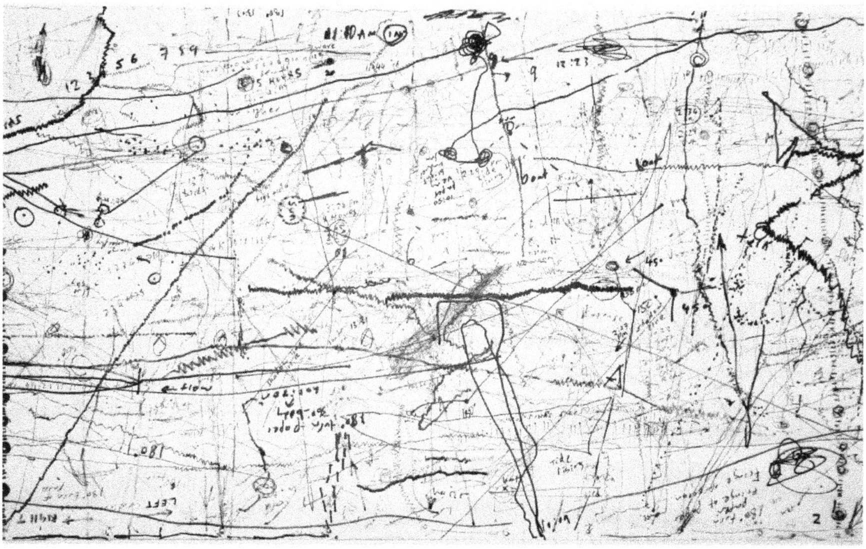

FIGURE 11.6 Peter Matthews, *5 Hours in the Pacific.* Mixed media on paper. © Peter Matthews.

physical and visual sensory relationship with body and ocean, ocean and body, body and universe' (Matthews 2015).

The sensory engagement presented in Matthews' drawing practice is one in which drawing not only extends the reach of the senses, but somehow becomes fused with them. The boundaries between bodily organ, drawing and the world become blurred, a grey area of interaction. The senses are not only an intermingled bouquet in themselves, but there is an intermingling beyond the bodily limits, in which we might be prompted to ask where does the sensory organs of sight and touch stop and the world begin. The art historian and theorist Norman Bryson describes drawing in general as 'an interlacing between inside and outside' of the body (Bryson 2003). While Bryson's essay refers to cognitive activity in drawing, how thoughts and ideas are bought into an external world, his observation could be equally relevant in terms of the body and senses: drawing as the interface between body and world. An idea we find readily articulated in Maurice Merleau-Ponty's concept of the 'chiasm', the meeting point between two entities, at the moment of touch, which is reciprocal and reflexive (Merleau-Ponty 1968).

In Matthews, the status of artist and subject is redefined. The artist's relationship to the object of study is reversed. The sea, no longer an image to be depicted, is now both an active agent in the artwork and a physical force to be contended with. In his drawings we see enacted the interrelationship between artist and subject, touching and meeting; Matthews sensing the sea, the environment in turn reflecting Matthews' waning strength and emotional state. The drawings embody and make visual the chiasm.

Conclusions

If we accept, as Michel Serres has argued, that the senses are interrelated and distinctions between them blurred (Connor 2005), can we conceive of our sensing organs extending beyond our bodily limits? Certainly we see and hear at a distance: sound waves travel from the source to us, light does the same, information is travelling through intervening space, yet we accept its immediacy unproblematically.

This very question is pondered by the feminist materialist philosophy of Karen Barad who coined the term intra-action to describe a coextensive contingent existent with the world. Barad is concerned with touch and touching, and on a quantum level we find it is deeply troubling, for it is no longer clear to see where one entity and another stop and start. Boundaries are blurred (Barad 2012). One insight into touch and relationship that Barad offers of particular relevance here is her discussion of 'prosthesis', which explores distinctions between where 'we' (our bodies) stop and where our tools begin (Barad 2007). For instance, she quotes Nils Bohr's example of a blind man feeling out a room with a stick. Imagine holding a stick. We can either touch the stick to appreciate its qualities, or use the stick as an extension of our hands to 'touch' the object of study for us (Barad 2007). The example prompts the question of where does the body stop and the stick begin? Is the stick part of the sensing organ? Or, returning to the issue of this chapter, if drawing is our metaphorical stick, does this make drawing itself a sense?

The significance of this distinction is that it strengthens an understanding of drawing not as skilled artisanal activity but as an approach to the world, facilitating meaningful engagement between body and world. In each of these artists we see drawing as a means of sensing; as a conduit or proxy, mediating between the body and the world. In Thopas we noted a working over the page, the scrutiny of his eye 'touching' the fabrics; in Bowen's perfomative mimesis the hand (re)enacts acts of touching on the page through drawing. More explicitly still, Matthews' drawing is a means of feeling the world, of touching it. In all cases drawing could be described as form of relationship builder, bridging between the body and the world, a sensory prosthesis, joined with the sense, enhancing their reach or grasp. Drawing as a medium shares much with the senses.

The examples given build a strong case that drawing can extend not only visual capacity but can also sharpen and refine other forms of sensory perception from hearing to touch. It is as if drawing offers a peculiar form of sensibility, finely tuned to the subtle distinctions of the objects of study. It has the capacity to see more closely (Ruskin 1857), touch more delicately (Berger 2007) and sensitize us to the subtle sounds of silence (Godfrey 2000). However, its benefits are not just quantitative, enabling us to see 'more' or 'better'. Drawing enhances the quality of sensory engagement.

We offer drawing as an inter-sense, a phenomena and practice which links or joins senses together. Perhaps drawing, in the way it enfolds the movement of our hand, the touch and sound of tool on surface, converts imagined into the actual and allows the 'other' to be mediated through the self. It makes us aware of new relationships between senses. We would not propose drawing as new sense or a freestanding sense in itself, but perhaps as a demi-sense, one that appeals to knowledge and experience from different, sometimes contradictory realms and in doing so holds both, or many senses, lightly in its fingertip grasp.

These examples also underscore contemporary thought that that senses of sight, touch, smell, taste and hearing are not discrete, autonomous operations but interrelated parts of a more holistic and pervasive sensory experience, as Serres and others have argued. In fact, viewing the drawings of these artists makes this palpable. We see how senses are synthesized, overlaid and integrated.

To conclude, the type of drawing we see exemplified in these artists is a practice which is responsive to the senses and co-extensive with lived experience. This drawing as demi-sense has proximity to other modes of sense and is situated within and across the senses. In acknowledging this new possibilities are opened up for artists and theorists which stretch our understanding of drawing and what it might be possible to do with it in an ever more interdisciplinary landscape.

References

Barad, K. (2007), *Meeting the Universe Halfway*. Durham: Duke University Press.

Barad, K. (2012), 'On Touching – The Inhuman That Therefore I Am'. *Differences: A Journal of Feminist Cultural Studies* 23:3. Durham: Duke University Press.

Berger, J. (2007), *Berger on Drawing*, edited by Jim Savage. Aghabullogue: Occasional Press.

Bowen, S. (2012), *Sian Bowen and Nova Zembla: Suspending the Ephemeral*. Amsterdam: Rijksmuseum.

Bryson, N. (2003), 'A Walk for a Walk's Sake'. In A. Newman and C. De Zegher (eds), *The Stage of Drawing Gesture and Act*. London: Tate; New York: The Drawing Center, pp. 149–158.

Casey, S. and G. Davies (2012), 'A Garland Of Thoughts: Ruskin and Contemporary Sight / Site Sensitive Drawing'. *TRACEY Drawing and Visualisation Research*. Loughborough: TRACEY.

Connor, S. (2005), 'Michel Serres' Five Senses'. In D. Howes (ed.), *Empire of the Senses: The Sensual Culture Reader*. Oxford: Berg, pp. 318–334.

Derrida, J. (1993), *Memoirs of the Blind: The Self- Portrait and Other Ruins*. Translated by Pascale-Anne Brault and Michael Naas. Chicago: University of Chicago Press.

Downs, A., et.al. (2007), *Drawing Now: Between the Lines of Contemporary Art* (Tracey). London: I.B. Taurus.

Eckhart, R. (2014), *Johannes Thopas: Deaf Dumb and Brilliant*. London: Paul Holberton Publishing.

Godfrey, T. (1990), *Drawing Today: Draughtsmen in the Eighties*. Oxford: Phaidon.

Godfrey, T. (2000), 'It Carries Its Own Time With It: The Recent Work of Sian Bowen'. In T. Godfrey (ed.). *Sian Bowen: Passage*. Nottingham: Angel Row Gallery; London: Hart Gallery.

Godfrey, T. (2007), 'To See Is To Touch, To Touch is To See'. in Gill Saunders (ed.), *Gaze*. London: V&A, pp. 71–77.

Katchadourian, N. (2010), *Sea Marks*. New York: The Drawing Center.

Lyons, L. (2009), *Delineating Disease: A System for Investigating Fibrodysplasia Ossificans Progressiva*. Doctoral thesis, Sheffield Hallam University.

Lyons, L. (2012), 'Drawing Your Way into Understanding'. *TRACEY Journal of Drawing and Visualisation Research: Drawing Knowledge*. Loughborough: TRACEY. Available at http://www.lboro.ac.uk/microsites/sota/tracey/journal/edu/2012/PDF/Lucy_Lyons-TRACEY-Journal-DK-2012.pdf (accessed 16 November 2015).

Maslen, M. and J. Southern (2011), *Drawing Projects: An Exploration of the Language of Drawing*. London: Blackdog.

Merleau-Ponty, M. (1968), *The Visible and the Invisible*. Chicago: Northwestern University Press.

Nasim, O. W. (2013), *Observing by Hand: Sketching the Nebulae in the Nineteenth Century*. Chicago: University of Chicago Press.

De Rijke, S. (2008), 'Drawing into Abstraction. Practices of Observation and Visualisation in the Work of Santiago Ramón y Cajal'. *Interdisciplinary Science Reviews* 33(4): 287–311.

Ruskin, J. (1997), *The Elements of Drawing*, edited by Bernard Dunstan. New York: Watson-Guptill.

Sacks, O. (2005), 'The Mind's Eye: What the Blind See'. In D. Howes (ed.), *Empire of the Senses: The Sensual Culture Reader*. Oxford: Berg, pp. 25–42.

Tal, G. (2010), 'The Gestural Language in Francisco Goya's Sleep of Reason Produces Monsters'. *Word & Image* 26(2): 115–127. London: Taylor & Francis.

Taylor, P. (ed.) (1960), *The Notebooks of Leonardo da Vinci*. London: Plume Books.

12

From Impressionism to Opticality: An Episode in the Sensory History of Art

Ian Heywood

Introduction

In the history of modern art different practices of and ideas about perception and making, and various ways of determining the nature, uses and meaning of the senses, have emerged in relation to different movements and the work of particular artists. Of particular importance for the visual arts is the character and significance of sight, but also the relationship between sight and touch. Better-known examples from the early years of modernism of changes in the way in which notions of vision took practical shape include the movements Impressionism, Cubism and Abstract Expressionism, and the work of artists like Édouard Manet, Paul Cézanne, Georg Braque, Pablo Picasso and Marcel Duchamp. Although often reviled by later avant-garde movements and frequently seen now as staid and unchallenging, Impressionism is without doubt very important not only for the history of modern visual art but also for that of modern sensory culture. It was in relation to Impressionism that some of the most influential ideas about the character and role of the sense of sight in modern painting were developed and applied.

Although at face value relatively simple, Impressionist thought and practice almost immediately gave rise to artistic and critical consequences still active and influential decades later. Out of this variegated historical legacy emerged the concept of 'opticality', part of the critical framework of formalist-modernism developed and vigorously defended by the American critic Clement Greenberg. For Greenberg, it was the fundamental guiding idea for the painting of Manet and the Impressionists, then taken up and developed by later painters, including Braque and Picasso during their

Cubist years. More specifically, his argument is usually thought to be that the most advanced tendencies in nineteenth-century painting set into motion painting's determined exploration of a particular kind of visual sensibility, a kind of seeing severely isolated from other senses, and directed only to the retinal or formal constituents of the visual field. Ultimately all that mattered to painting as a visual art were shapes and colours on a flat ground. According to Greenberg, this kind of 'purified' seeing lay at the core of the formalist–modernist movement that reached its zenith with post-war American abstract painting.

Widely questioned during the 1970s and 1980s, however, opticality became the touchstone for very different ideas about vision and visual art. While formalist–modernism was subjected to sustained attacks, many of these critiques – what is now a veritable 'antioptical' mainstream – have been dominated by similar ideas and concerns. As Michael Fried observes, 'Greenberg's overvaluing of opticality, an attitude he shares with his severest critic, Rosalind Krauss, bears witness to the lasting influence of Impressionism and its criticism on subsequent theorizing about modern art' (Fried 1996: 19).[1]

This chapter aims to revisit important episodes in these debates in order to clarify, separate and evaluate different interpretations of the concept of opticality and its implications for the study of sensory culture. Specifically, it will be argued that Greenberg's idea of opticality seeks to encapsulate, but ultimately confuses, two different ideas. The first, for which Greenberg has been justly criticized, is a restrictive teleology that seeks strenuously to isolate and decontextualize vision. The second, informed by Greenberg's acute critical analysis of the late paintings of Paul Cézanne, brings to light a fundamental historical aspect of the relationship between vision and touch, and between illusion and frank materiality in modern painting, a nexus with important philosophical and cultural implications.

Impressionism and Seeing

Whatever the validity of Greenberg's interpretation of modernism, it is clear that Impressionism is important as an example of an episode in the cultural history of the senses in which specific meanings and practices related to one or other sense have been devised and made concrete. In this case, the crucial idea is of vision, what it is to look at an aspect of the world in a particular way, specifically to look with the eye of a modern painter. It also encompasses the bodily, sensate action of painting, its techniques, and the ways not only the artist but also the artist's eventual audience should *see*.

The directness, relative straightforwardness and honesty of Impressionist technique mattered a great deal to contemporary painters. For Cezanne, for example, it was the means to rejuvenate modern painting, the imperative to 'become classical again by way of nature, that is, by way of sensation'.[2] Fried notes that for leading French critics of the 1880s and 1890s,

Impressionism 'simplified the art of painting', yet the seemingly unproblematic idea of an 'impression' proved from the first both mysterious and controversial. At its most basic, an impression is an instantaneous registering of visual sensations from the external world on the retina of the artist, particularly as an array of colours that could be rapidly recorded as spots, dashes or patches of paint. Impressionists often worked outdoors and from the life around them, using an array of vivid, 'pure' colours, leaving brush strokes clearly visible. They tried to capture the fleeting look of things, a chromatic display revealed at a glance. Elisabeth Reisner summarizes the point: 'To be avant-garde in the second half of the nineteenth century was in part to champion colour over line, but also to reject the tonal palette used in the academic *clair-obscur* method of painting' (Reisner in Buck et al. 2008: 49).

Yet sense terms often have more than one meaning. 'Impression' may also refer to tactile sensations and their results, for example, the marks or depressions imprinted on the skin or other pliable material by contact with a raised surface (Shiff 1984: 17). This second meaning relates to another topic discussed widely by Impressionist critics, the notion that the initial sensory impact of the external world is inevitably marked by the temperament and subjectivity of the artist. The impression is both objective when considered from the point of view of passively recorded sensations from the visible world, and subjective when thought about as a moment of active, individual reception, a duality that ran through much Impressionist theory and criticism.[3]

However rarefied the theory, having and responding to an impression became connected to a technique of making paintings which contrasted favourably, in the opinion of progressive artists and critics, with 'academicism', the stilted copying of old masters and a mechanical recording of visual detail, with its emphasis on linear outlines, chiaroscuro modelling and the static tableau compositions of traditional story-telling. Fried maintains that sympathetic contemporary critics realized that 'the new painting was addressed to the sense of sight virtually to the exclusion of other faculties [and] its basic assumptions were realist in that it sought to capture as directly and 'naively' as possible the truth of the painter's instantaneous impression, and that in particular instances (e.g. Monet's *Boulevard de Capucines*), the illusionistic effect was astonishing' (Fried 1996: 407).[4]

Turning to the painting itself, the emphasis on a surface built up of coloured dashes and patches tended to flatten it, demanding a new, shallower, mode of compositional articulation sometimes referred to as 'decorative'. Supporters welcomed the observational and practical techniques of Impressionism as a return to the essentials of painting. In retrospect, it can also be seen to have opened a new principle of painterly construction.

In sum, the critical success of impressionist ideas and techniques brought into prominence a certain idea of the primacy of spontaneous, receptive 'seeing'. The vision required to make Impressionist paintings was eventually associated, in part due to this specific mode of audience address, with a similar kind of spontaneous seeing needed to experience and judge them properly. Seeing in an Impressionist way became in principle available to everyone, not just artists making pictures.

Yet, if only by contrast, Impressionism raised the problem of other kinds of seeing. For example, it prompted questions about how realist and symbolist artists see. The idea of realism in art is far from simple, but minimally requires observing and recording the appearance of visible things as they are, not just the transient light they reflect or emit, and this implies that the artist must supplement retinal experience with what he or she knows or imagines. For symbolist artists and critics, Impressionistic seeing was excessively materialistic. What concerned them was feeling and internal psychic life, the different 'vision' characteristic of dream, reverie or hallucination. Take, for example, Paul Gaugin's famous criticism:

> The Impressionists study colour exclusively insofar as the decorative effect, but without freedom, retaining the shackles of verisimilitude . . . They heed only the eye and neglect the mysterious centres of thought, so falling into merely scientific reasoning. (Gaugin in Chipp 1968: 65)

Voicing ideas characteristic of other Symbolists, later echoed in Surrealism, Gaugin advised the young artist:

> [D]o not paint too much after nature. Art is an abstraction; derive this abstraction from nature while dreaming before it, and think more of the creation that will result than of nature. (60)

This kind of disagreement about the very nature and significance of the artist's act of seeing, even within painting, is characteristic of visual art in the modern period, reaching levels of intensity without parallel in the other arts, and rendering highly questionable any sweeping statement about the predominance of a simple, unitary ideology of the visual, an optical mainstream.

Seeing with Cézanne

The case of Paul Cézanne's painting and his opinions about it mark another important episode in the history and theory of the senses in modern visual art and culture. Cézanne has proved a notoriously difficult figure to pin down, in part because of the tensions that suffuse his work and views. He often expressed himself cryptically, seeming to provide support for many different versions of his painting project.[5] In this context we need to ask how Greenberg understood Cézanne's contribution to the evolution of opticality. It will emerge that this idea needs careful scrutiny. As Susan Stewart has argued:

> It is a cliché of contemporary culture to consider our lives as increasingly dominated by visuality. Yet if we review the history of our relation to the muses, we can in fact see that whereas a great shift seems to have taken place from the tactile to the visual, at the same time a residual desire to empathize with, and animate the visual through tactile means is everywhere apparent. (Stewart 2002: 171)

We will see below how Cézanne's fundamental revision of Impressionism required a demanding working out of a new relationship between vision and touch.

Cézanne had an impressionist concern for the appearance of nature, typically for much of his life working directly outdoors and believing strongly in the value of his own sensations, his unique way of seeing, rather than what convention required of a painter. It is worth noting that the now familiar idea that the individual's own way of seeing was something of significance and value first became prominent in the theory and criticism of late-nineteenth-century French painting. At issue was not just a purported fact of the physiological particularity of a painter's perceptual apparatus but the result and expression of the character of the artist as an artist. 'Seeing' refers to much more than simply passively received retinal phenomena.

While Cézanne borrowed aspects of his painting technique from the Impressionists, with their simplified palette, visible brush strokes, and a preference for colour over line and tonality, he was also a realist in his dedication – often expressed in his conversations and letters – to being true to nature 'itself', not just to his perception of it, and in his commitment to depicting everyday items and aspects of ordinary rural landscapes and life. Then again there was what might be called a symbolist or expressionist drive to realize a singular vision of the world.[6] Taken together with his realism, this might imply that he regarded his personal experience of nature as somehow part of nature.

Dissatisfied by the idea that colours are only retinal experiences, Cézanne sought to reunite them with things, to make colour intrinsic to their being. The experience of coloured things rather than of colour sensations is critical to our grasp of the world, in Cézanne's terms, it is a 'truth of nature'. Returning colour to the substance of things was Cezanne's way of repudiating the incorporeal pageant of Impressionism. Yet if colour is just as fundamental a property of things as size, solidity and texture this might suggest a return to tonally modulated local colour, the colour an object seems to be when viewed in isolation. What Cézanne does instead is build the volume of objects from planes of colour, pats and dabs of paint, in an insistently solid, blocky way that underscores the tactile materiality of the paintings themselves.[7] Greenberg describes the effect of this way of working as follows:

> The little overlapping rectangles of paint, laid on with no attempt to fuse their dividing edges, drew the depicted forms towards the surface while, at the same time, the modelling and contouring of these forms, as achieved by the paint dabs, pulled them back again into illusionistic depth. (Greenberg 1951/1993: 86)

Laurence Gowing observes that the textured surface of his paintings, the emphatic, purposeful facture, the flatness of material support and brushed deposits of pigment are arranged so as to matter in themselves, producing 'a new kind of intrinsic material unity, which links the picture not only with the material significance of objects, but also with the common consistency of the material world' (Gowing in Doran 2001: 183). The prominence of the marked surface, avoidance of conventional narrative or literary human interest, the 'gaucherie' or awkwardness of his drawing, and the sometimes disorienting departures from conventional pictorial space are informed by but also depart from the lessons of Impressionism.[8] Cumulatively these features redistribute attention across the whole surface of the painting. According to Greenberg, in the pictures of old masters

> the eye was lead through a rhythmically organized system of concavities and convexities, with manifold gradations of value simulating depth and volume marshalled around salient points of interest. (Greenberg 1993/1951: 85)

The eye of Cézanne's viewer, as it scans the picture plane, is released from its thrall to areas of narrative priority or expectations of compositional balance and harmony. Every sensation precipitated by the painting's surface matters, encouraging an open, interrogative scrutiny across the picture plane as edges are traced and volumes felt out.

For Greenberg the 'distension' of the picture plane pushes forward its 'weight', compacting its 'convexities and concavities together and threatening to fuse the heterogeneous content of the surface into a single image or form whose shape coincided with that of the canvas itself' (Greenberg 1961: 54). Cézanne's efforts to move away from Impressionism and back towards traditional 'sculptural' or 'tactile' values resulted ironically in a new structural emphasis on the picture as an object, with its flat, painted surface, shapes, colours, its material, multisensory presence. In Greenberg's telling formulation, Cézanne's self-imposed task was to relate the component parts of spatial illusion to 'a surface pattern endowed with even greater pictorial rights' (54). Departing dramatically from Cézanne's preferred terminology, Greenberg calls the salience of the organization of marks on a flat surface 'decorative.' Propelled to contradict some of his professed ideals by the demands of practice, Cézanne laid the foundations for the discoveries of Matisse and the Cubists. Although in no way exhaustive, many of Greenberg's insights into this aspect of Cezanne's practice are accurate and important.

Greenberg's Opticality

Where does Cézanne fit in the evolution of the idea of pictorial opticality? Greenberg presents Cézanne as driven by the logic of his method towards flatness and opticality, this despite his stated ambition to reconnect with the 'sculptural' tradition of the Old Masters and his realism. What, however, does Greenberg mean by 'opticality' in the case of Cézanne? Placing opticality into a historical context, he claims that by the middle of the nineteenth century all forward-looking painting was concerned to explore the differences between painting and sculpture. This tended to mean a greater emphasis on a surface composed of colour incidents over line, tonal modelling and the suggestion of a deep space in which the subject's imagination, a multisensory suggestibility, could wander at will. Hence the Impressionists rejected modelling not because of an overriding commitment to colour but because they were in pursuit of the 'purely and literally optical' (Greenberg 1993: 89). Yet Cézanne and later the Cubists turned away from Impressionism's opticality, or at least the idea of purely retinal experience. Despite seeking a renewal of objective and spatial integrity, they were driven by the very logic of their methods, suggests Greenberg, towards making paintings and ultimately collages that were unprecedentedly and decisively flat.

In sum, flatness and opticality are indeed Greenberg's two connected concerns. Minimally, at this point we might say that opticality is both a way of organizing the appearance of paintings and a way of looking at them, the two connected by the painting's mode of address. From Manet and Cézanne to Braque and Picasso, painterly effects of one kind or another, and in many cases representational 'content', are still present but conditioned for the viewer by an awareness that the experience of painterly space is an illusion produced by what a painting really is, a flat surface marked-up with pigment. Greenberg, however, elaborates the basic notion of opticality. We have already heard that an essential and unique condition of painting is the flatness of the support. Yet any mark put upon the flat surface causes an illusion of space, minimally the mark appears in front of the surface. The visual, pictorial illusion of space belongs to all painting, pre-modern and modern alike. The pre-modern painting invites the viewer to meander through an illusion of deep space, enjoying a range of narrative and sensory opportunities, typically not only visual but often also tactile. As Greenberg sees it, modern painters engaged in critical self-enquiry progressively sought to eliminate everything that might distract viewers from their awareness of the fact that the illusion of pictorial space is just that, an illusion generated by the devices and structures of painting, and one directed towards the ends of painting. Tactile and sculptural suggestions had to go. In the seminal essay 'Modernist Painting', Greenberg adds that the illusion of depth in modernist painting 'can be travelled through, literally and figuratively, only by the eye' (90). On this view of opticality, modernist painting calls for a way of looking entirely heedless of other sensory modes, bypassing the sensorium of the imagination, and shut off also from all cognitive, analytical and affective responses and projections. It is this reductive interpretation of opticality, and what often seems to be a deterministic teleology, views from which Greenberg insufficiently distanced himself, that have drawn most fire from his many critics.[9] Yet the syncretic view of opticality is logically distinct from a notion that more adroitly refers to the heightened awareness of certain structural preconditions of viewing invited by many modern paintings.[10]

Greenberg thus fails to distinguish between two different ideas to which he attaches the term 'opticality'. The first proposes a 'logic', uncovered by the practical enquiries of key painters seeking to rid their works of tactile, sculptural and narrative distractions, leading haltingly yet inexorably to paintings shorn of everything except the means of activating retinal phenomena. Such paintings appeal only to the abstraction of a bare, isolated sensory experience of vision. There is, however, a second, richer meaning of opticality. As we have seen, with Manet and Cézanne there emerges an idea of painting practice that explores the consequences of a way of making paintings that are assertively both spatially illusionistic and materially flat. Their works generate and articulate a point of tension between the literal surface, the materiality of paint and support, and the illusion of a human and natural space, and do so in particularly explicit and uncompromising ways. As Gowing astutely observes: 'We recognize form that is voluminous without being solid, colour that is luminous without light, representation that is apparently specific yet that specifies nothing' (Gowing in Doran 2001: 182). While these characteristics are plain to see in many of Cézanne's works, what matters is their significance.[11]

Martin Jay notes that Impressionism is often seen as a 'way station to the pure, self-referential art that is so often associated with high modernist formalism' (Jay 1993: 155). Qualifying this over-simplification, however, he notes that Impressionism's interest in the individual's bodily sense experience clearly distinguishes it from the disembodied, controlling gaze, or what he calls the 'hegemonic scopic regime of the modern era, Cartesian perspectivalism' (Jay 1993: 113). From the point of view of Jay's history of 'scopic regimes' Cézanne represents an important development in an alternative, critical discourse of sense unfolded by modern visual art. In Greenberg's story of the development of the optical concerns of modernist painting, however, Cézanne occupies an important if anomalous intermediate position between the Impressionists and post-war American abstraction. Despite its problems at the level of theory, Greenberg's critical analysis of Cézanne's practice suggests more fruitful possibilities, some of which have been explored above.

We have seen that Impressionism emphasized the role of direct sense perception, in this case the artist's act of looking at aspects of the visible world, but also the bodily and technical activity of the painter, a way of mixing and applying dots and dashes of coloured pigment, as he or she responded in the moment to sensations. It highlighted the artist's gaze, including the practical and critical scrutiny of the results of their actions, but it also suggested a way anyone might look 'as an Impressionist', not only at paintings, but at virtually any visible phenomenon. What Impressionism made of vision, the ways it changed ideas about looking, needs to be understood in relation to another sensory dimension of visual art, explored by artists before and after Impressionism, that is, the imagination's fierce appetite for non-visual sensory dimensions of the seen even when they are not literally present.

Like other important episodes in the history of art, then, Impressionism changed the way in which the visible and visibility mattered. In other words, it had an effect on ideas about the meaning of vision, the senses and a world to which we belong. How best to grasp the significance of Cézanne's painting for sight, touch and a level of human reality he pursued but which he felt constantly eluded him?

The response of Cézanne to Impressionist seeing and painterly practice was complex, artistically and theoretically. A frank, direct receptivity to the visual appearance of nature oriented him to a quotidian, material, embodied life-world, a world he sought, as he often put it, to 'realize' in the materials of paint.[12] Would it be fanciful to understand this as a desire to heed the entreaty of a forgotten, marginalized or fugitive life-world, a distinct realm of meaning, for recognition through the medium of the painter? By the standards of their time, Cézanne's paintings look severely stripped-back, as if he did not want anything to distract from their already 'plain' content – the mundane objects of still life, a simple Provençale landscape, some peasant card players – and their unadorned character as 'just paintings', their flat, marked-up surfaces undisguised by incident, drama, flashy technique or style. What Cézanne learned from the Impressionists was a kind of methodical realism, a commitment to the overriding importance of his sensations, albeit not sensations attended to as the ingredients of a chromatic spectacle but forming, in their simplicity and richness, a connection to a common human world inhabited, as phenomenologists were later to put it, 'prior' to its conceptualization as 'experience', with its puzzles about representation and subjectivity. Sensations lead Cézanne back to a world of exuberant appearance and wordless meaning, simultaneously familiar and elusive. If the Impressionists were realist in respect of their sensory experience, Cézanne's realist convictions about nature and art drove him towards the limits of the visible. In a reversal of older painting, spaces between objects in the foreground are not rendered as if 'empty' – smoothed, darkened, varnished over – but as surfaces in their own right, luminous and substantial. Heightened chromatic activity evenly distributed across the whole picture plane calls the attention of the viewer to the painted surface, but not at the expense of depth. A space of things is bound into the insistently asserted surface, denying the imagination of the viewer access to a virtual, immaterial space punctuated by a hierarchy of objects and narrative incidents. Greenberg suggests that the painterly importance of the marked-up surface gives it the potential to become important in itself, to claim independent pictorial rights. Despite himself, Cézanne was 'trying to give the picture surface its due as a physical entity' (Greenberg 1993[1951]: 86), but why, and what does this imperative mean?

Cézanne, Merleau-Ponty, Heidegger

In a recent book about the relevance of Hegel's philosophical aesthetics to pictorial modernism, the American philosopher Robert Pippin examines the approach of Maurice Merleau-Ponty and Martin Heidegger to Cézanne's paintings. From his discussion there emerge three different ways of thinking about the significance of early modern paintings, particularly works by Manet, Van Gogh and Cézanne, for our ideas of seeing and sensing.

Agreeing with Hegel that art can no longer provide human communities with a fundamental revelation of their identity and place in history, Heidegger maintained that it can still sometimes remind us of an inevitable human situation, a kind of self-questioning, a search for ultimate answers to questions posed by life about the meaning and purpose of the human being. In the modern period, such questioning is dominated by ideas about rationality, an ideal of 'fully self-reflexive and self-authorizing thought' (Pippin 2014: 115). Heidegger and many other recent thinkers have concluded that all such efforts must fail. The thinker is forced to concede that the ultimate ground is 'nothing'. What Heidegger calls 'Western metaphysics', a tradition of thought running from Plato to contemporary techno-science, disguises this bleak truth by its projective representations of a world that can gradually be rendered 'transparently visible' to reason. If authentic, reliable knowledge requires methods to objectify the world, removing merely individual variations in perception, meaning that what remains is necessarily subjective. Seen in this light, Cezanne's dissatisfaction with Impressionism, his objection to the ways in which subjective sensations of light and colour robbed the object of its proper dignity, independence and presence, takes on more importance. His response is to impart things with motionless, weighty, luminous solidity, conveying their restrained, indifferent comportment towards the viewer. In his late paintings these characteristics even applied to portraits and figure compositions.

For Merleau-Ponty, Cézanne is a lay phenomenologist who works doggedly to present in visual terms the happening of the world at a point 'before' habitual ways of thinking split it into the perceiving subject and the perceived object. This 'event', a moment of ontological disclosure, of being visible, is perceptually replete with colours, sounds, textures, smells and tastes. Yet perception is not something that happens to the sensing body. It is rather part of the body's lived presence in the world. We do not form a concept of an object – Cézanne's mountain, quarry, bowl of fruit or card players – by amalgamating different bits of sensory information. Rather our fundamental understanding of things is formed from this primary contact in which the sensing body and its world occur simultaneously. Sensations are never isolated, as a patch of colour or a single sound, but have a certain shape, juxtaposed to other shapes or sounds. They also appear against a visible, sensory background. In addition, sensations are never wholly abstract; to see blue is to see not just a colour but also the blue of the radiant sky or of a piece of closely woven cloth. The roundness of an object is that of an apple, a jug or a limb, not just roundness as such. When King Lear refers to the 'thick rotundity o'the world' he transfers to the globe of the earth just such a familiar, everyday roundness.

We have already seen how Greenberg and others have described the painterly structure of Cézanne's works, in particular the interlocking rectangles of reverberant colour that simultaneously establish form and emphasize the painting's surface. Summarizing what is at this point their more or less phenomenological approach to Cézanne, Pippin writes:

> For philosophers like Heidegger and Merleau-Ponty, the meaning of this painterly effect, the 'vibration', is some intimation of the object's actually coming into being, its 'birth', as if composing itself (not its coming into existence, but its taking intelligible form). (2014: 119)

Merleau-Ponty makes the point that in order to witness the 'coming-to-itself of the visible' the painting must be perceptually 'auto-figurative'. The occurrence of bare intelligibility requires that the painting gives itself pictorial form and frankly declares this to the viewer. In its own way and on its own terms, the painting re-enacts the material and perceptual happening of an elemental accessibility, it realizes meaningful things in the world by itself being realized in paint.

It is probable that for Heidegger, Cézanne's landscapes, still lives and late figure paintings suggested a less acquisitive and destructive relationship with being than that typical of modernity, albeit even then fading fast. Yet Heidegger finds their deepest significance in their paradoxical capacity to intimate a fundamental human dependency on a condition of bare meaningfulness that cannot be revealed, that is hidden by the dark, silent, refractory solidity of what he refers to as 'earth' (*Erde*). What they do reveal, what happens in and through them, is the visibility of the 'being at work', of meaningfulness. The emphasis here is on a duality, presence and presencing, that somehow 'realizes itself'. For Pippin, however, Cézanne's archetypally stripped-down works and the sumptuous austerity of his project, a dogged search for elemental meaningfulness, suggest something else, a historical condition in which there is a profound crisis of material and sensory intelligibility. For example, Cézanne's three *Bathers* pictures painted between 1884 and 1906, present quasi-amphibian creatures that strain at the limits of what is humanly recognizable. Formally they include moments where the means of painting bodies and limbs seem to break down.[13] For Pippin these and other late works are 'not a manifestation of any ontological truth as much as they are simply "what remains" as a possible level of shareable intelligibility in a situation of ever greater "worldlessness," or as

Heidegger himself says about animals, the world-poor contexts for such art' (127–128).

There is insufficient space here to pursue these arguments further. Briefly, however, it is worth considering whether Pippin's neo-Hegelian repudiation of Merleau-Ponty's and Heidegger's 'ontological' interpretations in favour of what seems to be a narrative of historical crisis and heroic failure is capable of saving the importance of Cézanne's work, and indeed of much of the pictorial modernism that came after. That is, Pippin praises Cézanne's unwavering conviction in the validity of his search, betraying 'no hint of scepticism or despair', and judges his late works to be 'extraordinarily powerful, effective paintings' (129) which keep open a question of fundamental importance, the possibility under modern conditions of mutual, bodily sensory intelligibility. Yet he also wants to say that what these paintings ultimately reveal is the inaccessibility of the vibrant human and natural reality that Cézanne sought. This needs to be set against not only the sheer quality of many of his late works as paintings but also their capacity to stand comparison with other high points in the tradition of painting as an art, and to spark and nourish further developments in pictorial modernism, notably from Cubism to Abstract Expressionism and beyond.

To conclude, it has been argued that Impressionism changed the ways in which practices of seeing were understood, both for painters and more generally. Yet the very idea of an impression is already as much tactile as it is purely visual or optical. The complex response of Cézanne to Impressionism has been outlined as well as Greenberg's controversial critical interpretations. The concept of opticality refers to both an emphasis on sight distorted in part by its isolation from other sensory and affective modes and also a more fruitful recognition of the importance for many modern painters of the duality of depth and surface, illusion and flatness, the virtual and an often-brutal material frankness. We have also seen something of how this insistence has been interpreted in the light of Cézanne's painting, with thinkers from a broadly phenomenological tradition like Merleau-Ponty and Heidegger evoking a moment of ontological disclosure, while a neo-Hegelian like Robert Pippin sets pictorial modernism in the context of a crisis of intelligibility and a social theory of meaning. While many questions remain I hope to have demonstrated the importance for the sensory history of art and culture of developments in concepts and practices of seeing that look place in and around early modernist painting.

Notes

1 See also Fried 1998: 58n. 25; Bois 1990: xvii; and Stephen Bann, 'Greenberg's Team', *Raritan* 13(4) (Spring 1994): 146, 160.

2 The remark is reported by Émile Bernard, 'Paul Cézanne', *L'Occident* 6 (July 1904): 24.

3 See Shiff 1984: pp. 14–26.
4 It was often said that the intellectual climate for Impressionism was influenced by French enthusiasm for positivism and its emphasis on the dependence of knowledge on direct observation. Yet, as Shiff points out, positivist philosophy also held that this kind of observation was the privilege of science, whereas artists should use their imagination to envisage a perfected or ideal world (Shiff 1984: 21–26).
5 See Doran 2001 and Danchev 2013.
6 Roger Fry saw Cézanne as 'expressive' rather than 'representational'. See Shiff 1984: 160.
7 Contrast Cézanne's approach with John Locke's famous distinction between the primary and secondary qualities of objects in Locke 1964: 189–190.
8 For a good example of the latter, see *Still Life With Plaster Cupid*, 1895, Courtauld Gallery, London.
9 See, for example, Krauss 1986. Also Fried 1998: 19–23.
10 Compare with Bois's distinction between 'two formalisms': one 'morphological' and the other 'structural or rhetorical' (Bois 1990: xvii–xx).
11 Among the more important and in some cases very ambitious interpretations of Cézanne are those of the philosophers Martin Heidegger, Maurice Merleau-Ponty (see discussion below), Giles Deleuze and Francois Lyotard. Deleuze discusses painting in *Francis Bacon: Logic of Sensation*, *What Is Philosophy?* and *Difference and Repetition*. For Lyotard, see *Des dispositifs pulsionnels* (1975), in particular 'Freud selon Cézanne'.
12 According to phenomenology, this kind of reassertion can be understood as a historical imperative called for by the ways the modern science, technology and the cultural outlook they sanction, equate intelligible, manipulable being with non-sensible, ultimately mathematical concepts. On the idea of the life-world as a constructed but pre-theoretical level of reality 'between' nature and human culture, see Husserl (1970).
13 See in particular passages in the foreground of the *Bathers (Les Grandes Baigneuses)* (1894–1905) in the National Gallery, London.

References

Bois, Y.-A. (1990), *Painting as Model*. Cambridge, MA: MIT Press.

Buck, S., J. House, E. Veglin van Claerbergen and B. Wright (eds) (2008), *The Courtauld Cézannes*. London: The Courtauld Gallery.

Chipp, H. B., P. Selz and J. C. Taylor (1984), *Theories of Modern Art: A Source Book By Artists and Critics*. Berkeley: University of California Press.

Danchev, A. (ed.) (2013), *The Letters of Paul Cézanne*. London: Thames and Hudson.

Doran, M. (ed.) (2001), *Conversations With Cézanne*, translated by J. L. Cochran. Berkeley: University of California Press.

Fried, M. (1996), *Manet's Modernism: The Face of Painting in the 1860s*. Chicago: University of Chicago Press.

Fried, M. (1998), *Art and Objecthood: Essays and Reviews*. Chicago: University of Chicago Press.

Greenberg, C. (1961), *Art and Culture*. Boston: Beacon Press.

Greenberg, C. (1993/1951), *The Collected Essays and Criticism*. Vol. 3, edited by John O'Brian. Chicago: Chicago University Press.
Husserl, E. (1970), *The Crisis of the European Sciences and Transcendental Phenomenology: An Introduction to Phenomenological Philosophy*, translated by D. Carr. Evanston: Northwestern University Press.
Jay, M. (1993), *Downcast Eyes: The Denigration of Vision in Twentieth-Century French Thought*. Berkeley: University of California Press.
Krauss, R. (1986), 'Antivision'. *October* 36 (Spring): 147–154.
Merleau-Ponty, M. (1994), *The Merleau-Ponty Aesthetics Reader*, edited by Galen A. Johnson. Evanston: Northwestern University Press.
Pippin, R. (2014), *After the Beautiful: Hegel and the Philosophy of Pictorial Modernism*. Chicago: University of Chicago Press.
Shiff, R. (1984), *Cézanne and the End of Impressionism*. Chicago: University of Chicago Press.
Stewart, S. (2002), *Poetry and the Fate of the Senses*. Chicago: University of Chicago Press.

13

A Choreography of the Senses – The Painter's Studio

Pip Dickens

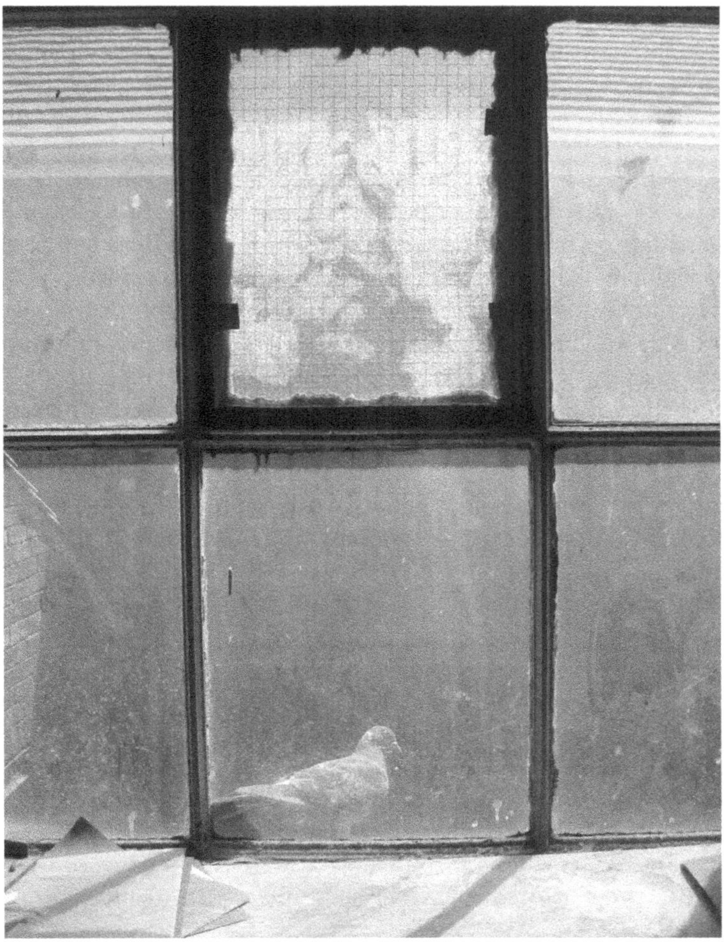

FIGURE 13.1 *Window in an artist's Leeds studio.* © Pip Dickens.

This chapter reflects on the painter's studio as an environment organized to control and adjust the senses. What kind of environment is this and what happens in there? How do such places limit, attune or free the senses to make artworks?

The idea of rhythm and movement as a kind of sense is also explored, together with the most commonly acknowledged senses (in Western society) – sight, touch, hearing, taste and smell. How do these operate in a painter's studio and to what degree might artists be conscious of them while making art? At what juncture may one sense override another and how does this happen if it is not a conscious instruction? While the senses tend to be placed in rank order, sight being primary, might this ranking vary in the context of artistic creation, determined, rather, by their usefulness in relation to making a specific work in a certain way or at a certain point?

Such questions cannot be unequivocally answered. Every artist has their own unique space, method of working and creative thought processes. This chapter attempts to provide glimpses, albeit through the veiled window of the studio, of what the senses contribute, how they are being organized and deployed, and if this process is directed consciously or subconsciously.

We might start from an assumption that a painter's studio is a space dedicated to the use of sight in order to make a visual image. In making paintings, however, it is the interplay between visual and haptic modes of awareness that is core. Also, the supposedly lower-ranking senses of smell and hearing may play larger parts than is commonly assumed.

In what follows, we will distinguish between different types of studio environments and how space, materials and objects are organized in order to compose sensory awareness. Smell, touch and hearing will be considered, as well as the notion of movement as a kind of bodily sense stimulating creative thinking and contributing to the phenomena of flow.[1] For example, the feeling of 'being in the zone' amplifies some modes of sensory awareness while others seem to diminish or disappear. In conclusion, it will be proposed that some form of 'choreography of the senses' is facilitated by the studio, organizing specific senses in relation to the demands of the activity or work taking place.

Out of This World

In recent years (2009–2012) a number of publications and broadcasts have focused on artist interviews specifically about their work environment.[2] Hossein Amirsadeghi, author of *Sanctuary: Britain's Artists and Their Studios*, gained access to approximately 120 artists' studios in the United Kingdom in order to find out what these places are really like. In 2009 artist Susan Aldworth interviewed Amirsadeghi for a BBC Radio 4 programme *A Room for a View: The Artist's Studio*:

> Aldworth asks: 'Do you think you can be an artist if you don't have an art studio?'
>
> Amirsadeghi replies: 'I think not, from my experience, because every artist I have ever seen has had a studio even if they work in different conceptual art/new mediums but even they need the cloistered environment, if you will, of the art studio . . . they are portals . . . it's like the cupboard in Narnia – it's a bit of a letdown when you do actually walk into the studios – they are mostly pretty decrepit, and hard, and cold, and uncomfortable, and unfriendly and you wonder how do these people spend not just hours but days on end incarcerating themselves in there.' (Aldworth 2013)

Clearly, there is curiosity about what goes on in these private spaces and what they are like. Their functions vary. Some are shared with other artists. Others become a platform for sociability or promotion; Courbet, Turner and Warhol used their studios for such purposes. More commonly, however, studios are relatively invisible and inaccessible, 'out of this world', a world apart. They can take the form of co-operatives, community studios, individual spaces or spaces lent to artists by galleries, but they remain spaces of focus, for thinking and making with as little interruption from the outside world as possible.

Artists describe the studio in multifarious ways: a room of privilege, a sanctuary, luridly a 'chamber of death' (because of the volume of destroyed work).[3] Its physical structure may be that of a cell or small room, an attic, a barn, a bedroom or a defunct industrial building. As a space organized and controlled by the artist the studio is meant to regulate or enhance sensory experience in relation to the pressures and opportunities of external factors and circumstances. Moreover, this orchestration sometimes has a significant effect on the artist's experience of time. Many artists acknowledge that awareness of the passage of time in the studio is distinct, and when conditions are right, the artist can undergo an intensity of focus that is almost magical.

Some spaces are deliberately isolated from the world, without telephones, doorbells or obvious entrances. Windows may be modified to restrict looking out or looking in. These physical interventions secure a degree of privacy and provide clues to what kind of environment an artist may be attempting to create and how it impacts on physical, sensory experience and, ultimately, the work. Artist and critic Robert Storr reflects on artists' studios in his paper *A Room of One's Own, a Mind of One's Own*:

> The bottom line is that artists work where they can and how they can. Accordingly the announcement 'I am going to the studio' can mean going to the: living room, a bedroom, the basement, the attic, an attached or

> free-standing garage, a coach house in the back of a grand old house, a storefront downstairs or down the block from your apartment, the floor of a warehouse, the sublet corner of a floor of a warehouse, the classroom of a vacant school that has been turned over to artists by enlightened city officials, a room in an office building on its way to becoming a residential building, a cubicle within a subdivided factory in a neighbourhood that light industry has left for good, a cubicle in a subdivided factory so toxic as a result of the previous manufacturing of goods or storage of materials that no one has figured out how to clean it up if the site were razed, which no one is going to pay for unless enlightened city officials force them to or a very rich or a very gullible client shows up with a plan to gentrify the whole area or without telling future tenants that they will forever be inhaling noxious fumes and drinking water infused with carcinogens. Naturally, there are other possibilities. (Jacob and Grabner 2010: 49)

Artists frequently find themselves uprooted from their studio, sometimes to find better working environments, sometimes involuntarily. This uprooting stirs up the senses like a hornet's nest; resuming organization and a sense of rhythm within the working environment can take many months as studios usually contain not just tools and materials but also habitual arrangements and conventions, some directly relevant to daily patterns of sensory experience.

The requirement for a dedicated space is not merely about the practicalities of making. The need to step back from the world, away even from the very influences the artwork draws upon, in order to consider and respond to them is important. As a place of retreat the studio has symbolic value; windows, doors and portals are separation devices or boundaries and have been used to describe the artist's distinct viewpoint:

> The condition of the window implies a boundary between the perceiver and the perceived. It establishes as a condition for perception a formal separation between a subject who sees the world and the world that is seen, and in so doing it sets the stage, as it were, for that retreat or withdrawal of the self from the world which characterizes the dawn of the modern age. Ensconced behind the window the self becomes an observing subject, a spectator, as against a world which becomes a spectacle, an object of vision. Almost two centuries before Descartes will establish the philosophical grounds of a consciousness, a self, separated from the world, the imaginal eye of the artist has already prepared the space for that achievement. With the condition of a window, the 'twofold flight from the earth into the universe and from the world into the self,' which Hannah Arendt says characterizes our modern alienation, has a beginning. (Romanyshyn 1989: 42)

By creating a space between herself and a world whose claims to reality often take the form of imperious demands, the studio becomes a place of distanced focus, quiet contemplation, a laboratory and test bed, somewhere to conjure with and test new perspectives or aspects of the external world. Most importantly it is a place in which, initially at least, prior to the process of 'working through', anything goes. Nothing is certain, nothing is wrong, nothing is taboo. A process of physical immersion calling upon directed, sustained perception is of critical importance.

The influence of the senses on studio organization is reflected in how artists prepare and place material, things like furniture, paints, brushes and other equipment. In the act of painting, touch and sight are paramount but the practical ordering of things helps to enhance and focus sensory activity in general, just as an operating theatre or a laboratory will have its systems and protocols. This may include specific placement of things to enhance sensory reception, reduce distraction and increase focus. Such fastidiousness makes possible, for example, not having to look away from the work while putting down one tool and picking up another up.

The studio set up is in one way designed for optimum sensory activity. Faced with inadequate lighting the artist may struggle to identify a colour tone value. In response, she may need to change the angle at which what light there is hits the surface of the canvas or to move in for a closer look. Sensory practices may be required to make adjustments through a compensatory 'tweak'.

Patrick Heron's studio in Cornwall had no wall windows – the light entered through a huge skylight – yet he spoke of arriving in the studio in the morning and moving all of his paintings on to different walls:

> One of the things I find myself doing is altering the positions of everything on the walls so that it doesn't look as it did the night before. One wants to get a new view . . . the other factor is the light in every square foot of the walls, of any room actually, is very different. (*Artists on Film: Scenes from Working Lives* 1998)

This is a kind of understanding that senses, and sensitively understands, that a colour has an appearance that, if moved into the brighter light of say a gallery, would be very different. A solution might be to install better lighting but this is not always possible. A studio based in an old factory may have many large windows letting in vast amounts of light that constantly varies throughout daylight hours and where no amount of artificial lighting will have consistent effect until the hours of relative darkness. Painters have often aspired to achieve the ideal that is the cool stability of north light.

Eric Fischl, when interviewed in *Inside the Painter's Studio*, talks about the light problems of his bespoke studio:

> And then, the lighting . . . I don't understand lighting, and the architect didn't understand it. It's not great light for morning painting because [the sun] rakes through. But it works okay for starting around [late morning] and for the rest of the day it's okay. It's not that I think of myself

> as painting with 'natural' light – I don't think of specific light – I paint sometimes in artificial light, sometimes natural light. It can get rather dark in here, and I'm still painting as though it weren't. So I might have [built the studio] differently. (Fig 2009: 63)

Understood in a positive light, such challenges expand or refine the sensory repertoire, habits and practices of perception. A variety of compensatory adjustments and solutions, sensory skills, accrue while looking, touching, making and appraising. The painter Joan Mitchell, when interviewed by Yves Michaud in 1986, stated:

> I often paint during the night but I have nothing to do with night. I like the light. I prefer the daylight. I also work in the afternoon; I check what I have done the night before. Certain colours change enormously with electric light. (Stiles and Selz 1996: 33)

In sum, then, artists attempt to create environments that allow for focus, separation, privacy and concerted time in order to create. Studios are pragmatically organized not only to facilitate the making of works but also to stimulate and focus the activity of specific senses.

Smell as a Gauge

In the painter's studio smell might be considered the least important of the senses but there is no doubt that studios do smell, and smell may sometimes contribute towards the working environment. Like a kitchen or a laboratory, the odour of wood, white spirit, oil paint, varnish and resin tell you where you are: for the painter it is the smell of industry, of creation, reassuring and informative. Odours identify materials and processes: the smell of rabbit-skin glue (a canvas is being sized); the smell of cut wood (a new stretcher made); the smell of linseed oil (a painting in progress). The musty, damp smell of winter air in an unheated studio is in stark contrast to the summer odour of warm dust floating in fingers of light, of timbers cracking, releasing their moisture into the air and the slow gas-building smell of chemicals in glass bottles and tins slowly heating in the sunlight. Odours also inform. As in a kitchen or laboratory, the smell of burning, of something having gone off, the fact of recognition when a sniff identifies a material in an unmarked tin, for example, all provide indications, evidence. Smell answers queries and tests, it checks and confirms. The French perfumier Jean-Claude Ellena's description of his studio both contrasts with that of the painting studio but also reveals parallels. He points out how he downgrades sight in favour of the sense of smell:

> A visitor looking at my desk would find it littered with dozens of tightly sealed little bottles, test-blotter-holders shaped like windmills, a worn

> file filled with a hundred formulae, a pot of colouring, pencils, boxes of junk, a photo frame. Still, it can't be called a mess so long as I know where to find the formula for the draft I stopped working on a few months back, the grey crayon that I need, the box with the worn pencil rubber and the paper clips, not to mention my glasses – the ones for reading and the ones for distances. For me this 'mess' is connected to memory. When everything is organised, I forget.
>
> Behind the desk . . . is a chair that I use . . . everything is within reach by shuffling a few steps. From there, I can look out at the Mediterranean. Actually, when I'm lost in smells and formulae, I don't see anything, but I know the sea is there. I just have to stop smelling, stop writing and look up for a moment to appreciate it. (Ellena 2012: 62)

Ellena is commenting on both conscious and unconscious sensory ordering. For the perfumier or olfactory expert, smell must trump vision, although what smell conjures up in the sensory imagination may dramatically exceed odour. Equally, painting may also exceed the 'purely visual' particularly through powerful, involuntary sensory associations with depicted things and settings in the real world; the fragrant rose; the plump, appetizing peach; the lustrous silk drape.

The Magic Touch

> 'God, but it's beautiful!' He fixed it on the wall at once, with a nail in each corner and then feasted his eyes upon it for hours. His hands began to tremble and his cheeks grew hotter and hotter as he looked at his work and wondered how he could possibly have shown such mastery. He must have had genius then, he reflected. Could his brain and his eyes and his hands have changed in the meantime? (*The Masterpiece*, Émile Zola 1886: 248)

Sight operates at a variety of distances and angles from a painting, but physical touch is inevitably direct contact. The brush, knife or stick, whatever delivers the paint, while not having the cutaneous receptor-value of skin, is an extension instrument that has sensorial qualities of its own.

Brushes and bristles of different shapes, density, length, material and weight bend, hold, release, deposit and drip the medium they carry. Fingers test, sometimes they paint, and even the mouth may blow upon the surface of the painting, depositing pigments, dust or detritus. How each instrument and medium is deployed contributes vital visual information to a painting: from a distance; gently or with force; on a flat or tilted surface and so on. For the painter, touches and gestures are made and contact 'recorded' in mark making evidenced through facture, colour and material deposits. The results can usually be identified as such, and in the era of modern and contemporary painting artists have often devoted time to un-learning formal training in order to discover new ways of touching surfaces with paint using tools and methods of their own devising:

The British painter Jason Martin, when asked about his process, responded:

> I chase an enlightened space. There is a curiosity and a fascination with the improbable events I generate with my bespoke brushes. You have an oversized brush and move it around in a number of ways that are unrepeatable. There's always something happening that you can't recreate. I'm always experimenting with paint with the intention of balancing chance and intention. I'm caught between deliberation and abandon . . . [and] the oils are made on the wall and my mixed media and pigment works on the flat. Both approaches demand choreography of sorts, repeatedly going over a surface and refining many movements. (Amirsadeghi 2012: 132)

Control, choreography, movement and repetition are all present in Martin's process not only of painting onto a surface but in the rotation and placement of works around the studio. Using the brush is a sensory negotiation between how it feels, what kind of shape of mark is deposited, how ambient light might hit and 'charge' the textured traces and how eye and mind respond to a particular expression.

For painting it is touch – the laying down of marks and materials, of layers, skins and textures– that constitutes a specific visual language. The components are highly specific. One mark successfully executed in one portion of a canvas if replicated at another point might fail to deliver. Even the 'feel' of paint itself can matter. The American painter Bill Jensen explains how the paint he makes from pigment feels different, each colour recognizable through its particular weight and texture:

> I really like the feeling handmade paints have. Every colour should have a different texture because every colour is a different pigment. You can almost paint blindfold because of the differences in texture. So with a very simple recipe, I can make my own colour, my own paint . . . I also like the process of stirring . . . it's like how the Japanese master carpenters love sharpening their tools – it's all meditation about the work. I love the whole painting process; I love to do the whole thing. (Fig 2009:114)

As Jensen points out, the rigour and skill of preparing materials and wielding tools is something that is particularly revered in other cultures, Japan, in particular, which formally acknowledges mastery of advanced craft skills. Japanese *katagami* stencil cutters will spend a decade mastering sharp knives and metal punches in order to cut by hand highly decorative and complex mulberry paper stencils used to decorate kimono fabric. These artisans are considered national treasures, honing over many years hand–eye skills in order to cut the stencils with absolute precision. Often a complete design is made in one sitting – a staggering performance – ensuring that the continuity of the pattern or design is safeguarded through a singular rhythmic 'episode' of cutting. It would be easy to suggest that such designs be made using laser technology, but that would be to misunderstand what is at stake, that is, a process of embodied sensitivity and control important in its own right.

In painting practice, then, seeing and touching interact but the balance between them varies. The canvas is a virtual skin which is constantly touched; movements may be jabbing, cutting, scribbling, scumbling, scrubbing, scraping, smoothing, layering, brushing, sanding and sealing. Paint goes on and comes off in an intimate process of physical contact and manipulation.

When discussing a work in progress, painters frequently talk about how a small percentage of a painting is 'working well' at a particular stage of its making and yet what frequently happens is the obliteration of these hard-won successes in pursuit of a more distant, uncertain goals. The painter must step back, move away and appraise the detail against the whole. The value of this motion towards and away from the painting is significant. The break from absorption, often intimately structured by touch, is necessary in order to assess what has taken place from a different visual, physical or intellectual standpoint. A rhythmic to-and-fro movement responds to the tension between engagement and detachment, a pattern maintained until the work is complete.

Sound and Silence

In the studio, the sounds and rhythms of work being made – the pacing up and down, the scumbling of a brush across the canvas, the scrape of knife mixing colour on a palette, the sawing of wood, the hammering of nails, the movement of paintings around the studio – such sounds are the reliable echoes of work in progress and the rhythm of concentration, audible reassurance that work is going well or at least going on. Studios sometimes need to be quiet, but at others the sounds of the external world, connecting with the rhythms of cities or countryside provide an audible backdrop, by turns stimulating, comforting, disturbing or informative. Like the internal sounds of the studio, external noises tend to ebb and flow through awareness. Some painters make full use of the sound just beyond the studio but still need to withdraw in order to reflect and act upon stimuli. The Scottish-born painter Thomas Lawson describes his studio thus:

> These rooms are in a building on a busy thoroughfare in a complex and thriving city. Art is made of the noise and distraction of the street, the passing signs, multiple voices, the endless cacophony of the city. But it can only be brought to fruition at some remove from all that, and my workspace is in the back of the building, withdrawn from the hurly-burly. Back there I reflect, make notes, begin to order my thoughts, and

> in time bring things into shape, give them form and colour. (Jacob and Grabner 2010: 121)

Many artists, while fully engaged in painting, seem to become oblivious to sound. It is only when concentration is broken that there is a realization of somehow having 'been away'. This experience of immersion is what the artist strives for, craves even, but it is not something that can be switched on or off at will.

The disappearance of sound is an instance of a constantly adjusted balance between different sensory modes. Dore Ashton relates a visit to the painter Philip Guston:

> Some years ago Guston and I made plans to have dinner together. I was to meet him at his studio. When I arrived he was painting and reluctant to leave off. 'I'll take a nap,' I told him. 'Wake me up when you are ready.'
>
> I opened my eyes after an hour or so. He was still painting, standing almost on top of the canvas, lost in it, too close really to see it, his only reality the innate feel of the material he was using. As I awoke he made a stroke on the canvas, then turned to me, confused, almost laughing because he was confused, and said with a certain humorous helplessness, 'Where is it?' (Ashton 1976: 105)

Guston's departure is not just about lack of hearing but total disengagement from clock time. Once Guston returns to it, his sense of confusion is masked by humour, indicating a resumed self-awareness and public recognition that he has been in control at one level, yet out of control at another.

Pacing, Prowling and Puttering

> All truly great thoughts are conceived while walking.
>
> (*Twilight of the Idols, or, How to Philosophise with a Hammer*, Friedrich Nietzsche 1888)

Is rhythmic bodily movement another kind of sense? Many studies have been concerned with how movement combined with rhythm – walking and/or pacing – stimulates thought and creativity.

In 2014, Stanford education and psychology researchers examined and compared creativity levels of people who were sedentary or walking, and the results revealed that, on average, creativity increased by 60 per cent through movement (Schwartz 2014). Moreover, the study found it irrelevant where the walking took place. Oppezzo comments: 'I thought walking outside would blow everything out of the water, but walking on a treadmill in a small, boring room still had strong results, which surprised me' (Wong 2014).

The importance of moving as an aid to concentration and creative thinking in the arts has often been noted:

> While he composed [F. Scott] Fitzgerald tended to pace around the room, trying words and phrases aloud, impelled by the urgency of putting language into motion. (Churchwell 2013: 17)

Perhaps an even better known example is the poet William Wordsworth, famed for striding out on long walks across Britain and in Europe. Most intriguing is the platform he had constructed in his small garden at Dove Cottage in the Lake District, an elevated flattening with a mountain view accessed by steps from the back of the cottage. On this small platform, Wordsworth would pace up and down, talking aloud, creating poems, editing lines, using the sound of words, aloud, carried along at a pace, in rhythm. His sister, Dorothy, captured these words as they bounced through the air, fixing them with ink to paper.[4]

Pacing and movement in Jackson Pollock's abstract action paintings reveal parallels in a visual context. The production of large canvases, some of which were made *en plein air*, stepping out of the studio into the landscape:

> But Pollock wanted instinctively to begin at the beginning. The strange war dance he performed went back to the most primitive ritual; beside it, the cave paintings of Altamira or Lascaux are incomparably sophisticated. Yet this primitivism was in no way faked. It sprang from a real need, an almost physical need to come at painting as if no one had ever painted before . . . 'on the floor I am more at ease. I feel nearer, more part of the painting, since this way I can walk round it, work from the four sides and literally be in the painting.' (Jacob and Grabner 2010: 75)

The contemporary artist Michael Smith talks of his tendency for puttering 'a kind of running in place' as he describes it. 'I embrace distraction', he comments. Smith moves about the studio space touching things, walking, postponing starting the work in hand. This act of putting things off by using petty distractions may be a form of limbering up, mentally, creatively, and through seeing and touching, in readiness for conscious focus in the work (Jacob and Grabner 2010: 28).

As proposed by Oppezzo, the notion of moving while thinking creatively is not bound to a specific environment. The British painter Katy Moran provides this example where thinking and moving while swimming has provided a creative solution for a problematic painting:

> I had made a painting, and there were interesting parts of it, but it wasn't working as a whole. I was doing my lengths [swimming] and I thought, I could take the painting off the canvas and cut it up, cut it in half, and then start playing around with those two half bits of canvas . . . That

> just came to me when I was swimming. I don't know if I would have thought of it if I'd been in the studio looking at the work. (Amirsadeghi 2012: 158)

Recent debate about teaching painting has touched on the importance of movement as an aid to creative thinking. Some undergraduate fine-art courses (including at Lancaster University) take students beyond the campus, walking and climbing or engaging in the urban environment through psycho-geographical approaches to mapping and seeing. Encounters with new terrains provide a release from the confines and formality of the studio environment. Moreover, these peripatetic forays into unfamiliar external environments facilitate an important, qualitative, change of intellectual tempo what Dougal McKenzie describes as 'slow thinking'.[5]

The idea of rhythmic motion also has application to a longer-term view of dedication to a practice. Creating or crafting must be practised frequently or the quality of the skilled performance flounders. A rhythm of application, effort and rest assures continuity and level of expertise. The importance of sustained focus and continuity in the long-term is identified in Mihaly Csikszentmihalyi's phrase 'optimal experience':

> It is what a painter feels when the colours on the canvas begin to set up a magnetic tension with each other, and a new *thing*, a living form, takes shape in front of the astonished creator . . . The best moments usually occur when a person's body or mind is stretched to its limits in a voluntary effort to accomplish something difficult and worthwhile. (Csikszentmihayli 2002: 3)

Zola describes the very same experience in his novel *The Masterpiece* when his protagonist, Claude Lantier, on stepping back from his masterpiece, is astonished at what has been accomplished: his cheeks get hotter, his hands shake and his heart beats faster.

Csikszentmihalyi's (1990) well-known idea of 'flow' identifies how the aim of a sense of mastery, which has to do with focus and being 'in the moment', can only be achieved by consistent effort and application. Further, he proposes that artists re-order consciousness and the senses in order to match them with their intentions. Training focus in this way to achieve the 'optimal experience' is a combining of differentiation – separation and qualities of uniqueness – with integration, union of ideas and communicating them to others. If achieved, a feeling of 'ecstasy for no apparent reason' is sometimes experienced, particularly when a goal is achieved using discipline and skills, as opposed to chance or serendipity alone.

The British abstract painter William Hayter, when interviewed on film by the BBC in his Paris studio in 1964 about making paintings, stated:

> The brush begins to move itself in a sort of rhythmic fashion and rhythm is involved in all these things clearly it is in the whole business of living

> and of heartbeat and circulation . . . things sort of take off by itself. It can hardly be said to be uncontrolled because there is quite clearly something controlling it but one isn't entirely conscious of that. There are other moments when one becomes conscious in a curious sort of way in which absolute certainty is necessary but doesn't mean they [the paintings] must be done painfully and meticulously even. They have to be done very spontaneously and very freely but they must be right and they should be right to the thickness of a hair or the whole thing will fall apart. (*Artists on Film: Scenes from Working Lives* 1998)

For the painter, then, being in this quality zone is something of a tightrope walk between discipline and control of consciousness and being open to new possibilities.

Csikszentmihalyi defines 'optimal experience' as 'flow' and claims that it is something that may seem effortless when attained, but actually requires mental and physical rigour. When it is experienced, the sensation is as if a magical entity carries one forward in free flow, that there is a sense of escape from any thoughts or anxieties other than the task in hand.

Csikszentmihalyi also discusses the idea of transformation of time:

> One of the most common descriptions of optimal experience is that time no longer seems to pass the way it ordinarily does. The objective, external duration we measure with reference to outside events like night and day, or the orderly progression of clocks, is rendered irrelevant by the rhythms dictated by the activity . . . it is not clear whether this dimension of flow is just an epiphenomenon – a by-product of the intense concentration required for the activity at hand – or whether it is something that contributes in its own right to the positive quality of experience. (Csikszentmihayli 2002: 66–67)

To conclude, the studio plays an important role as the physical portal the artist enters in order to attain and control these experiences. It is often central to the process of making art. It is not a place for sensory isolation but rather attunement and coordination. It is where the senses can be organized and orchestrated, where touch and vision interchange, where odours question or reassure, and where hearing is stimulated by or quietens sound.

Senses supposedly of lower rank, such as smell and hearing, contribute qualitatively to experience and labour. The physical arrangements of the studio help optimize senses and skills. Bodily movement aids creative thinking and also assists in focusing the senses through a form of rhythmic concentration.[6] Embodied knowledge and intellection interact, testing and innovating new thoughts and ideas. When all aspects work in concert, an 'optimal experience' can be achieved, and the experience of being 'in the zone' can produce an almost magical sense of controlled freedom. A coveted by-product of this is the feeling of having been away from the world, and oneself, in order to make work and have ideas. Ultimately, the successful organization of such spaces facilitates a stepping aside from quotidian concerns and self-awareness in order to enter an empyreal place where, as Deleuze reminds us, the senses are sovereign (Deleuze 1981).

Notes

1 The word 'flow' in this context is the term introduced by psychologist Mihaly Csikszentmihalyi to describe attaining a state of being 'in the zone', achieved through concentration or absorption in a task.

2 Recent publications and broadcasts into artists' studios include: *The Studio Reader: On the Space of Artists, Sanctuary* and *Inside the Painter's Studio.* Radio and TV broadcasts include the BBC TV series *What Do Artists Do All Day?* and most recently, *A Room for a View: The Artist's Studio*, BBC Radio 4.

3 'Chamber of death' is a phrase describing the studio of the main character in Émile Zola's novel *The Masterpiece.* The story is a fictional, semi-autobiographical reflection on Zola's friendship with Paul Cézanne. The main protagonist, Claude Lantier, is thought to be a composite character of Zola's friends Claude Monet, Édouard Manet as well as Paul Cézanne.

4 *Journals of Dorothy Wordsworth*, 1897.

5 D. McKenzie 2015, *Step Away From The Screen, Please (Or, The Painting Student On The Road To Tarascon)*, Teaching Painting – A Conference, 29–30 October 2015, Manchester School of Art, Manchester Metropolitan University/Whitworth Art Gallery, Manchester.

6 An idea thoroughly explored in Richard Sennett's book *The Craftsman.*

References

Aldworth, S. (2013), *A Room for a View: The Artist's Studio.* London: BBC.

Amirsadeghi, H. (2012), *Sanctuary: Britain's Artists and their Studios.* London: Thames & Hudson.

Artists on Film: Scenes from Working Lives (1998), [Film]: BBC 4 Collections.

Ashton, D. (1976), *A Critical Study of Philip Guston.* Berkeley, Los Angeles, Oxford: Oxford University Press.

Churchwell, S. (2013), *Careless People: Murder, Mayhem and the Invention of The Great Gatsby.* London: Hachette Digital.

Csikszentmihayli, M. (1990/2002), *Flow: The Classic Work on How to Achieve Happiness.* London: Random House.

Deleuze, G. (1981), *Francis Bacon: Logique de la Sensation.* Paris: Editions de la Difference.

Ellena, J. C. (2012), *The Diary of a Nose: A Year in the Life of a Perfumier.* London: Particular Books.

Fig, J. (2009), *Inside the Painter's Studio.* New York: Princeton Architectural Press.

Jacob, M. J. and M. Grabner (2010), *The Studio Reader: On the Space of Artist.* Chicago and London: The University of Chicago Press.

McKenzie, D. (2015), *Step Away From The Screen, Please (Or, The Painting Student On The Road To Tarascon)*. Manchester School of Art, unpublished conference paper.

Romanyshyn, R. D. (1989), *Technology as Symptom and Dream*. London: Routledge.

Schwartz, D. L. and M. Oppezzo (2014), 'Give Your Ideas Some Legs: The Positive Effect of Walking'. *Journal of Experimental Psychology: Learning, Memory and Cognition* 40(4): 1142–1152.

Sennett, R. (2008), *The Craftsman*. Penguin Group: London.

Stiles, K. and P. Selz (1996), *Theories and Documents of Contemporary Art*. Los Angeles and London: University of California Press.

Wong, M. (2014), *Stanford Report*. Available at http://news.stanford.edu/news/2014/april/walking-vs-sitting-042414.html (accessed 16 July 2015).

Wordsworth, D. (1897), *Journals of Dorothy Wordsworth*, edited by William Knight. London: Macmillan.

Zola, E. (2008), *The Masterpiece*, edited by Roger Pearson and translated by Thomas Walton. Oxford: Oxford University Press.

Index

For Product Safety Concerns and Information please contact our EU
representative GPSR@taylorandfrancis.com
Taylor & Francis Verlag GmbH, Kaufingerstraße 24, 80331 München, Germany

www.ingramcontent.com/pod-product-compliance
Ingram Content Group UK Ltd.
Pitfield, Milton Keynes, MK11 3LW, UK
UKHW010958180926
475701UK00004B/434

* 9 7 8 1 3 5 0 0 8 0 1 0 2 *